DEEP LEARNING IN BIOLOGY AND MEDICINE

DEEP LEARNING IN BIOLOGY AND MEDICINE

Editors

Davide Bacciu
University of Pisa, Italy

Paulo J. G. Lisboa
Liverpool John Moores University, UK

Alfredo Vellido
Universitat Politècnica de Catalunya, Spain

World Scientific

NEW JERSEY • LONDON • SINGAPORE • BEIJING • SHANGHAI • HONG KONG • TAIPEI • CHENNAI • TOKYO

Published by

World Scientific Publishing Europe Ltd.

57 Shelton Street, Covent Garden, London WC2H 9HE

Head office: 5 Toh Tuck Link, Singapore 596224

USA office: 27 Warren Street, Suite 401-402, Hackensack, NJ 07601

Library of Congress Cataloging-in-Publication Data
Names: Bacciu, Davide, editor. | Lisboa, P. J. G. (Paulo J. G.), 1958– editor. |
    Vellido, Alfredo, editor.
Title: Deep learning in biology and medicine / editors, Davide Bacciu, University of Pisa, Italy,
    Paulo J. G. Lisboa, Liverpool John Moores University, UK,
    Alfredo Vellido, Universitat Politècnica de Catalunya, Spain.
Description: New Jersey : World Scientific, [2022] | Includes bibliographical references and index.
Identifiers: LCCN 2021036691 | ISBN 9781800610934 (hardcover) |
    ISBN 9781800610941 (ebook) | ISBN 9781800610958 (ebook other)
Subjects: LCSH: Medical informatics. | Artificial intelligence--Medical applications | Bioinformatics.
Classification: LCC R858 .D43412 2022 | DDC 610.285--dc23
LC record available at https://lccn.loc.gov/2021036691

British Library Cataloguing-in-Publication Data
A catalogue record for this book is available from the British Library.

For any available supplementary material, please visit
https://www.worldscientific.com/worldscibooks/10.1142/Q0322#t=suppl

Desk Editors: Christina Ramalingam/Michael Beale/Shi Ying Koe

Typeset by Stallion Press
Email: enquiries@stallionpress.com

Preface

Current life sciences, including biology, medicine and biochemistry are data-centric research fields for which Deep Learning methods and technologies are delivering groundbreaking performances, becoming crucial to address challenges of high impact for societal welfare and wellbeing.

This book provides an accessible and organic collection of Deep Learning essays concerning the life sciences, with a focus on bioinformatics and medicine. It caters for a wide readership, ranging from machine learning practitioners and data scientists seeking methodological knowledge to address biomedical applications to life science specialists in search of a gentle reference for advanced data analytics.

The book is contributed by internationally renowned experts, covering foundational methodologies for a wide range of life sciences problems, including electronic health record processing, diagnostic imaging, text processing, as well as omics-data processing. This survey of consolidated problems is complemented by a selection of advanced applications, including cheminformatics and biomedical interaction network analysis. A modern and mindful approach to the use of data-driven methodologies in the life sciences also needs careful consideration of the associated societal, ethical, legal and transparency challenges, which are covered in the concluding chapters of this book.

About the Editors

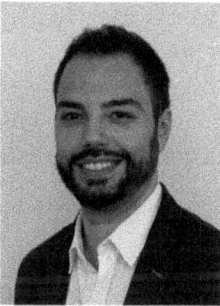

Davide Bacciu is an Associate Professor at the Department of Computer Science, University of Pisa, where he heads the Pervasive Artificial Intelligence Laboratory. Previously, he was a Visiting Researcher at the Neural Computation Research Group, Liverpool John Moores University, in 2007–2008 and at the Cognitive Robotic Systems Laboratory, Orebro University, in 2012. He holds a Ph.D. in Computer Science and Engineering from the IMT Lucca Institute for Advanced Studies, for which he has been awarded the 2009 E.R. Caianiello Prize for the best Italian Ph.D. thesis on neural networks. He has co-authored over 120 research works on (deep) neural networks, generative learning, Bayesian models, learning for graphs, continual learning, and distributed and embedded learning systems. He has been the coordinator of several European, national and industrial research projects. Currently, he is Secretary and Board Member of the Italian Association for Artificial Intelligence, a Senior Member of the IEEE and a member of the IEEE CIS Neural Networks Technical Committee. He is the Associate Editor of the *IEEE Transactions on Neural Networks and Learning Systems*. He chairs the IEEE CIS Task Force on Learning for Structured Data and the Bioinformatics workgroup of the CLAIRE COVID-19 initiative.

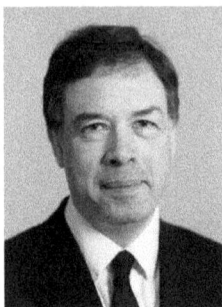

Paulo J. G. Lisboa is the Professor and co-Director of the School of Computer Science and Mathematics at Liverpool John Moores University. He is past Chair of the Horizon 2020 Advisory Group for Societal Challenge 1: Health, Demographic Change and Wellbeing, the world's largest coordinated research programme in health, and of the Healthcare Technologies Professional Network and JA Lodge Prize Committee in the Institution of Engineering and Technology. He is a long-time advocate of interpretable machine learning with over 250 peer-reviewed publications. In 1992, he edited the first book on applications of neural networks. He studied mathematical physics at Liverpool University where he took a Ph.D. in particle physics in 1983. He was appointed Chair of Industrial Mathematics at Liverpool John Moores University in 1996, becoming Head of Graduate School and Head of Department of Applied Mathematics.

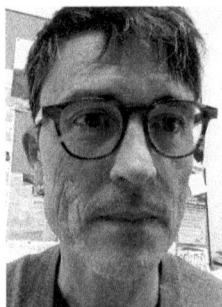

Alfredo Vellido is an Associate Professor and former Ramón y Cajal fellow at the Department of Computer Science, Universitat Politècnica de Catalunya (UPC BarcelonaTech) in Barcelona, Spain. Currently coordinator of the Health, Wellbeing and Inclusion area of the Intelligent Data Science and Artificial Intelligence (IDEAI-UPC) Research Center and Chair of the Task Force on Medical Data Analysis for the IEEE-Computational Intelligence Society Data Mining and Big Data Analytics Technical Committee. He is also a member of the CIBER-BBN Spanish network and the Big Data, Inteligencia Artificial (BIGSEN) Group of the Spanish Nephrology Society. He was awarded a Ph.D. in neural computation from Liverpool John Moores University (Liverpool, UK) in 2000. He has devoted a good share of the last 25 years to research in medical applications of machine learning.

Acknowledgements

This work has been more or less willingly supported by several research programmes and funds who have allowed me to navigate through the perils of untenured waters to the point where I could safely dedicate to this amazing editorial venture. So, thank you (with no grant number). I need to thank all friends, students and colleagues of the Computational Intelligence and Machine Learning Group at the University of Pisa, who always make daily work a pleasure. This book really owes a great deal of debt to some very important people in my life: to the late Antonina Starita, mentor and friend, who introduced me to the challenges of machine learning applications to health and medicine; to Paulo Lisboa, whom I share this venture with, for having kept me on research's tracks when I needed so; to Giulia, who keeps me on track with everything else; and to Dalia who delivers the right amount of daily noise and shocks to shift me off my routines.

Davide Bacciu

Contents

https://doi.org/10.1142/9781800610941_0001

Chapter 1

Introduction

Davide Bacciu[*,§], Paulo J. G. Lisboa[†,¶], and Alfredo Vellido[‡,||]

*Department of Computer Science, University of Pisa,
Lungarno Antonio Pacinotti, 43, 56126 Pisa PI, Italy
†School of Computer Science and Mathematics, Liverpool John Moores
University, Byrom St., Liverpool L3 3AF, UK
‡Computer Science Department, IDEAI-UPC Research Center,
Universitat Politècnica de Catalunya — UPC BarcelonaTech
C. Jordi Girona, 1-3, Barcelona 08034, Spain
§davide.bacciu@unipi.it
¶p.j.lisboa@ljmu.ac.uk
||avellido@cs.upc.edu

The vast community of the life sciences encompasses research fields studying all aspects of the processes underlying and sustaining life, including biology, genetics, chemistry and medicine. In their modern interpretations, these large and diverse fields of study all share a common trait: their daily research and professional activities generate large amounts of digitized data comprising noisy, heterogeneous and often interrelated information. Such a data deluge has necessarily shifted attention towards data-driven or data-informed activities and processes, provoking a transformational effect on these fields, and as a result, producing novel developments, such as personalized medicine, intelligent molecule design, multi-omics, to name a few. The availability of data-driven computational models capable of processing, making sense of and exploiting such information is a key enabler to the progress of the life science field. This book is intended to provide an organic introduction to a groundbreaking data-driven methodology, deep learning, and to its manifold applications across the whole field. This chapter provides a high-level introduction to deep learning and reflects on the issues and challenges underlying the application of deep learning models to the life sciences. We conclude by providing a key to reading the technical essays in the book.

1. Deep Learning

Providing accurate and universally agreed boundaries for the deep learning realm has become an increasingly challenging task. In its early stages, this area could be characterized as a thriving research topic within the artificial neural network field, where deep learning was providing the necessary machinery to train neural architectures organized in multi-layered hierarchies of hidden neurons, enabling sophisticated multi-stage feature extraction from raw input data. Therefore, it was a natural extension of existing shallow artificial neural networks. Since then, the term has evolved to become a byword for machine learning and even artificial intelligence. From a more grounded perspective, deep learning can be considered an umbrella term for a set of methodologies, models and algorithms allowing efficient and effective representation learning from complex raw data. It uses powerful neural function approximators as key ingredients of articulated adaptive systems integrating heterogeneous concepts and components from artificial neural networks, probabilistic and generative learning, optimization, kernel methods and, lately, even knowledge-based and reasoning systems. The breadth of the deep learning models covered by this book will be coherent with such a wide and general definition of the field.

Autoencoders are among the first architectures investigated in deep learning. They can be characterized as unsupervised neural models trained to reconstruct their inputs by jointly learning two mappings, one from the input space to a latent space and another from the latent space back to the input space. During training, the latent space learns general features about the input that help achieve a good reconstruction. The key to learning meaningful latent space representations is that of constraining the autoencoder by enforcing sparse activations in the hidden neurons or by penalizing sensitivity to random or infinitesimal changes to the input information.[1] Such constrained autoencoders are an excellent example of representation learning: their learned latent space can be interpreted as a manifold, that is, a lower-dimensional subspace with local Euclidean properties. High-dimensional and complex input data can be projected onto such manifold for visualization purposes to ease manipulation of the information content or to simplify the learning of downstream predictive tasks. More recently, Variational Auto Encoders (VAEs)[2] have provided a generative framework for autoencoder training, where the latent space can be constrained to behave according to known prior distributions (typically as simple as a single Gaussian). VAEs can learn an effective generative model of the original input data by leveraging the learned latent space. As such, they can be used to sample new data points coherent with the original input dataset.

Convolutional Neural Networks (CNNs)[3] are neural architectures which have developed heavily in the field of computer vision. The key ingredient of this model are the parameterized filters (kernels) which are applied to an input sample (often an image) through a convolution operator. By virtue of the convolutions, they enforce a weight sharing scheme in which, for instance, the same parameterized filter is applied to every pixel in the image. This, compared to the dense approach in classical multi-layer perceptrons, offers considerable advantages both in terms of robustness to image transformations as well as in terms of computational and model complexity. Convolutional layers are often interleaved with pooling layers to provide coarser representations of the original signal. CNNs have found wide application in machine vision tasks, both in terms of predicting properties of the full images (e.g., scene and image recognition) as well as performing pixel-level predictions (e.g., object recognition and semantic segmentation). Their use has also been extended to video processing, typically considering time as an additional dimension for the convolutional operators.

Gated recurrent networks are the standard deep learning paradigm to deal with sequential data processing. Long short-term memory (LSTM)[4] and Gated Recurrent Unit (GRU)[5] networks are the most popular members of this family of models. They share the underlying intuition that, in order to learn long-term dependencies between observations in an input sequence, one can leverage gating units to determine which portion of the input history can be stored in the dynamic memory of the recurrent neuron. The same gating units can then be used to control the amount of information shared by the recurrent neuron with the rest of the network. Applications of gated recurrent networks are numerous, including natural language processing (sequence of words), multivariate time series prediction (sequences of observations in time), behavior recognition (sequence of actions) and, of course, bioinformatics (genomic or proteomic sequences).

Apart from the foundational models above, within this book, we will also consider more recent deep learning models. This is the case, for instance, of deep graph networks (DGNs),[6] learning models that can operate on data of structured nature. This is articulated compound data made of atomic information entities, typically attached to the nodes, bound by some relationship represented by the edges of the structure. DGNs provide means to process input information that is of structured nature, but they also allow us to generate predictions that are themselves graph-structured.

2. Deep Learning in Biology and Medicine

One of the keys to the success of deep learning approaches has been the ability to provide models capable of achieving groundbreaking predictive performances on a variety of data-intensive applications, working mostly on raw and heterogeneous information and relying on little prior knowledge about the task at hand. Medicine, genetics, biology and chemistry, i.e. the life sciences, are among the most data-rich research fields where deep learning can play an essential role in addressing challenges that have an impact on societal welfare and well-being.[7] We briefly discuss what we believe to be the fundamental keys to the success and main shortcomings of deep learning when applied to the life sciences.

The ability to process raw data is an essential feature when dealing with life science data. Noise is an inherent feature in the measurement of a physical quantity, but biological data-generating processes are characterized by an increased level of stochasticity with respect to artificial processes. Engineering strong and general features on such low signal-to-noise-ratio data is a challenging task that is better tackled by deep learning models through their ability to learn to adaptively filter out irrelevant data variations by developing the most task-efficient and robust representation of input information directly from raw observations.

Life science applications require dealing with complex data, often of multi-modal nature. The neural machinery underlying deep learning models is particularly well-suited to deal with such heterogeneous data, mainly thanks to their ability as non-parametric universal approximators. This flexibility and generality allows one to design effective predictors with minimal *a priori* knowledge as regards the data-generating process and its distribution. At the same time, the ability to frame such neural machinery within an overall probabilistic scheme (see discussion in Section 1) also allows learning distributions and sampling processes over complex data, yielding models that can generate new samples that are highly realistic. This last feature is of paramount importance in medicine, where sample scarcity is often an issue in rare diseases or due to the invasive/costly nature of the exams.

Deep learning models and techniques are characterized by superior computational efficiency and higher degree of parallelism when compared to other machine learning methodologies, e.g., kernel methods, which reflect in efficient implementations made available by the most popular deep learning frameworks. Such scalability is another desirable property when realizing life science applications which often require dealing with high-dimensional data. This is typically the case for diagnostic imaging, where images themselves are high-resolution, high-dimensional objects, often involving measurements in multiple channels/spectra or following a time evolution (e.g., in functional imaging). More broadly, multi-omics techniques require the ability to work with high-dimensional samples. Low latency requirements can also play a role in biomedical applications, for instance, when considering the identification of potentially life-critical events in fast streaming data, such as physiological sensors and monitors.

The application of deep learning within the scope of the life sciences also has shortcomings which can, in general, be reconciled with the scarce insight available into the learned models. This can be a limiting factor due to the difficulty in explaining the decision process underlying a prediction to the domain expert who is ultimately responsible (also legally) for putting into actions the model outputs (e.g., by determining the therapeutic plan following the outcome of an automated diagnostic exam). Similarly, the lack of insights into the learned model can exacerbate the risk of developing models affected by bias and confounders in the data,[8] which can yield predictions of poor generalization capabilities (to new hardware, to minority cohorts, etc.) and that can even pose discriminatory threats. Finally, deep neural networks are known to lack robustness to adversarial attacks,[9] which are samples maliciously crafted to induce a prediction error. As it will be shown in the concluding chapters of this book, though, the research community is actively working to propose solutions to such intepretability, discriminatory and security threats.

3. Book Outline

The book is organized to follow a progression from more consolidated and traditional applications of intelligent information processing systems to biomedical problems, to more recent research themes at the crossroads between modern machine learning and the life sciences. We conclude by broadening the discussion to social, ethical and legal implications underlying the adoption of deep learning technologies in biology and medicine, which are often discussed under the unifying term of Trustworthy Artificial Intelligence.[10]

Chapter 2 provides a comprehensive view over the field of *deep learning for medical imaging* by introducing a taxonomy of the general deep learning strategies considered in the literature. This broad discussion is complemented by a close-up analysis on applications to brain imaging which provides an extensive review of the most relevant works in the field along with a clearly organized index of associated datasets. Finally, it identifies the key challenges to be addressed in order to ease applicability of deep imaging methods in clinical practice.

Chapter 3 focuses on *the evolution of mining electronic health records in the era of deep learning*, discussing their key role as a stepping stone upon which to build truly personalized diagnostics, therapeutics and care. Electronic health records (EHRs) capture snapshots of people's health, accumulated in massive storehouses of structured and unstructured data which provide not only unparalleled opportunities but also challenges for predictive and exploratory techniques built to leverage deep learning models. The chapter takes pace from surveying the origins and evolution of EHRs to their current status. Then, it reviews the main deep learning applications to the analysis of EHRs, considering broad classes of supervised and unsupervised tasks involving disease prediction, disease phenotyping, patient stratification and clinical note understanding.

Chapter 4 expands on the topic of understanding human language by providing a progressive introduction to the use of *natural language technologies in the biomedical domain*. The chapter starts with a gentle introduction to the main concepts and methods of the Natural Language Processing (NLP) field. It then takes a deep dive into NLP applications to the life sciences. The methodological survey is well complemented by an accurate index of available resources, including both linguistic corpora, software libraries, as well as pretrained linguistic models, both general-purpose and domain-specific.

Chapter 5 takes a vertical route towards the introduction of an approach for *metabolically driven latent space learning for gene expression data*. The chapter discusses how deep generative models provide an effective unsupervised approach to gain novel insights into the structure of gene expression data. In particular, it focuses on the how the neural representation learned by the model can be constrained based on *a priori* knowledge made available under the form of a metabolic model.

Chapter 6 focuses on *deep learning in cheminformatics* and addresses a long-standing research field at the crossroads between computer science and chemistry. It discusses how chemical compounds find their natural computational representation as graph-structured data, where atoms and their properties are encoded by the vertices of the molecular graph, while edges represent atomic bonds and their characteristics. By building on such a representation, the chapter introduces the lively field of deep learning for the adaptive processing of structured data, which encompasses learning models capable of processing information in its rich structured representation. Then it moves to analysing two relevant applications in the cheminformatics landscape: property prediction from molecular structures and *de novo* drug design by generative deep learning models.

Chapter 7 focuses on *deep learning methods for network biology* which, in a sense, naturally complements the discussion on structured data analysis in Chapter 6 by introducing the use of larger-scale graphs, i.e. the networks, in modelling the complexity of the interactions underlying biological processes. The chapter begins by providing the necessary foundations of network science and ground concepts of system biology to allow entering the field. Then it provides a detailed survey of publicly available biological networks and associated resources, such as data collections and libraries. The chapter concludes by a detailed survey of the literature on deep learning approaches tackling relevant network biology tasks, including prediction of protein–protein interactions, gene–disease association and network–pharmacology applications.

Chapter 8 shifts focus from applications-driven challenges towards a human-centred perspective by elaborating upon *the need for interpretable and explainable deep learning in medicine and healthcare.* The discussion revolves around three motivating facets: investigating fundamental aspects such as to what extent data should be at the core of healthcare research, assessing whether deep learning is an adequate paradigm in data-centred medical applications, and concluding with a discussion and a survey on interpretability and explainability in the medical context.

Chapter 9 concludes this book with a critical analysis of *ethical, societal and legal issues in deep learning for healthcare.* The chapter not only praises the importance of AI ethics but also examines the theme from a practical perspective, analysing the implications of the ethical and legal guidelines for deep learning in healthcare. Particular focus is given to the European guidelines on Trustworthy AI, and the implementation of the associated AI application lifecycle. The chapter concludes with a technical close-up on aspects pertaining to bias, fairness and privacy in deep learning.

References

1. P. Vincent, H. Larochelle, I. Lajoie, Y. Bengio, and P.-A. Manzagol, Stacked denoising autoencoders: Learning useful representations in a deep network with a local denoising criterion. *J. Mach. Learn. Res.,* **11**, 3371–3408 (2010).
2. D. P. Kingma and M. Welling. Auto-encoding variational bayes. In *2nd International Conference on Learning Representations, ICLR 2014, Banff, AB, Canada, April 14-16, 2014, Conference Track Proceedings* (2014).
3. Y. LeCun and Y. Bengio, Convolutional networks for images, speech, and time series. In *The Handbook of Brain Theory and Neural Networks*, pp. 255–258. MIT Press, Cambridge, MA, USA (1998).

4. S. Hochreiter and J. Schmidhuber, Long short-term memory, *Neural Comput.*, **9**(8), 1735–1780 (1997).

5. J. Chung, C. Gulcehre, K. Cho, and Y. Bengio. Empirical evaluation of gated recurrent neural networks on sequence modeling. In *NIPS 2014 Workshop on Deep Learning* (2014).

6. D. Bacciu, F. Errica, A. Micheli, and M. Podda, A gentle introduction to deep learning for graphs, *Neural Network*, **129**, 203–221 (2020).

7. D. Bacciu, P. Lisboa, J. D. Martín, R. Stoean, and A. Vellido. Bioinformatics and medicine in the era of deep learning. In *26th European Symposium on Artificial Neural Networks, ESANN 2018, Bruges, Belgium, April 25–27, 2018* (2018).

8. E. Ferrari, A. Retico, and D. Bacciu, Measuring the effects of confounders in medical supervised classification problems: The confounding index (CI), *Artif. Intell. Med.*, **103**, 101804 (2020).

9. B. Biggio and F. Roli, Wild patterns: Ten years after the rise of adversarial machine learning, *Pattern Recognit.*, **84**, 317–331 (2018).

10. L. Floridi, Establishing the rules for building trustworthy AI, *Nat. Mach. Intell.*, **1**, 261–262 (2019).

Chapter 2

Deep Learning for Medical Imaging

Jose Bernal[*,†,‡], Kaisar Kushibar[*,†,§], Albert Clèrigues[*,†,¶],
Arnau Oliver[*,‖], and Xavier Lladó[*,†,**]

*Institute of Computer Vision and Robotics,
Universitat de Girona, Girona 17003, Spain*
‡*jose.bernal@udg.edu*
§*kaisar.kushibar@udg.edu*
¶*albert.clerigues@udg.edu*
‖*arnau.oliver@udg.edu*
***llado@eia.udg.edu*

Deep learning has attracted the attention of researchers in the last few
years due to its impressive performance on a plethora of computer vision
tasks; and medical image analysis is no exception. In this chapter, we
discuss the general deep learning strategies that have been considered in
medical imaging; widespread preprocessing, processing, and postprocessing schemes; their targets and applications; and discuss key challenges
to address in the future for easing their applicability in clinical practice.

1. Introduction

Machine learning technologies have become part of our daily lives:
from intelligent systems recommending products and services[1] to
complex natural language processors installed in smartphones capable of understanding questions and answering them accordingly.[2]

---

*Equal contribution.
†All authors were affiliated to the Institute of Computer Vision and Robotics at
the Universitat de Girona when the manuscript was conceived.

In the medical domain, these intelligent systems permit supporting and easing medical decision-making in sensible, intricate, and time-consuming tasks, primarily diagnostics,[3] which not so long ago were unaddressable, such as automatic breast cancer screening,[4] skin lesion classification,[5] cardiac structure segmentation and diagnosis,[6] segmentation and identification of retinal landmark and pathologies,[7] histopathology image analysis,[8] and brain segmentation.[9]

A branch of machine learning, referred to as deep learning, has become a hot topic due to its astonishing performance in a myriad of computer vision applications.[10–14] Although early applications of deep learning in medical image analysis date back to the 1990s,[15–17] the lack of sufficient and correctly labelled data, computational power limitations, and reduced interpretability discouraged researchers to continue developing such deep learning techniques. With the diffusion of graphic processing units,[18] improvements in imaging, and efforts for collecting and processing vast amounts of data, this research area has rekindled and expanded considerably, as depicted in Figure 1.

Deep learning in medical imaging has been extensively reviewed in the recent years.[19–26] In this chapter, we aim to outline widespread

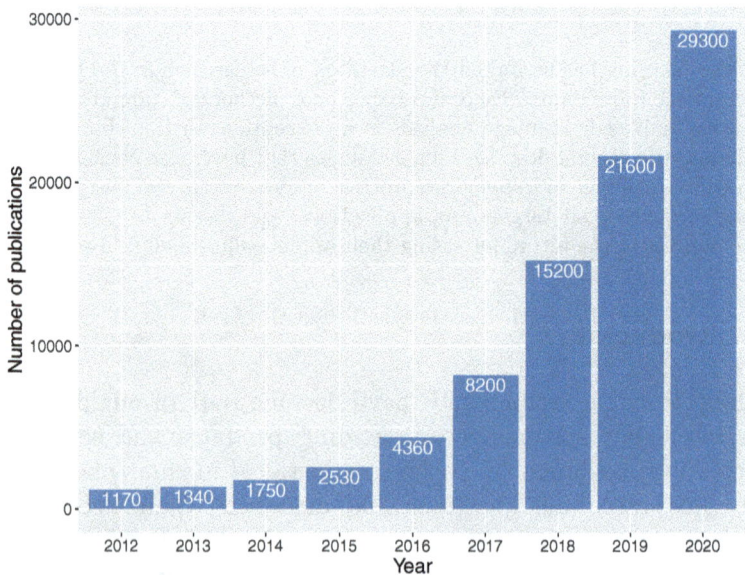

Fig. 1. Number of publications per year between 2012 and 2020 according to Google Scholar using deep learning in medical imaging. Keywords: deep learning and medical imaging. (Queried: December 20th, 2020).

strategies in the medical domain (Section 2), describe specific applications for brain image analysis (Section 3), and discuss current challenges and future directions (Section 4). We intend to cover works in this field published between 2012 and 2020.

2. Taxonomy of Deep Learning Strategies for Medical Image Analysis

In this section, we describe, at a general level, deep learning strategies used for medical image analysis. As illustrated in Figure 2, we categorise them based on their input and output dimensionality, input sources, network interconnection, sources of contextual information, and training schemes.

2.1. *Input dimensionality*

Deep learning strategies can be classified into 2D, 2.5D, and 3D based on their input dimensionality, as illustrated in Figure 3. Two-dimensional convolutional neural networks process 2D information extracted from a single orthogonal plane (e.g., axial, sagittal, or coronal). These types of networks are widely found in the literature since their baselines were firstly introduced for natural image processing,[10–12, 27] they can be easily adapted to work with different imaging techniques, and they are computationally less demanding than their 2.5D and 3D versions. Ulas *et al.*[28] processed 4D dynamic contrast-enhanced magnetic resonance images (2D+time) using a 2D architecture with multiple channels (a channel per time point) to compute quantitative scores of blood brain barrier dysfunction.

Triplanar (also known as 2.5D) architectures receive 2D inputs from the three orthogonal views (e.g., axial, sagittal, and coronal).[29–34] This aspect makes them appealing as they are less demanding than 3D networks due to the use of 2D kernels and incorporate additional implicit contextual information that may lead to improved performance compared to 2D networks.

3D networks could be used to exploit 3D volumetric data directly. Although they are considerably more computationally demanding than the other two variants and are restricted to 3D acquisitions, they integrate additional contextual information compared to 2D and 2.5D architectures that may result in enhanced performance.

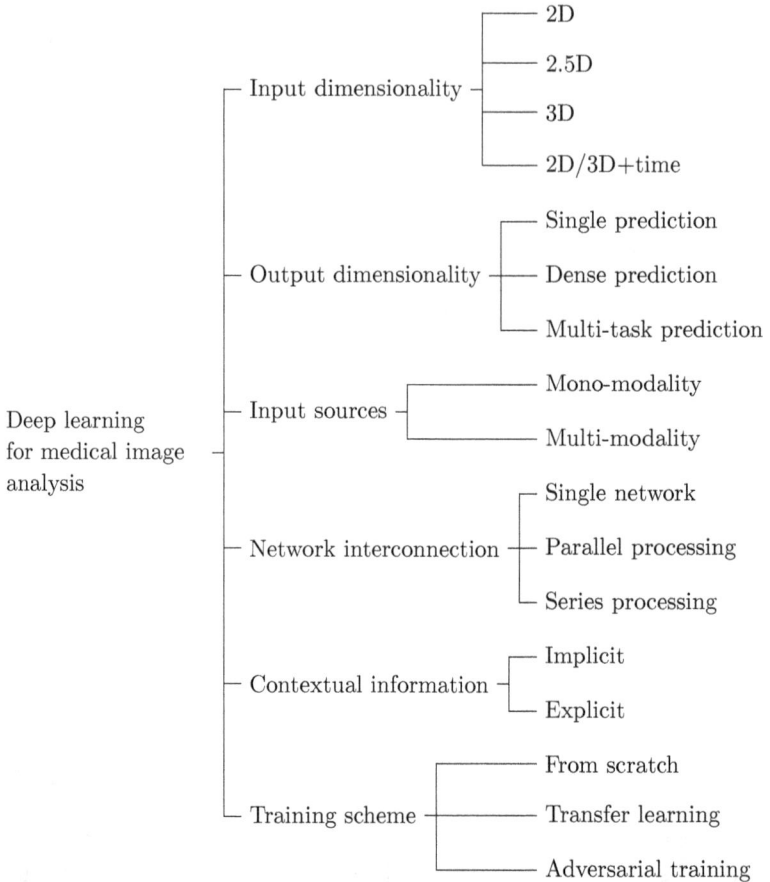

Fig. 2.   Taxonomy of deep learning strategies for medical image analysis.

Of note, 3D networks tend to outperform their 2D analogues, but performance differences may not be significant.[35] Moreover, in particular scenarios in which imaging varies, 2D networks may be more useful.[35]

2.2. *Output dimensionality*

Pioneering works in deep learning for medical image analysis produced a single label for a given input (classification networks). Authors would extract features through convolutional layers, concatenate and flatten them into a one-dimensional feature vector and

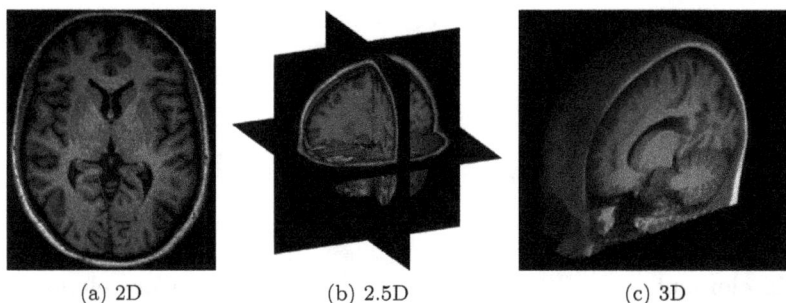

(a) 2D   (b) 2.5D   (c) 3D

Fig. 3. Examples of input dimensionalities in brain magnetic resonance imaging. 2D and 2.5D models obtain information from a single plane or multiple planes using two-dimensional kernels, respectively. 3D models analyse volumetric data directly using 3D kernels.

pass them through fully connected layers to mine them and infer the content of the input and predict the corresponding label. Nonetheless, such a processing strategy would be inconvenient and computationally demanding (time and memory) for tasks in which every voxel is to be processed, e.g., segmentation or image generation, since the network would need to process as many inputs as voxels in the analysed scans.

Authors have looked into faster ways to dense prediction to overcome this issue. The widespread approximation, referred to as fully convolutional neural networks,[36] consists of using 1×1 convolutions ($1 \times 1 \times 1$ for 3D processing)[37] instead of the fully connected modules.[38–48] These modules act as embedded multi-layer perceptrons which may enhance the discriminant and representation power of the entire model.[27,37] Furthermore, authors consider upsampling or upconvolution layers to enlarge the cardinality of the output.[35,38,40,42,49–53]

The prevalent architecture pattern in convolutional neural networks is the U-shape as it combines both the aforementioned strategies. U-Nets contain a contracting path, performing consecutive convolution and downsampling operations, and an expansive path, carrying successive upsampling and convolutions, as shown in Figure 4. In this way, it is possible to output a patch with the same dimensions as the input while reducing response times. Additionally, U-Nets incorporate skip or residual connections that merge feature maps from higher-resolution layers with deconvolved maps to

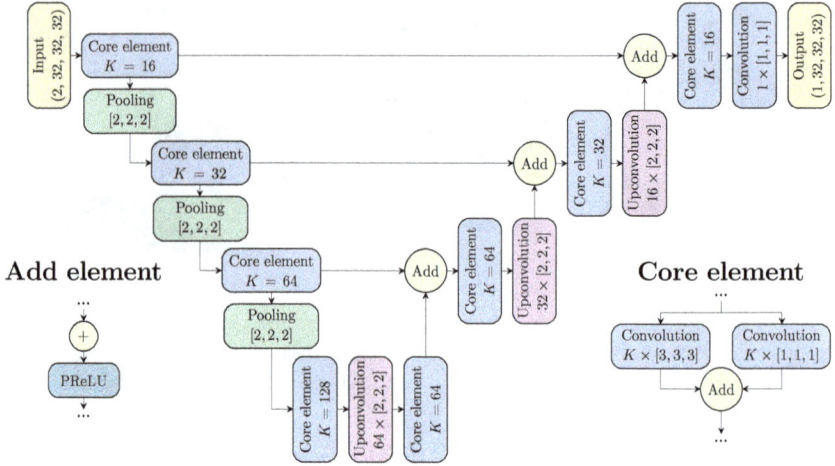

Fig. 4.   Example of a U-Net.[60] U-Nets contain an encoding and a decoding path. The encoding path performs consecutive convolution and downsampling until a certain level is reached (latent space). The decoding path carries successive upsampling and convolutions to output an image of the same size as that of the input. Additionally, U-Nets incorporate skip/residual connections to merge feature maps from higher-resolution layers with deconvolved maps.

preserve localisation details and improve back-propagation.[11,49,54] The combination of the feature maps has been carried out up to now by concatenating[38,40,41,55–57] or adding them.[50,58,59] Note that the latter strategy helps to reduce the number of trainable parameters of the network.

Extracted features can also be used for addressing multiple yet related tasks at once, thus producing multiple outputs. Le *et al.*[61] and van der Voort[34] used a single encoding–decoding network to segment and classify regions of interest. In both cases, classification used features from the latent space. On the one hand, multi-task prediction may increase the effectiveness of the model since multiple losses would propagate through the network during training.[61] On the other hand, these types of models can only be trained when enough data of multiple tasks are available.

2.3.   *Input sources and modalities*

Networks can incorporate information coming from various modalities and sources — when available. Such a multi-modal information fusion may help the networks to discriminate better between classes.[62,63] The union can occur either right at the beginning or before prediction, referred to as early and late fusion, respectively.[64]

Some successful cases of networks incorporating multiple modalities and information sources include the combination of features from magnetic resonance imaging and positron–emission tomography in a late fusion fashion to discern among Alzheimer's disease, mild cognitive impaired, and normal control subjects;[65] the fusion of T1-w, T2-w, and fractional anisotropy for improving baby brain tissue segmentation;[35,63] and their suitability for building modality-invariant latent spaces for synthesising missing modalities or inpainting white matter hyperintensities onto normal-appearing tissue.[66,67]

2.4. *Network interconnection*

Automatic feature extraction is a key process that networks learn based on the inputs and outputs. The more the valuable information they capture from the inputs, the better the response. However, at some point during training, networks converge to a set of filters and stop learning from thereon. Different networks can be arranged in parallel or series to capture comprehensive and potentially complementary features that may result in improved performance due to the information fusion.[68]

Parallel data processing consists of multiple networks that process variants of the same target area, in which features or responses are later merged prior to producing a final verdict, as illustrated in Figure 5(a). Information fusion can take place before each network produces its individual response — feature level — or afterwards — response level. Evidently, a main drawback of these kinds of approaches is their increased computational cost. Some relevant architectures performing parallel data processing are the multi-scale or multi-resolution networks[42,45,68,69] which process versions of the same region of interest at different scales; multi-view networks[30,70] which process data from different anatomical planes (e.g., 2.5D architectures); and some multi-modality networks which process data from multiple modalities separately.[35] Moeskops *et al.*[68] and Kamnitsas *et al.*[42] present both qualitative and quantitative examples of the significant improvement that these networks may have over their independent data processing analogues for brain segmentation tasks.

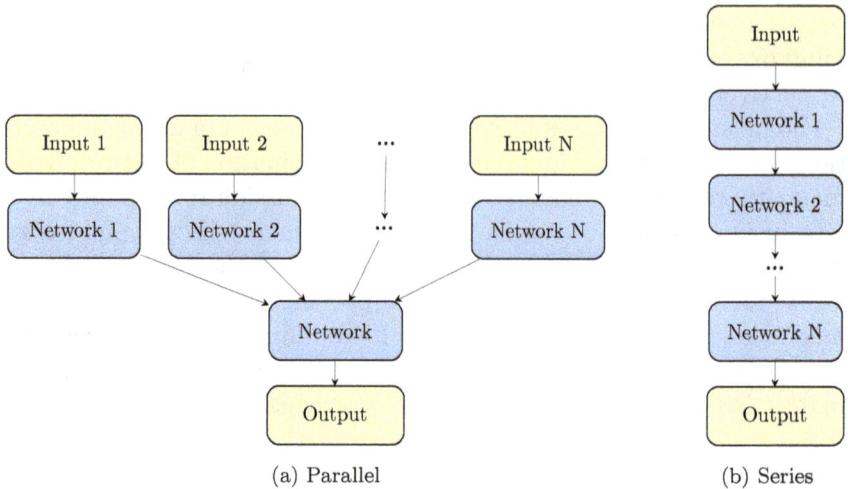

(a) Parallel   (b) Series

Fig. 5. Parallel (a) and series data (b) processing. In the former, multiple networks process variants of the same target area. In the latter, a network is fed with the output of another one to process, correct, smooth, or refine the final response.

In series, also referred to in the literature as cascaded, data processing is typically used as a refinement strategy.[44, 71–77] However, some works have used this approximation to perform one task after another (e.g., segmentation after skull stripping).[41, 78, 79] The approach consists of feeding the output of one network to another one to process, correct, smooth, or refine the final response, as shown in Figure 5(b). These networks have been successfully considered for segmenting liver and, subsequently, segmenting liver lesions in computed tomography,[41] refining multi-organ segmentation results in computed tomography,[75] and multiple sclerosis lesion segmentation.[73, 80] In most cases, cascaded models performed better than their single model analogues.

2.5. *Contextual information*

Most of the strategies found in the literature do not process entire input acquisitions at once. Instead, authors commonly extract patches out of the inputs, process them with the networks independently, and, once processed, merge them together to obtain the output of the whole image. The patch content provides networks with contextual information which they can use to perform their tasks appropriately. On the one side, the larger the patch size, the more the implicit contextual information the network receives and, in some cases, the better the performance of the network.[35, 42, 44] On the other hand, the larger the patch size, the more the trainable parameters, the slower the processing, and the more the data required to train the network correctly. Regardless of the approximation, the patchwise strategies dispense with relevant contextual information which could help to enhance the overall performance.[81] To overcome the aforementioned limitations, convolutional neural networks have been recently equipped with explicit information.

Outstanding applications of explicit contextual information comprise the use of Cartesian or spectral coordinates[82–84] in the works of Ghafoorian *et al.*[64, 85] and Wachinger *et al.*[79] and the use of atlas-based segmentation priors in the works of Kushibar *et al.*[86] and Jia *et al.*[87] Note that the incorporation of explicit information may help to better discern among structures and hemispheres, as illustrated in Figure 6, but it may also increase the computational complexity (e.g., due to registration).

2.6. *Training schemes*

Deep learning methods can be trained from scratch for the particular task of interest. This training scheme is widespread in the literature. However, its implementation requires researchers to either have enough samples for training or augment the available ones appropriately, which is not ideal in the medical field since training samples sizes are typically small and heterogeneous. Alternative training schemes can be used to cope with the afore issue, such as adversarial training or transfer learning.

Adversarial training[88] leverage networks that compete between themselves, as illustrated in Figure 7(a). In generative adversarial training, one network learns the underlying structure of the training data and generates samples from its distribution (the generator) and another one judges whether incoming data are synthetic or not (the discriminator). While the generator's task is to create synthetic data of such quality that they fool the discriminator, the task of the discriminator is to find characteristics in the data that help it to discern between fake and real images. Note that the generator is of particular interest in medical image analysis where data is particularly

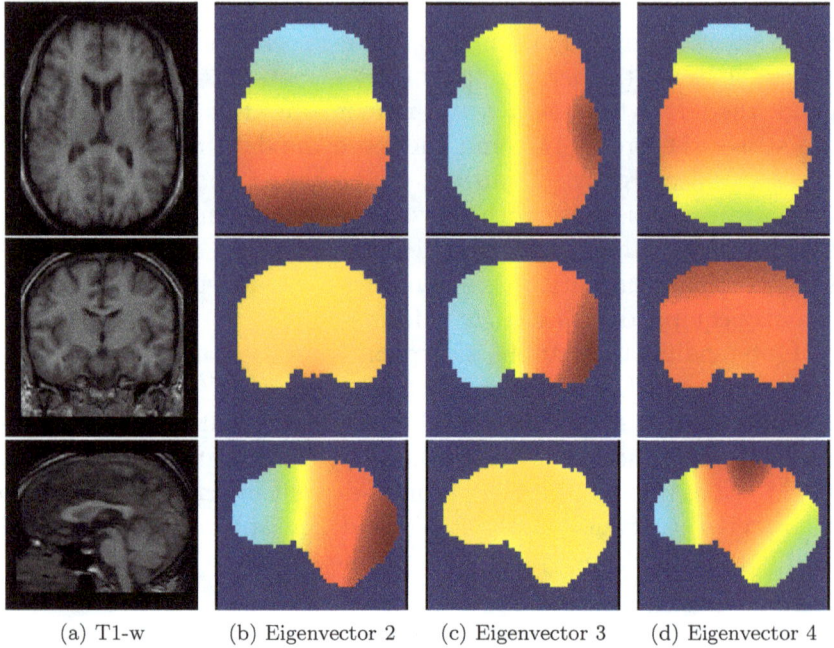

| (a) T1-w | (b) Eigenvector 2 | (c) Eigenvector 3 | (d) Eigenvector 4 |

Fig. 6.   Spectral coordinates as explicit contextual information. This coordinate system within the intracranial volume permits distinction between left and right hemispheres, anterior and posterior, and superior and inferior.

scarce.[21] Two fruitful applications of these networks are the generation of realistic magnetic resonance scans from brain anatomy and tumour segmentation maps while protecting patient information[89] and domain-shift resilient segmentation networks using cycle generative adversarial networks.[90] In domain-invariant training, models can be trained to perform well on two or more related and heterogeneous sets of data by penalising them for extracting different features,[91–93] as illustrated in Figure 7(b). The key advantage is that models learn to extract features that are invariant to the heterogeneity present in the training cases.

In transfer learning, the knowledge stored in pre-trained networks is used in a different but related task.[93–95] Commonly, part of a network is used as a general feature extractor (convolutional layers) and the rest (fully convolutional layers) fine-tuned to the new problem,[96–102] as depicted in Figure 8. This strategy fastens training, enables applying deep architectures using relatively small datasets,

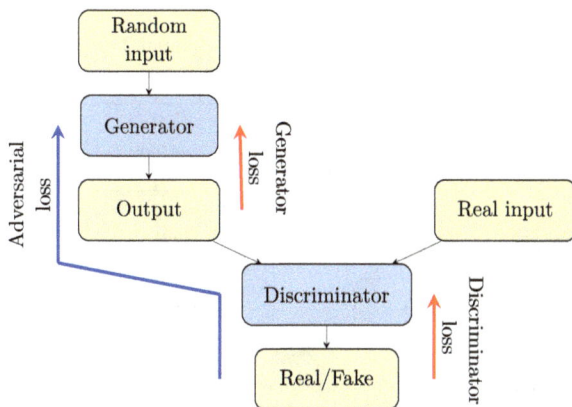

(a) Generative adversarial training

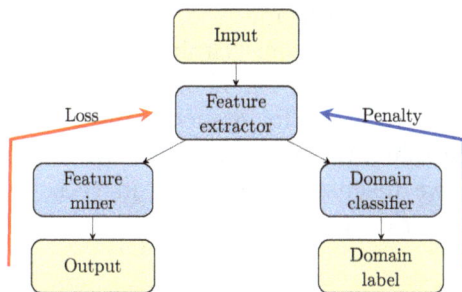

(b) Domain invariant training

Fig. 7.   Adversarial training leverage networks that compete between themselves, e.g., a generator and a discriminator.[88] In generative adversarial training, the generator's task is to create synthetic data of such quality that they fool the discriminator whereas that of the discriminator is to find characteristics in the data that help it to discern between fake and real images. In domain-invariant training, the feature extractor is penalised for extracting different features for different inputs.

and, potentially, reduces the number of training samples needed for training.

3.   Applications in Brain Image Analysis

Along with pathology-related image analysis, brain image analysis is a primary area of development of deep learning in medicine.[20] In this section, we focused on those works. We searched for published

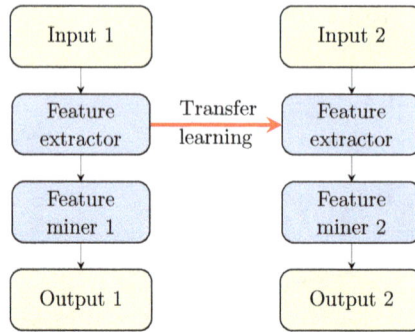

Fig. 8.   In transfer learning, part of a network previously trained for addressing a certain task is transferred to another one.

journal papers between 2012 and 2020 in brain image analysis. Our search keywords were as follows: "Brain", "Medical image analysis", "Deep learning", "Convolutional neural networks". We used Elsevier and IEEE Xplore to perform such a task. Processing pipelines comprise preprocessing, processing, and postprocessing.[25] In the following sections, we discuss our findings in these aspects for brain image analysis using deep learning.

3.1.   *Preprocessing*

A summary of preprocessing strategies commonly used in the literature is presented in Figure 9. Brain acquisitions may incorporate regions that are of no particular significance for the task of interest, such as scalp, skull, cerebellum, eyes, among others. Their presence may compromise not only the entire analysis[103, 104] but also their inaccurate removal.[105–107] We found out that the stripping of skull and cerebellum was carried out in approximately 48% of the articles we reviewed, making it the most common preprocessing step. Note that this figure might be higher than reported here as public datasets coming from popular challenges may be preprocessed beforehand. Popular methods for non-brain region stripping are as follows: the Brain Extraction Tool (BET)[108, 109] as part of the FSL toolbox, Robust Brain Extraction (ROBEX),[110] Learning Algorithm for Brain Extraction and Labeling (LABEL)[111] for pediatric brain extraction, Brain Extraction based on nonlocal Segmentation Technique (BEaST).[112]

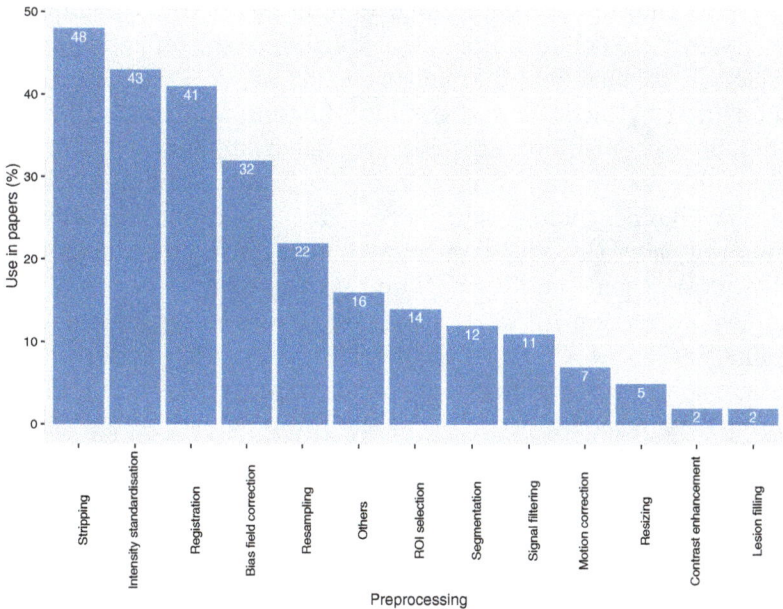

Fig. 9.   Use of preprocessing strategies for brain image analysis. Numbers indicate their occurrence in revised journal papers. Stripping: Skull and cerebellum stripping. Intensity standardisation: z-score, min–max normalisation, histogram matching. Signal filtering: low-pass, band-pass, and high-pass filtering. ROI selection: manual cropping of the ROI.

Data harmonisation, the process of standardising acquisitions possibly coming from different scanners (various vendors), was also a big part of the processing pipelines in the literature. In particular, we observed that intensity standardisation, registration and resampling were applied in 43%, 41% and 22% of the journal papers in our review, respectively. Intensity standardisation was carried out using the z-score (zero mean, unit variance), intensity rescaling (e.g., from 0 to 1), histogram matching,[113, 114] and intensity clipping. However, more recent intensity standardisation techniques, such as segmentation-based standardisation,[115] white stripe[116] or Removal of Artificial Voxel Effect by Linear regression (RAVEL)[117] have not been considered yet. Both registration and resampling were mainly applied for realigning scans in dynamic or functional acquisitions or bringing all modalities and scans to a standard space (e.g., a reference scan from the cohort).

Due to the nature or prolonged duration of the scanning process, magnetic resonance imaging acquisitions are prone to imaging artefacts, e.g., bias field inhomogeneity, noise, and truncation artefacts caused by intrinsic and extrinsic factors. Moreover, functional or dynamic acquisitions are also affected by temporal distortions, for example, as a result of motion during k-space sampling. Spatial intensity inhomogeneities were corrected in 32% of the revised works, commonly using the non-parametric non-uniform intensity normalisation (N3)[118] and N4ITK.[119] Note that careful application of these bias field correction methods is needed to avoid any side effects on the analysis, as explained in the work of Valdés-Hernández *et al.*[120] Spatial signal filtering, including low-pass, band-pass, and high-pass filtering, was considered in 11% of the reviewed articles and motion correction, applicable in functional or dynamic acquisitions, was used in 7% of papers.

3.2. *Processing tasks*

For each paper, we analysed the target, the processing task (e.g., classification and segmentation), the number of considered datasets and their availability, whether the authors carried out cross-dataset assessments, and whether the authors considered transfer learning or trained a network from scratch. We condensed all of those details in Table 1.

The medical community has made publicly available datasets and challenges[a] to allow researchers to compare their works under the same evaluation framework and directives. Most of these available datasets are focused around segmentation and classification tasks. This fact might explain why the majority of the works (approximately 73%) of deep learning-based applications for brain image analysis were centred around these two tasks. The remaining 27% was distributed as follows: 7% for regression, 7% for detection, 3% for generation, and the rest for image enhancement, prediction, registration, retrieval, and superresolution.

---

[a]Refer to the following link for more information: https://grand-challenge.org/challenges/.

Table 1. Journal articles in brain magnetic resonance image analysis published between Jan 2012 and Jan 2020. In the datasets column, the number in parenthesis indicates the number of datasets. Private refers to either clinical or private data collections. AD: Alzheimer's disease. MS: Multiple sclerosis. ADHD: Attention deficit hyperactivity disorder.

Article	Target	Datasets (n)	Cross dataset tests?	Training
Classification				
Afzal et al.[137]	AD	Public (1)	No	Transfer learning
Ahmed et al.[138]	AD	Public (1), private (1)	Yes	Transfer learning
Basaia et al.[139]	AD	Public (1), private (1)	No	Scratch
Chaddad et al.[140]	AD/Gender/Age	Public (3)	No	Scratch
Chesching et al.[141]	Brain dysmaturation	Private (1)	No	Scratch
Eitel et al.[142]	AD	Public (1), private (1)	No	Transfer learning
Feng et al.[143]	AD	Public (1)	No	Scratch
Graham et al.[144]	Quality control	Public (1), private (1)	Yes	Scratch
Huang et al.[145]	Functional network	Public (1)	No	Scratch
Hu et al.[136]	Biological sex	Public (1)	No	Scratch
Kam et al.[146]	AD	Public (1)	No	Scratch
Lee et al.[147]	AD	Public (1)	Yes	Scratch
Liu et al.[148]	AD	Public (3)	No	Scratch
Liu et al.[149]	AD	Public (4)	No	Scratch
Liu et al.[150]	Landmark	Public (3)	Yes	Scratch
Li et al.[151]	Functional network	Public (1)	No	Scratch
Maleki et al.[152]	MS lesion	Private (1)	No	Scratch
Minaee et al.[153]	Lesion	Private (1)	No	Scratch
Ren et al.[154]	AD	Public (1)	No	Scratch
Sarraf et al.[155]	AD	Public (1)	No	Scratch
Suk et al.[65]	AD	Public (1)	No	Scratch
Sultan et al.[156]	Tumour	Public (2)	No	Scratch
Wang et al.[157]	ADHD/ Schizophrenia	Public (1), private (1)	No	Scratch
Yuan et al.[158]	Biological sex	Public (6)	Yes	Scratch
Yue et al.[159]	AD	Public (2)	No	Scratch

(*Continued*)

Table 1. (*Continued*)

Article	Target	Datasets (n)	Cross dataset tests?	Training
Zhang et al.[160]	Gyri/Sulci signal	Public (1), private (1)	No	Scratch
Zhao et al.[161]	Functional network	Public (1)	No	Scratch
Zou et al.[162]	ADHD	Public (1)	No	Scratch
Segmentation				
Agn et al.[163]	Tumour	Public (1)	No	Scratch
Aslani et al.[133]	MS lesion	Public (1), private (1)	No	Scratch
Atlason et al.[125]	Lesion	Public (1), private (1)	No	Scratch
Bao et al.[129]	Structure/Lesion	Public (2)	No	Scratch
Bernal et al.[35]	Tissue	Public (3)	No	Scratch
Birenbaum & Greenspan[31]	MS lesion	Public (1)	No	Scratch
Brosch et al.[40]	MS lesion	Public (2), private (1)	No	Transfer learning
Chen et al.[76]	Tissue	Public (1)	No	Scratch
Chen et al.[164]	Tumour	Public (1)	No	Scratch
Clèrigues et al.[58]	Lesion	Public (1)	No	Scratch
de Brebisson et al.[165]	Brain structure	Public (1)	No	Scratch
Deng et al.[166]	Tissue	Public (2), private (1)	No	Scratch
Ding et al.[167]	Tumour	Public (1)	No	Scratch
Ding et al.[168]	Tumour	Public (1)	No	Scratch
Dolz et al.[45]	Sub-cortical structure	Public (2)	Yes	Scratch
Dolz et al.[169]	Tissue	Public (2)	No	Scratch
Enguehard et al.[170]	Tissue	Public (1)	No	Scratch
Ghafoorian et al.[64]	Lesion	Private (1)	No	Scratch
Ghafoorian et al.[97]	Lesion	Private (1)	Yes	Transfer learning
Guerrero et al.[50]	Lesion	Private (1)	No	Scratch
Havaei et al.[44]	Tumour	Public (1)	No	Scratch
Hou et al.[171] 2018	Tissue	Public (3)	No	Scratch
Hu et al.[172]	Tumour	Public (3)	No	Scratch

Table 1. (*Continued*)

Article	Target	Datasets (n)	Cross dataset tests?	Training
Huo et al.[90]	Skull	Private (1)	No	Scratch
Huo et al.[135]	Brain structure	Public (11)	Yes	Scratch
Kamnitsas et al.[42]	Lesion	Public (2), private (1)	No	Scratch
Kleesiek et al.[128]	Skull	Public (3), private (1)	Yes	Scratch
Kushibar et al.[86]	Sub-cortical structure	Public (2)	No	Scratch
Kushibar et al.[98]	Sub-cortical structure	Public (2)	Yes	Transfer learning
Li et al.[173]	Brain structure	Private (1)	No	Scratch
Li et al.[174]	Tumour	Public (1)	No	Scratch
Li et al.[175]	Lesion	Public (1)	No	Scratch
Lyksborg et al.[30]	Tumour	Public (2)	No	Scratch
Mehta et al.[70]	Sub-cortical structure	Public (5)	No	Scratch
Milletari et al.[176]	Brain structure	Private (2)	No	Scratch
Moeskops et al.[68]	Tissue	Public (3)	No	Scratch
Moeskops et al.[177]	Tissue and lesion	Public (1), private (2)	No	Scratch
Morrison et al.[178]	Cerebral microbleed	Private (1)	No	Scratch
Nair et al.[179]	MS lesion	Private (1)	No	Scratch
Nie et al.[180]	Tissue	Public (1), private (1)	No	Scratch
Pereira et al.[127]	Tumour	Public (2)	No	Scratch
Pereira et al.[181]	Lesion	Public (4)	No	Scratch
Rajchl et al.[130]	Whole-brain	Private (1)	No	Scratch
Razzak et al.[182]	Tumour	Public (2)	No	Scratch
Roy et al.[183]	Brain structure	Public (9)	Yes	Transfer learning
Salehi et al.[184]	Skull	Public (2), private (1)	No	Scratch
Schirmer et al.[185]	Lesion	Private (1)	Yes	Scratch
Shakeri et al.[131]	Sub-cortical structure	Public (1), private (1)	No	Scratch
Shao et al.[186]	Ventricle	Public (1), private (1)	No	Scratch
Shi et al.[187]	Vessel wall	Private (2)	Yes	Scratch
Stollenga et al.[188]	Tissue	Public (1)	No	Scratch

(*Continued*)

Table 1.   (*Continued*)

Article	Target	Datasets (n)	Cross dataset tests?	Training
Thyreau et al. 2018[189]	Hippocampus	Public (5)	No	Scratch
Valverde et al.[73]	MS lesion	Public (1), private (1)	No	Scratch
Valverde et al.[99]	MS lesion	Public (1), private (1)	Yes	Transfer learning
Wachinger et al.[79]	Sub-cortical structure	Public (1)	No	Scratch
Wang et al.[190]	Tissue	Public (3)	Yes	Scratch
Wang et al.[191]	Tumour	Public (1)	No	Scratch
Wang et al.[192]	Whole-brain/Tumour	Public (1), private (1)	No	Transfer learning
Xue et al.[126]	Lesion	Public (1), private (2)	Yes	Scratch
Zhang et al.[63]	Tissue	Private (1)	No	Scratch
Zhao and Jia[69]	Tumour	Public (1)	No	Scratch

Detection

Article	Target	Datasets (n)	Cross dataset tests?	Training
Alansary et al.[132]	Landmark	Public (1)	No	Scratch
Basher et al.[134]	Hippocampus	Public (2)	No	Scratch
Chauvin et al.[193]	Landmark	Public (4)	No	Scratch
Dou et al.[39]	Cerebral microbleed	Private (1)	No	Scratch
Ghafoorian et al.[85]	Lacune	Private (2)	No	Scratch
Liu et al.[194]	Cerebral microbleed	Private (4)	No	Scratch
McKinley et al.[195]	MS lesion	Private (1)	No	Scratch
Salem et al.[56]	MS lesion	Private (1)	No	Scratch
Zhang et al.[196]	Landmark	Private (1)	No	Scratch

Regression

Article	Target	Datasets (n)	Cross dataset tests?	Training
Bollmann et al.[197]	Quantitative imaging	Private (3)	No	Scratch
Cole et al.[198]	Age	Private (4)	Yes	Scratch
Dubost et al.[199]	Perivascular spaces	Private (1)	No	Scratch
Li et al.[200]	Quantitative imaging	Public (1), private (1)	No	Scratch
Mårtensson et al.[201]	Visual rating	Public (1), private (1)	No	Scratch

Table 1. (*Continued*)

Article	Target	Datasets (n)	Cross dataset tests?	Training
Salehi *et al.*[202]	Head pose	Public (1), private (1)	No	Scratch
Ulas *et al.*[28]	Quantitative imaging	Private (1)	No	Scratch
Wei *et al.*[203]	Quantitative imaging	Private (3)	Yes	Scratch
Yoon *et al.*[204]	Quantitative imaging	Private (1)	No	Scratch
Registration				
Balakrishnan *et al.*[55]	Whole-brain	Public (8)	No	Scratch
Yang *et al.*[205]	Whole-brain	Public (6)	Yes	Scratch
Generation				
Chartsias *et al.*[66]	Modality	Public (3)	No	Scratch
Han *et al.*[206]	Tumour	Public (1)	No	Scratch
Salem *et al.*[67]	Lesion	Public (1), private (1)	No	Scratch
Xiang *et al.*[207]	Whole-brain	Private (1)	No	Scratch
Prediction				
Hong *et al.*[208]	Quantitative imaging	Private (1)	No	Scratch
Liu *et al.*[209]	Tumour	Private (1)	No	Scratch
Enhancement				
Jung *et al.*[210]	Perivascular spaces	Private (1)	No	Scratch
Ran *et al.*[211]	Skull	Private (2)	No	Scratch
Others				
Du *et al.*[212]	Whole-brain	Public (4)	Yes	Scratch
Gu *et al.*[213]	Image	Private (1)	No	Scratch
Swati *et al.*[214]	Tumour	Public (1)	No	Transfer learning

A downfall of these public challenges is that algorithms are usually tweaked to perform the best on these specific datasets (tending to a clear overfitting), but they may not behave as well on unseen ones with possibly different acquisition protocols, imaging quality, target populations, among other key factors.[121] Cross-dataset evaluations become an appropriate and necessary tool for addressing this issue and demonstrate quantitatively how generalisable and, ultimately, how applicable to real-life scenarios are the proposals. From our literature revision, we noted that less than a fifth of the works performed such types of assessments. Even in cases where datasets were available, such as tissue, sub-cortical structure, tumour, and white matter hyperintensity segmentation, researchers tended to omit them (approximately 90%).

Current approaches towards diminishing the repercussions of the domain shift problem and improving the applicability of deep learning in clinical practice are transfer learning and domain-invariant training,[122, 123] as discussed in Section 2.6. During our literature revision, we spotted four promising ways of using these strategies: (1) transfer learning to reduce the number of cases needed to fully train a network[40, 96] by initially training the network on identity mapping and then on the task of interest; (2) domain-invariant training to force networks to learn domain-invariant features[92] by penalising them for extracting different features for different domains;[91] (3) transfer learning to adapt a legacy model to a few cases with possibly varying acquisition conditions through fine-tuning;[96–99] (4) contrast-agnostic training to enable models to be robust to intensity variations and perform well on potentially unseen modalities without the need of retraining or fine-tuning.[124] Nonetheless, we observed that these techniques are not widespread in the literature. In fact, less than 10% of the works made use of these training strategies.

3.3. *Postprocessing*

Postprocessing consists of refining results provided by the deep learning model. In our revision, approximately 36% of the works considered postprocessing and it was applied for transforming probability maps into hard segmentation maps (e.g., through thresholding),[39, 40, 58, 73, 125–127] filtering spurious and relatively small or large regions,[44, 45, 67, 73, 86, 98, 128] smoothing segmentation maps (e.g., to fill holes),[30, 42, 52, 79, 129–131] or reaching a final verdict (e.g., by means of majority voting).[77, 132–136]

4. Challenges and Future Directions

Despite the recent success of deep learning methods for medical image analysis, there are still issues to be addressed prior to deploying them for routine clinical practice. We have identified the following key challenges that should be tackled in the future: retrospective data harmonisation, data availability, generalisation, information fusion limitations, and interpretability.

4.1. *Imaging challenges*

Medical imaging acquisition devices suffer to a lesser or greater extent from intrinsic and extrinsic imaging artefacts. For example, due to the nature of the acquisition process, magnetic resonance imaging is prone to Rician noise[215]; bias field inhomogeneity depends on the position of the receiver coil with respect to the object to image; k-space undersampling may produce ringing artefacts[216]; and motion may introduce distortion of low and high frequencies.[217, 218] Such distortions degrade the image quality and create variability that may prevent algorithms from performing as effectively as they would on "clean data".

Retrospective image enhancement may help to reduce training–testing variations. Conventional approaches leverage *a priori* information about the noise or artefacts to enhance the image. We think that deep learning can have a considerable impact in this regard as networks would learn statistics that help reduce these imaging artefacts directly from the input data. Examples of recently proposed deep learning techniques comprise magnetic resonance imaging motion artefact correction,[219, 220] magnetic resonance imaging denoising[221, 222] and low-dose computed tomography denoising.[223, 224] Nonetheless, the applicability of these techniques as the preprocessing step needs to be quantitatively assessed for the particular task of interest.

Data harmonisation may help reduce variation between training and testing domains. Research on this topic is needed to further improve both harmonisation and subsequent processing.[225] Also, the use of domain adaptation techniques, e.g., by means of transfer learning or image synthesis, can help mitigate the performance deterioration when switching image domains.[96, 123] In some cases, even a single case can allow trained models to perform similar to fully trained ones on another domain.[98, 99] These approaches are not yet widespread in the literature nor are cross-dataset evaluations. We think that more work should be done in these ways to examine how practical — not how intricate — deep learning-based solutions are.

4.2. *Deep learning challenges*

Deep learning techniques present several drawbacks and issues that are intrinsic to their nature: generalisation, information fusion limitations, and interpretability. Deep learning systems make an implicit assumption that a slow parameter tuning while minimising a loss function over a small collection of training images allows them to generalise well to other, possibly never seen, samples. Although this assumption may hold true for various fields, it does not for medical image analysis where large, heterogeneous and well-labelled datasets are typically scarce. Although valuable publicly available datasets have been released in the recent years, more ground truth is needed not only for training networks in such a way they generalise better but also for the sake of reproducibility. Further development on image synthesis or data augmentation could help overcome these limitations.[124, 218] Additionally, more frameworks for testing generalisability blindly are needed. To our knowledge, the Medical Image Segmentation Decathlon[b] and the six-month infant brain magnetic resonance imaging segmentation challenge[c] currently allow assessing the generalisability and robustness to imaging variations and processing tasks.

Information fusion implies processing imaging data along with personal, clinical, and/or genetic data from the patient.[226, 227] While deep learning techniques are extremely well-suited for analysis of natural signals, such as images, they are limited with other types

---

[b]More information at http://medicaldecathlon.com.
[c]More information at http://iseg2019.web.unc.edu/.

of data such as single numbers or text. Ongoing research focuses on the best and optimal ways to integrate these kinds of data into deep learning systems, which could predict clinical patient outcomes or improve treatment decisions.[226–228]

Another issue present in deep learning is the lack of interpretability.[227, 229–231] These kinds of systems train a model with large amounts of data to identify and learn image patterns that are needed to approximate the desired output. A trained model essentially consists of a huge number of learned parameters that regulate the mathematical operations that will be performed on the input image to produce the model output. It is not trivial to understand why or how a deep learning model outputs a certain result by looking at the values of trained parameters or the intermediate operations. Several techniques have been developed with the goal of reaching some level of understanding on how or why the network is reaching the specific outputs. For example, recently proposed techniques[223, 232] try to visualise what areas of the input image have been more influential and informative to reach the output result. Moreover, the output of deep learning systems is usually given without any measure of uncertainty or confidence of the results. This often results in obviously inaccurate or erroneous outputs given with the same level of confidence as the correct ones. Estimation of the certainty or confidence of deep learning methods[233] would increase their reliability and improve their accuracy.[179]

References

1. S. Zhang, L. Yao, A. Sun, and Y. Tay, Deep learning based recommender system: A survey and new perspectives, *ACM Comput. Surv. (CSUR)* **52**(1), 1–38 (2019).
2. A. Bouziane, D. Bouchiha, N. Doumi, and M. Malki, Question answering systems: Survey and trends, *Procedia Comput. Sci.* **73**, 366–375 (2015).
3. X. Liu, L. Faes, A. U. Kale, S. K. Wagner, D. J. Fu, A. Bruynseels, T. Mahendiran, G. Moraes, M. Shamdas, C. Kern, *et al.*, A comparison of deep learning performance against health-care professionals in detecting diseases from medical imaging: A systematic review and meta-analysis, *Lancet Digit. Health* **1**(6), e271–e297 (2019).

4. S. M. McKinney, M. Sieniek, V. Godbole, J. Godwin, N. Antropova, H. Ashrafian, T. Back, M. Chesus, G. C. Corrado, A. Darzi, *et al.*, International evaluation of an AI system for breast cancer screening, *Nature* **577**(7788), 89–94 (2020).

5. A. Esteva, B. Kuprel, R. A. Novoa, J. Ko, S. M. Swetter, H. M. Blau, and S. Thrun, Dermatologist-level classification of skin cancer with deep neural networks, *Nature* **542**(7639), 115–118 (2017).

6. O. Bernard, A. Lalande, C. Zotti, F. Cervenansky, X. Yang, P.-A. Heng, I. Cetin, K. Lekadir, O. Camara, M. A. G. Ballester, *et al.*, Deep learning techniques for automatic MRI cardiac multi-structures segmentation and diagnosis: Is the problem solved?, *IEEE Trans. Med. Imag.* **37**(11), 2514–2525 (2018).

7. M. Badar, M. Haris, and A. Fatima, Application of deep learning for retinal image analysis: A review, *Comput. Sci. Rev.* **35**, 100203 (2020).

8. D. Komura and S. Ishikawa, Machine learning methods for histopathological image analysis, *Comput. Struct. Biotechnol. J.* **16**, 34–42 (2018).

9. Z. Akkus, A. Galimzianova, A. Hoogi, D. L. Rubin, and B. J. Erickson, Deep learning for brain MRI segmentation: State of the art and future directions, *J. Digit. Imag.* **30**(4), 449–459 (2017).

10. A. Krizhevsky, I. Sutskever, and G. E. Hinton. Imagenet classification with deep convolutional neural networks. In *Advances in Neural Information Processing Systems*, pp. 1097–1105 (2012).

11. K. He, X. Zhang, S. Ren, and J. Sun. Deep residual learning for image recognition. In *Proceedings of the IEEE Conference on Computer Vision and Pattern Recognition*, pp. 770–778 (2016).

12. C. Szegedy, S. Ioffe, V. Vanhoucke, and A. A. Alemi. Inception-v4, Inception-ResNet and the impact of residual connections on learning. In *Proceedings of the Thirty-First AAAI Conference on Artificial Intelligence, February 4-9, 2017, San Francisco, California, USA.*, pp. 4278–4284 (2017).

13. H. Noh, S. Hong, and B. Han. Learning deconvolution network for semantic segmentation. In *Proceedings of the IEEE International Conference on Computer Vision*, pp. 1520–1528 (2015).

14. S. Ioffe and C. Szegedy. Batch normalization: Accelerating deep network training by reducing internal covariate shift. In *Proceedings of The 32nd International Conference on Machine Learning*, pp. 448–456 (2015).

15. A. Hasegawa, S.-C. B. Lo, M. T. Freedman, and S. K. Mun. Convolution neural-network-based detection of lung structures. In *Medical Imaging 1994*, pp. 654–662 (1994).

16. S.-C. Lo, S.-L. Lou, J.-S. Lin, M. T. Freedman, M. V. Chien, and S. K. Mun, Artificial convolution neural network techniques and applications for lung nodule detection, *IEEE Trans. Med. Imag.* **14**(4), 711–718 (1995).

17. B. Sahiner, H.-P. Chan, N. Petrick, D. Wei, M. A. Helvie, D. D. Adler, and M. M. Goodsitt, Classification of mass and normal breast tissue: A convolution neural network classifier with spatial domain and texture images, *IEEE Trans. Med. Imag.* **15**(5), 598–610 (1996).

18. A. Eklund, P. Dufort, D. Forsberg, and S. M. LaConte, Medical image processing on the GPU–past, present and future, *Med. Imag. Anal.* **17**(8), 1073–1094 (2013).

19. D. Shen, G. Wu, and H.-I. Suk, Deep learning in medical image analysis, *Ann. Rev. Biomed. Eng.* **19**, 221–248 (2017).

20. G. Litjens, T. Kooi, B. E. Bejnordi, A. A. A. Setio, F. Ciompi, M. Ghafoorian, J. A. van der Laak, B. van Ginneken, and C. I. Sánchez, A survey on deep learning in medical image analysis, *Med. Imag. Anal.* **42**, 60–88 (2017).

21. X. Yi, E. Walia, and P. Babyn, Generative adversarial network in medical imaging: A review, *Med. Imag. Anal.* **58**, 101552 (2019).

22. A. S. Lundervold and A. Lundervold, An overview of deep learning in medical imaging focusing on MRI, *Zeitschrift für Medizinische Physik* **29**(2), 102–127 (2019).

23. V. Cheplygina, M. de Bruijne, and J. P. Pluim, Not-so-supervised: A survey of semi-supervised, multi-instance, and transfer learning in medical image analysis, *Med. Imag. Anal.* **54**, 280–296 (2019).

24. G. Litjens, F. Ciompi, J. M. Wolterink, B. D. de Vos, T. Leiner, J. Teuwen, and I. Išgum, State-of-the-art deep learning in cardiovascular image analysis, *JACC: Cardiovasc. Imag.* **12**(8), 1549–1565 (2019).

25. J. Bernal, K. Kushibar, D. S. Asfaw, S. Valverde, A. Oliver, R. Martí, and X. Lladó, Deep convolutional neural networks for brain image analysis on magnetic resonance imaging: A review, *Artif. Intell. Med.* **95**, 64–81 (2019).

26. G. Zhu, B. Jiang, L. Tong, Y. Xie, G. Zaharchuk, and M. Wintermark, Applications of deep learning to neuro-imaging techniques, *Front. Neurol.* **10**, 869 (2019).

27. C. Szegedy, W. Liu, Y. Jia, P. Sermanet, S. Reed, D. Anguelov, D. Erhan, V. Vanhoucke, and A. Rabinovich. Going deeper with convolutions. In *Proceedings of the IEEE Conference on Computer Vision and Pattern Recognition*, pp. 1–9 (2015).

28. C. Ulas, D. Das, M. J. Thrippleton, M. D. C. Valdes Hernandez, P. A. Armitage, S. D. Makin, J. M. Wardlaw, and B. H. Menze, Convolutional neural networks for direct inference of pharmacokinetic parameters: Application to stroke dynamic contrast-enhanced MRI, *Front. Neurol.* **9**, 1147 (2019).

29. H. R. Roth, L. Lu, A. Seff, K. M. Cherry, J. Hoffman, S. Wang, J. Liu, E. Turkbey, and R. M. Summers. A new 2.5 D representation for lymph node detection using random sets of deep convolutional neural network observations. In *International Conference on Medical Image Computing and Computer-Assisted Intervention*, pp. 520–527 (2014).

30. M. Lyksborg, O. Puonti, M. Agn, and R. Larsen. An ensemble of 2D convolutional neural networks for tumor segmentation. In *Scandinavian Conference on Image Analysis*, pp. 201–211 (2015).

31. A. Birenbaum and H. Greenspan. Longitudinal multiple sclerosis lesion segmentation using multi-view convolutional neural networks. In *Deep Learning and Data Labeling for Medical Applications*, pp. 58–67. Springer (2016).

32. H. R. Roth, Y. Wang, J. Yao, L. Lu, J. E. Burns, and R. M. Summers. Deep convolutional networks for automated detection of posterior-element fractures on spine CT. In *Medical Imaging 2016: Computer-Aided Diagnosis*, Vol. 9785, p. 97850P (2016).

33. J. Yun, J. Park, D. Yu, J. Yi, M. Lee, H. J. Park, J.-G. Lee, J. B. Seo, and N. Kim, Improvement of fully automated airway segmentation on volumetric computed tomographic images using a 2.5 dimensional convolutional neural net, *Med. Imag. Anal.* **51**, 13–20 (2019).

34. S. R. van der Voort, F. Incekara, M. M. Wijnenga, G. Kapsas, R. Gahrmann, J. W. Schouten, R. N. Tewarie, G. J. Lycklama, P. C. Hamer, R. S. Eijgelaar, *et al.*, WHO 2016 subtyping and automated segmentation of glioma using multi-task deep learning, *coRR.* **abs/2010.04425** (2020).

35. J. Bernal, K. Kushibar, M. Cabezas, S. Valverde, A. Oliver, and X. Lladó, Quantitative analysis of patch-based fully convolutional neural networks for tissue segmentation on brain magnetic resonance imaging, *IEEE Access* **7**, 89986–90002 (2019).

36. J. Long, E. Shelhamer, and T. Darrell. Fully convolutional networks for semantic segmentation. In *Proceedings of the IEEE Conference on Computer Vision and Pattern Recognition*, pp. 3431–3440 (2015).

37. M. Lin, Q. Chen, and S. Yan, Network in network, *coRR.* **abs/1312.4400** (2013).

38. Ö. Çiçek, A. Abdulkadir, S. S. Lienkamp, T. Brox, and O. Ronneberger. 3D U-Net: Learning dense volumetric segmentation from sparse annotation. In *International Conference on Medical Image Computing and Computer-Assisted Intervention*, pp. 424–432 (2016).

39. Q. Dou, H. Chen, L. Yu, L. Zhao, J. Qin, D. Wang, V. C. Mok, L. Shi, and P.-A. Heng, Automatic detection of cerebral microbleeds from MR images via 3D convolutional neural networks, *IEEE Trans. Med. Imag.* **35**(5), 1182–1195 (2016).

40. T. Brosch, L. Y. Tang, Y. Yoo, D. K. Li, A. Traboulsee, and R. Tam, Deep 3D convolutional encoder networks with shortcuts for multiscale feature integration applied to multiple sclerosis lesion segmentation, *IEEE Trans. Med. Imag.* **35**(5), 1229–1239 (2016).

41. P. F. Christ, M. E. A. Elshaer, F. Ettlinger, S. Tatavarty, M. Bickel, P. Bilic, M. Rempfler, M. Armbruster, F. Hofmann, M. D'Anastasi, *et al.* Automatic liver and lesion segmentation in CT using cascaded fully convolutional neural networks and 3D conditional random fields. In *International Conference on Medical Image Computing and Computer-Assisted Intervention*, pp. 415–423 (2016).

42. K. Kamnitsas, C. Ledig, V. F. Newcombe, J. P. Simpson, A. D. Kane, D. K. Menon, D. Rueckert, and B. Glocker, Efficient multi-scale 3D CNN with fully connected CRF for accurate brain lesion segmentation, *Med. Imag. Anal.* **36**, 61–78 (2017).

43. A. G. Roy, S. Conjeti, S. P. K. Karri, D. Sheet, A. Katouzian, C. Wachinger, and N. Navab, ReLayNet: Retinal layer and fluid segmentation of macular optical coherence tomography using fully convolutional networks, *Biomed. Opt. Express* **8**(8), 3627–3642 (2017).

44. M. Havaei, A. Davy, D. Warde-Farley, A. Biard, A. Courville, Y. Bengio, C. Pal, P.-M. Jodoin, and H. Larochelle, Brain tumor segmentation with deep neural networks, *Med. Imag. Anal.* **35**, 18–31 (2017).

45. J. Dolz, C. Desrosiers, and I. B. Ayed, 3D fully convolutional networks for subcortical segmentation in MRI: A large-scale study, *NeuroImage* **170**, 456–470 (2018).

46. A. G. Roy, N. Navab, and C. Wachinger, Concurrent spatial and channel "squeeze & excitation" in fully convolutional networks. In *International Conference on Medical Image Computing and Computer-Assisted Intervention*, pp. 421–429 (2018).

47. H. Oda, H. R. Roth, K. K. Bhatia, M. Oda, T. Kitasaka, S. Iwano, H. Homma, H. Takabatake, M. Mori, H. Natori, *et al.* Dense volumetric detection and segmentation of mediastinal lymph nodes in chest CT images. In *Medical Imaging 2018: Computer-Aided Diagnosis*, Vol. 10575, p. 1057502 (2018).

48. M. Khened, V. A. Kollerathu, and G. Krishnamurthi, Fully convolutional multi-scale residual DenseNets for cardiac segmentation and automated cardiac diagnosis using ensemble of classifiers, *Med. Imag. Anal.* **51**, 21–45 (2019).

49. F. Milletari, N. Navab, and S.-A. Ahmadi. V-net: Fully convolutional neural networks for volumetric medical image segmentation. In *2016 Fourth International Conference on 3D Vision (3DV)*, pp. 565–571 (2016).

50. R. Guerrero, C. Qin, O. Oktay, C. Bowles, L. Chen, R. Joules, R. Wolz, M. d. C. Valdés-Hernández, D. Dickie, J. Wardlaw, *et al.*, White matter hyperintensity and stroke lesion segmentation and differentiation using convolutional neural networks, *NeuroImage: Clin.* **17**, 918–934 (2018).

51. X. Li, H. Chen, X. Qi, Q. Dou, C.-W. Fu, and P.-A. Heng, H-DenseUNet: Hybrid densely connected UNet for liver and tumor segmentation from CT volumes, *IEEE Trans. Med.Imag.* **37**(12), 2663–2674 (2018).

52. J. Hu, H. Wang, S. Gao, M. Bao, T. Liu, Y. Wang, and J. Zhang, S-UNet: A bridge-style U-Net framework with a saliency mechanism for retinal vessel segmentation, *IEEE Access* **7**, 174167–174177 (2019).

53. C. Ye, W. Wang, S. Zhang, and K. Wang, Multi-depth fusion network for whole-heart CT image segmentation, *IEEE Access* **7**, 23421–23429 (2019).

54. L. Yu, X. Yang, H. Chen, J. Qin, and P. A. Heng. Volumetric ConvNets with mixed residual connections for automated prostate segmentation from 3D MR images. In *Thirty-first AAAI Conference on Artificial Intelligence* (2017).

55. G. Balakrishnan, A. Zhao, M. R. Sabuncu, J. Guttag, and A. V. Dalca, VoxelMorph: A learning framework for deformable medical image registration, *IEEE Trans. Med. Imag.* **38**(8), 1788–1800 (2019).

56. M. Salem, S. Valverde, M. Cabezas, D. Pareto, A. Oliver, J. Salvi, À. Rovira, and X. Lladó, A fully convolutional neural network for new T2-w lesion detection in multiple sclerosis, *NeuroImage: Clin.* **25**, 102149 (2020).

57. F. Isensee, P. F. Jaeger, S. A. Kohl, J. Petersen, and K. H. Maier-Hein, nnu-net: A self-configuring method for deep learning-based biomedical image segmentation, *Nat. Methods* pp. 1–9 (2020).

58. A. Clèrigues, S. Valverde, J. Bernal, J. Freixenet, A. Oliver, and X. Lladó, Acute ischemic stroke lesion core segmentation in CT perfusion images using fully convolutional neural networks, *Comput. Biol. Med.* **115**, 103487 (2019).

59. A. Clèrigues, S. Valverde, J. Bernal, J. Freixenet, A. Oliver, and X. Lladó, Acute and sub-acute stroke lesion segmentation from multimodal MRI, *Comput. Methods Programs Biomed.* p. 105521 (2020).

60. O. Ronneberger, P. Fischer, and T. Brox. U-net: Convolutional networks for biomedical image segmentation. In *International Conference*

on *Medical Image Computing and Computer-Assisted Intervention*, pp. 234–241 (2015).

61. T.-L.-T. Le, N. Thome, S. Bernard, V. Bismuth, F. Patoureaux, *et al.* Multitask classification and segmentation for cancer diagnosis in mammography. In *International Conference on Medical Imaging with Deep Learning–Extended Abstract Track* (2019).

62. S. Spasov, L. Passamonti, A. Duggento, P. Liò, N. Toschi, A. D. N. Initiative, *et al.*, A parameter-efficient deep learning approach to predict conversion from mild cognitive impairment to Alzheimer's disease, *Neuroimage* **189**, 276–287 (2019).

63. W. Zhang, R. Li, H. Deng, L. Wang, W. Lin, S. Ji, and D. Shen, Deep convolutional neural networks for multi-modality isointense infant brain image segmentation, *NeuroImage* **108**, 214–224 (2015).

64. M. Ghafoorian, N. Karssemeijer, T. Heskes, I. W. van Uden, C. I. Sanchez, G. Litjens, F.-E. de Leeuw, B. van Ginneken, E. Marchiori, and B. Platel, Location sensitive deep convolutional neural networks for segmentation of white matter hyperintensities, *Sci. Rep.* **7**(1), 1–12 (2017).

65. H.-I. Suk, S.-W. Lee, D. Shen, Alzheimer's Disease Neuroimaging Initiative, *et al.*, Hierarchical feature representation and multimodal fusion with deep learning for AD/MCI diagnosis, *NeuroImage* **101**, 569–582 (2014).

66. A. Chartsias, T. Joyce, M. V. Giuffrida, and S. A. Tsaftaris, Multimodal MR synthesis via modality-invariant latent representation, *IEEE Trans. Med. Imag.* **37**(3), 803–814 (2017).

67. M. Salem, S. Valverde, M. Cabezas, D. Pareto, A. Oliver, J. Salvi, À. Rovira, and X. Lladó, Multiple sclerosis lesion synthesis in MRI using an encoder-decoder U-NET, *IEEE Access* **7**, 25171–25184 (2019).

68. P. Moeskops, M. A. Viergever, A. M. Mendrik, L. S. De Vries, M. J. Benders, and I. Išgum, Automatic segmentation of MR brain images with a convolutional neural network, *IEEE Trans Med. Imag.* **35**(5), 1252–1261 (2016).

69. L. Zhao and K. Jia, Multiscale CNNs for brain tumor segmentation and diagnosis, *Comput. Math. Methods Med.* **2016** (2016).

70. R. Mehta, A. Majumdar, and J. Sivaswamy, BrainSegNet: a convolutional neural network architecture for automated segmentation of human brain structures, *J. Med. Imag.* **4**(2), 024003 (2017).

71. S. Hussain, S. M. Anwar, and M. Majid. Brain tumor segmentation using cascaded deep convolutional neural network. In *2017 39th Annual International Conference of the IEEE Engineering in Medicine and Biology Society (EMBC)*, pp. 1998–2001 (2017).

72. Y. He, A. Carass, Y. Yun, C. Zhao, B. M. Jedynak, S. D. Solomon, S. Saidha, P. A. Calabresi, and J. L. Prince. Towards topological correct segmentation of macular OCT from cascaded FCNs. In *Fetal, Infant and Ophthalmic Medical Image Analysis*, pp. 202–209. Springer (2017).

73. S. Valverde, M. Cabezas, E. Roura, S. González-Villà, D. Pareto, J. C. Vilanova, L. Ramió-Torrentà, À. Rovira, A. Oliver, and X. Lladó, Improving automated multiple sclerosis lesion segmentation with a cascaded 3D convolutional neural network approach, *NeuroImage* **155**, 159–168 (2017).

74. R. Janssens, G. Zeng, and G. Zheng. Fully automatic segmentation of lumbar vertebrae from CT images using cascaded 3D fully convolutional networks. In *2018 IEEE 15th International Symposium on Biomedical Imaging (ISBI 2018)*, pp. 893–897 (2018).

75. H. R. Roth, H. Oda, X. Zhou, N. Shimizu, Y. Yang, Y. Hayashi, M. Oda, M. Fujiwara, K. Misawa, and K. Mori, An application of cascaded 3D fully convolutional networks for medical image segmentation, *Comput. Med. Imag. Graph.* **66**, 90–99 (2018).

76. H. Chen, Q. Dou, L. Yu, J. Qin, and P.-A. Heng, VoxResNet: Deep voxelwise residual networks for brain segmentation from 3D MR images, *NeuroImage* **170**, 446–455 (2018).

77. M. Liu, D. Cheng, K. Wang, Y. Wang, A. D. N. Initiative, *et al.*, Multi-modality cascaded convolutional neural networks for Alzheimer's disease diagnosis, *Neuroinformatics* **16**(3–4), 295–308 (2018).

78. K. Bahrami, I. Rekik, F. Shi, and D. Shen. Joint reconstruction and segmentation of 7T-like MR images from 3T MRI based on cascaded convolutional neural networks. In *International Conference on Medical Image Computing and Computer-Assisted Intervention*, pp. 764–772 (2017).

79. C. Wachinger, M. Reuter, and T. Klein, DeepNAT: Deep convolutional neural network for segmenting neuroanatomy, *NeuroImage* **170**, 434–445 (2018).

80. O. Commowick, A. Istace, M. Kain, B. Laurent, F. Leray, M. Simon, S. C. Pop, P. Girard, R. Ameli, J.-C. Ferré, *et al.*, Objective evaluation of multiple sclerosis lesion segmentation using a data management and processing infrastructure, *Sci. Rep.* **8**(1), 1–17 (2018).

81. G. A. Reina, R. Panchumarthy, S. P. Thakur, A. Bastidas, and S. Bakas, Systematic evaluation of image tiling adverse effects on deep learning semantic segmentation, *Front. Neurosci.* **14**, 65 (2020).

82. H. Lombaert, J. Sporring, and K. Siddiqi. Diffeomorphic spectral matching of cortical surfaces. In *International Conference on Information Processing in Medical Imaging*, pp. 376–389 (2013).

83. C. Wachinger, M. Brennan, G. Sharp, and P. Golland. On the importance of location and features for the patch-based segmentation of parotid glands. In *MICCAI Workshop on Image-Guided Adaptive Radiation Therapy* (2014).
84. C. Wachinger, M. Brennan, G. C. Sharp, and P. Golland, Efficient descriptor-based segmentation of parotid glands with nonlocal means, *IEEE Trans. Biomed. Eng.* **64**(7), 1492–1502 (2016).
85. M. Ghafoorian, N. Karssemeijer, T. Heskes, M. Bergkamp, J. Wissink, J. Obels, K. Keizer, F.-E. de Leeuw, B. van Ginneken, E. Marchiori, *et al.*, Deep multi-scale location-aware 3D convolutional neural networks for automated detection of lacunes of presumed vascular origin, *NeuroImage: Clin.* **14**, 391–399 (2017).
86. K. Kushibar, S. Valverde, S. González-Villà, J. Bernal, M. Cabezas, A. Oliver, and X. Lladó, Automated sub-cortical brain structure segmentation combining spatial and deep convolutional features, *Med. Imag. Anal.* **48**, 177–186 (2018).
87. H. Jia, Y. Xia, Y. Song, W. Cai, M. Fulham, and D. D. Feng, Atlas registration and ensemble deep convolutional neural network-based prostate segmentation using magnetic resonance imaging, *Neurocomputing* **275**, 1358–1369 (2018).
88. I. Goodfellow, J. Pouget-Abadie, M. Mirza, B. Xu, D. Warde-Farley, S. Ozair, A. Courville, and Y. Bengio. Generative adversarial nets. In *Advances in Neural Information Processing Systems*, pp. 2672–2680 (2014).
89. H.-C. Shin, N. A. Tenenholtz, J. K. Rogers, C. G. Schwarz, M. L. Senjem, J. L. Gunter, K. P. Andriole, and M. Michalski. Medical image synthesis for data augmentation and anonymization using generative adversarial networks. In *International Workshop on Simulation and Synthesis in Medical Imaging*, pp. 1–11 (2018).
90. Y. Huo, Z. Xu, H. Moon, S. Bao, A. Assad, T. K. Moyo, M. R. Savona, R. G. Abramson, and B. A. Landman, Synseg-net: Synthetic segmentation without target modality ground truth, *IEEE Trans. Med. Imag.* **38**(4), 1016–1025 (2018).
91. Y. Ganin and V. Lempitsky. Unsupervised domain adaptation by backpropagation. In *International Conference on Machine Learning*, pp. 1180–1189 (2015).
92. K. Kamnitsas, C. Baumgartner, C. Ledig, V. Newcombe, J. Simpson, A. Kane, D. Menon, A. Nori, A. Criminisi, D. Rueckert, *et al.* Unsupervised domain adaptation in brain lesion segmentation with adversarial networks. In *International Conference on Information Processing in Medical Imaging*, pp. 597–609 (2017).

93. C. S. Perone, P. Ballester, R. C. Barros, and J. Cohen-Adad, Unsupervised domain adaptation for medical imaging segmentation with self-ensembling, *NeuroImage* **194**, 1–11 (2019).
94. J. Yosinski, J. Clune, Y. Bengio, and H. Lipson. How transferable are features in deep neural networks? In *Advances in Neural Information Processing Systems*, pp. 3320–3328 (2014).
95. A. R. Zamir, A. Sax, W. Shen, L. J. Guibas, J. Malik, and S. Savarese. Taskonomy: Disentangling task transfer learning. In *IEEE Conference on Computer Vision and Pattern Recognition*, pp. 3712–3722 (2018).
96. N. Tajbakhsh, J. Y. Shin, S. R. Gurudu, R. T. Hurst, C. B. Kendall, M. B. Gotway, and J. Liang, Convolutional neural networks for medical image analysis: Full training or fine tuning?, *IEEE Trans. Med. Imag.* **35**(5), 1299–1312 (2016).
97. M. Ghafoorian, A. Mehrtash, T. Kapur, N. Karssemeijer, E. Marchiori, M. Pesteie, C. R. Guttmann, F.-E. de Leeuw, C. M. Tempany, B. van Ginneken, *et al.* Transfer learning for domain adaptation in MRI: Application in brain lesion segmentation. In *International Conference on Medical Image Computing and Computer-Assisted Intervention*, pp. 516–524 (2017).
98. K. Kushibar, S. Valverde, S. González-Villà, J. Bernal, M. Cabezas, A. Oliver, and X. Lladó, Supervised domain adaptation for automatic sub-cortical brain structure segmentation with minimal user interaction, *Sci. Rep.* **9**(1), 1–15 (2019).
99. S. Valverde, M. Salem, M. Cabezas, D. Pareto, J. C. Vilanova, L. Ramió-Torrentà, À. Rovira, J. Salvi, A. Oliver, and X. Lladó, One-shot domain adaptation in multiple sclerosis lesion segmentation using convolutional neural networks, *NeuroImage: Clin.* **21**, 101638 (2019).
100. C. Mazo, J. Bernal, M. Trujillo, and E. Alegre, Transfer learning for classification of cardiovascular tissues in histological images, *Comput. Methods Programs Biomed.* **165**, 69–76 (2018).
101. D. Chaves, L. Fernández-Robles, J. Bernal, E. Alegre, and M. Trujillo, Automatic characterisation of chars from the combustion of pulverised coals using machine vision, *Powder Technol.* **338**, 110–118 (2018).
102. A. Rehman, S. Naz, M. I. Razzak, F. Akram, and M. Imran, A deep learning-based framework for automatic brain tumors classification using transfer learning, *Circuits Syst. Signal Process.* **39**(2), 757–775 (2020).
103. J. Acosta-Cabronero, G. B. Williams, J. M. Pereira, G. Pengas, and P. J. Nestor, The impact of skull-stripping and radio-frequency bias correction on grey-matter segmentation for voxel-based morphometry, *NeuroImage* **39**(4), 1654–1665 (2008).

104. V. Popescu, M. Battaglini, W. Hoogstrate, S. C. Verfaillie, I. Sluimer, R. A. van Schijndel, B. W. van Dijk, K. S. Cover, D. L. Knol, M. Jenkinson, *et al.*, Optimizing parameter choice for FSL-Brain Extraction Tool (BET) on 3D T1 images in multiple sclerosis, *NeuroImage* **61**(4), 1484–1494 (2012).

105. J.-M. Lee, U. Yoon, S. H. Nam, J.-H. Kim, I.-Y. Kim, and S. I. Kim, Evaluation of automated and semi-automated skull-stripping algorithms using similarity index and segmentation error, *Comput. Biol. Med.* **33**(6), 495–507 (2003).

106. S. A. Sadananthan, W. Zheng, M. W. Chee, and V. Zagorodnov, Skull stripping using graph cuts, *NeuroImage* **49**(1), 225–239 (2010).

107. K. Nakamura, S. F. Eskildsen, S. Narayanan, D. L. Arnold, D. L. Collins, Alzheimer's Disease Neuroimaging Initiative, *et al.*, Improving the SIENA performance using BEaST brain extraction, *PloS One* **13**(9) (2018).

108. S. M. Smith, Fast robust automated brain extraction, *Hum. Brain Mapp.* **17**(3), 143–155 (2002).

109. M. Jenkinson, M. Pechaud, S. Smith, *et al.* BET2: MR-based estimation of brain, skull and scalp surfaces. In *Eleventh Annual Meeting of the Organization for Human Brain Mapping*, Vol. 17, p. 167 (2005).

110. J. E. Iglesias, C.-Y. Liu, P. M. Thompson, and Z. Tu, Robust brain extraction across datasets and comparison with publicly available methods, *IEEE Trans. Med. Imag.* **30**(9), 1617–1634 (2011).

111. F. Shi, L. Wang, Y. Dai, J. H. Gilmore, W. Lin, and D. Shen, LABEL: Pediatric brain extraction using learning-based meta-algorithm, *NeuroImage* **62**(3), 1975–1986 (2012).

112. S. F. Eskildsen, P. Coupé, V. Fonov, J. V. Manjón, K. K. Leung, N. Guizard, S. N. Wassef, L. R. Østergaard, D. L. Collins, Alzheimer's Disease Neuroimaging Initiative, *et al.*, BEaST: Brain extraction based on nonlocal segmentation technique, *NeuroImage* **59**(3), 2362–2373 (2012).

113. L. G. Nyúl and J. K. Udupa, On standardizing the MR image intensity scale, *Magnet. Reson. Med.: Off. J. Int. Soc. Magnet. Reson. Med.* **42**(6), 1072–1081 (1999).

114. M. Shah, Y. Xiao, N. Subbanna, S. Francis, D. L. Arnold, D. L. Collins, and T. Arbel, Evaluating intensity normalization on MRIs of human brain with multiple sclerosis, *Med. Imag. Anal.* **15**(2), 267–282 (2011).

115. J. C. Reinhold, B. E. Dewey, A. Carass, and J. L. Prince, Evaluating the impact of intensity normalization on MR image synthesis. In *Medical Imaging 2019: Image Processing*, Vol. 10949, p. 109493H (2019).

116. R. T. Shinohara, E. M. Sweeney, J. Goldsmith, N. Shiee, F. J. Mateen, P. A. Calabresi, S. Jarso, D. L. Pham, D. S. Reich, C. M. Crainiceanu, *et al.*, Statistical normalization techniques for magnetic resonance imaging, *NeuroImage: Clin.* **6**, 9–19 (2014).

117. J.-P. Fortin, E. M. Sweeney, J. Muschelli, C. M. Crainiceanu, R. T. Shinohara, Alzheimer's Disease Neuroimaging Initiative, *et al.*, Removing inter-subject technical variability in magnetic resonance imaging studies, *NeuroImage* **132**, 198–212 (2016).

118. J. G. Sled, A. P. Zijdenbos, and A. C. Evans, A nonparametric method for automatic correction of intensity nonuniformity in MRI data, *IEEE Trans. Med. Imag.* **17**(1), 87–97 (1998).

119. N. J. Tustison, B. B. Avants, P. A. Cook, Y. Zheng, A. Egan, P. A. Yushkevich, and J. C. Gee, N4ITK: Improved N3 bias correction, *IEEE Trans. Med. Imag.* **29**(6), 1310–1320 (2010).

120. M. D. C. V. Hernández, V. González-Castro, D. T. Ghandour, X. Wang, F. Doubal, S. M. Maniega, P. A. Armitage, and J. M. Wardlaw, On the computational assessment of white matter hyperintensity progression: Difficulties in method selection and bias field correction performance on images with significant white matter pathology, *Neuroradiology* **58**(5), 475–485 (2016).

121. L. Maier-Hein, M. Eisenmann, A. Reinke, S. Onogur, M. Stankovic, P. Scholz, T. Arbel, H. Bogunovic, A. P. Bradley, A. Carass, *et al.*, Why rankings of biomedical image analysis competitions should be interpreted with care, *Nat. Commun.* **9**(1), 1–13 (2018).

122. M. Wang and W. Deng, Deep visual domain adaptation: A survey, *Neurocomputing* **312**, 135–153 (2018).

123. A. Choudhary, L. Tong, Y. Zhu, and M. D. Wang, Advancing medical imaging informatics by deep learning-based domain adaptation, *Yearb. Med. Inform.* **29**(1), 129 (2020).

124. B. Billot, D. Greve, K. Van Leemput, B. Fischl, J. E. Iglesias, and A. V. Dalca, A learning strategy for contrast-agnostic MRI segmentation, *coRR.* **abs/2003.01995** (2020).

125. H. E. Atlason, A. Love, S. Sigurdsson, V. Gudnason, and L. M. Ellingsen, SegAE: unsupervised white matter lesion segmentation from brain MRIs using a CNN autoencoder, *NeuroImage: Clin.* **24**, 102085 (2019).

126. Y. Xue, F. G. Farhat, O. Boukrina, A. Barrett, J. R. Binder, U. W. Roshan, and W. W. Graves, A multi-path 2.5 dimensional convolutional neural network system for segmenting stroke lesions in brain MRI images, *NeuroImage: Clin.* **25**, 102118 (2020).

127. S. Pereira, A. Pinto, V. Alves, and C. A. Silva, Brain tumor segmentation using convolutional neural networks in MRI images, *IEEE Trans. Med. Imag.* **35**(5), 1240–1251 (2016).

128. J. Kleesiek, G. Urban, A. Hubert, D. Schwarz, K. Maier-Hein, M. Bendszus, and A. Biller, Deep MRI brain extraction: A 3D convolutional neural network for skull stripping, *NeuroImage* **129**, 460–469 (2016).

129. S. Bao, P. Wang, T. C. Mok, and A. C. Chung, 3D Randomized connection network with graph-based label inference, *IEEE Trans. Imag. Process.* **27**(8), 3883–3892 (2018).

130. M. Rajchl, M. C. Lee, O. Oktay, K. Kamnitsas, J. Passerat-Palmbach, W. Bai, M. Damodaram, M. A. Rutherford, J. V. Hajnal, B. Kainz, *et al.*, Deepcut: Object segmentation from bounding box annotations using convolutional neural networks, *IEEE Trans. Med. Imag.* **36**(2), 674–683 (2016).

131. M. Shakeri, S. Tsogkas, E. Ferrante, S. Lippe, S. Kadoury, N. Paragios, and I. Kokkinos. Sub-cortical brain structure segmentation using F-CNN's. In *2016 IEEE 13th International Symposium on Biomedical Imaging (ISBI)*, pp. 269–272 (2016).

132. A. Alansary, O. Oktay, Y. Li, L. Le Folgoc, B. Hou, G. Vaillant, K. Kamnitsas, A. Vlontzos, B. Glocker, B. Kainz, *et al.*, Evaluating reinforcement learning agents for anatomical landmark detection, *Med. Imag. Analy.* **53**, 156–164 (2019).

133. S. Aslani, M. Dayan, L. Storelli, M. Filippi, V. Murino, M. A. Rocca, and D. Sona, Multi-branch convolutional neural network for multiple sclerosis lesion segmentation, *NeuroImage* **196**, 1–15 (2019).

134. A. Basher, K. Y. Choi, J. J. Lee, B. Lee, B. C. Kim, K. H. Lee, and H. Y. Jung, Hippocampus localization using a two-stage ensemble hough convolutional neural network, *IEEE Access* **7**, 73436–73447 (2019).

135. Y. Huo, Z. Xu, Y. Xiong, K. Aboud, P. Parvathaneni, S. Bao, C. Bermudez, S. M. Resnick, L. E. Cutting, and B. A. Landman, 3D whole brain segmentation using spatially localized atlas network tiles, *NeuroImage* **194**, 105–119 (2019).

136. D. Hu, Z. Luo, and L. Zhao, Gender identification based on human brain structural MRI with a multi-layer 3D convolution extreme learning machine, *Cognit. Comput. Syst.* **1**(4), 91–96 (2019).

137. S. Afzal, M. Maqsood, F. Nazir, U. Khan, F. Aadil, K. M. Awan, I. Mehmood, and O.-Y. Song, A data augmentation-based framework to handle class imbalance problem for Alzheimer's stage detection, *IEEE Access* **7**, 115528–115539 (2019).

138. S. Ahmed, K. Y. Choi, J. J. Lee, B. C. Kim, G.-R. Kwon, K. H. Lee, and H. Y. Jung, Ensembles of patch-based classifiers for diagnosis of Alzheimer diseases, *IEEE Access* **7**, 73373–73383 (2019).

139. S. Basaia, F. Agosta, L. Wagner, E. Canu, G. Magnani, R. Santangelo, M. Filippi, Alzheimer's Disease Neuroimaging Initiative, *et al.*,

Automated classification of Alzheimer's disease and mild cognitive impairment using a single MRI and deep neural networks, *NeuroImage: Clin.* **21**, 101645 (2019).

140. A. Chaddad, M. Toews, C. Desrosiers, and T. Niazi, Deep radiomic analysis based on modeling information flow in convolutional neural networks, *IEEE Access* **7**, 97242–97252 (2019).

141. R. Ceschin, A. Zahner, W. Reynolds, J. Gaesser, G. Zuccoli, C. W. Lo, V. Gopalakrishnan, and A. Panigrahy, A computational framework for the detection of subcortical brain dysmaturation in neonatal MRI using 3D convolutional neural networks, *NeuroImage* **178**, 183–197 (2018).

142. F. Eitel, E. Soehler, J. Bellmann-Strobl, A. U. Brandt, K. Ruprecht, R. M. Giess, J. Kuchling, S. Asseyer, M. Weygandt, J.-D. Haynes, *et al.*, Uncovering convolutional neural network decisions for diagnosing multiple sclerosis on conventional MRI using layer-wise relevance propagation, *NeuroImage: Clin.* **24**, 102003 (2019).

143. C. Feng, A. Elazab, P. Yang, T. Wang, F. Zhou, H. Hu, X. Xiao, and B. Lei, Deep learning framework for Alzheimer's disease diagnosis via 3D-CNN and FSBi-LSTM, *IEEE Access* **7**, 63605–63618 (2019).

144. M. S. Graham, I. Drobnjak, and H. Zhang, A supervised learning approach for diffusion MRI quality control with minimal training data, *NeuroImage* **178**, 668–676 (2018).

145. H. Huang, X. Hu, Y. Zhao, M. Makkie, Q. Dong, S. Zhao, L. Guo, and T. Liu, Modeling task fMRI data via deep convolutional autoencoder, *IEEE Trans. Med. Imag.* **37**(7), 1551–1561 (2017).

146. T.-E. Kam, H. Zhang, Z. Jiao, and D. Shen, Deep learning of static and dynamic brain functional networks for early MCI detection, *IEEE Trans. Med. Imag.* **39**(2), 478–487 (2019).

147. E. Lee, J.-S. Choi, M. Kim, H.-I. Suk, A. D. N. Initiative, *et al.*, Toward an interpretable Alzheimer's disease diagnostic model with regional abnormality representation via deep learning, *NeuroImage* **202**, 116113 (2019).

148. M. Liu, J. Zhang, D. Nie, P.-T. Yap, and D. Shen, Anatomical landmark based deep feature representation for MR images in brain disease diagnosis, *IEEE J. Biomed. Health Informat.* **22**(5), 1476–1485 (2018).

149. M. Liu, J. Zhang, E. Adeli, and D. Shen, Joint classification and regression via deep multi-task multi-channel learning for Alzheimer's disease diagnosis, *IEEE Trans. Biomed. Eng.* **66**(5), 1195–1206 (2018).

150. M. Liu, J. Zhang, E. Adeli, and D. Shen, Landmark-based deep multi-instance learning for brain disease diagnosis, *Med. Imag. Anal.* **43**, 157–168 (2018).

151. H. Li and Y. Fan, Interpretable, highly accurate brain decoding of subtly distinct brain states from functional MRI using intrinsic functional networks and long short-term memory recurrent neural networks, *NeuroImage* **202**, 116059 (2019).

152. M. Maleki, M. Teshnehlab, and M. Nabavi, Diagnosis of multiple sclerosis (MS) using convolutional neural network (CNN) from MRIs, *Glob. J. Med. Plant Res.* **1**(1), 50–54 (2012).

153. S. Minaee, Y. Wang, A. Aygar, S. Chung, X. Wang, Y. W. Lui, E. Fieremans, S. Flanagan, and J. Rath, MTBI identification from diffusion MR images using bag of adversarial visual features, *IEEE Trans. Med. Imag.* **38**(11), 2545–2555 (2019).

154. F. Ren, C. Yang, Q. Qiu, N. Zeng, C. Cai, C. Hou, and Q. Zou, Exploiting discriminative regions of brain slices based on 2D CNNs for Alzheimer's disease classification, *IEEE Access* (2019).

155. S. Sarraf, D. D. Desouza, J. A. Anderson, and C. Saverino, MCADNNet: Recognizing stages of cognitive impairment through efficient convolutional fMRI and MRI neural network topology models, *IEEE Access* **7**, 155584–155600 (2019).

156. H. H. Sultan, N. M. Salem, and W. Al-Atabany, Multi-classification of brain tumor images using deep neural network, *IEEE Access* **7**, 69215–69225 (2019).

157. Z. Wang, Y. Sun, Q. Shen, and L. Cao, Dilated 3D convolutional neural networks for brain MRI data classification, *IEEE Access* **7**, 134388–134398 (2019).

158. L. Yuan, X. Wei, H. Shen, L.-L. Zeng, and D. Hu, Multi-center brain imaging classification using a novel 3D CNN approach, *IEEE Access* **6**, 49925–49934 (2018).

159. L. Yue, X. Gong, J. Li, H. Ji, M. Li, and A. K. Nandi, Hierarchical feature extraction for early Alzheimer's disease diagnosis, *IEEE Access* **7**, 93752–93760 (2019).

160. S. Zhang, H. Liu, H. Huang, Y. Zhao, X. Jiang, B. Bowers, L. Guo, X. Hu, M. Sanchez, and T. Liu, Deep learning models unveiled functional difference between cortical gyri and sulci, *IEEE Trans. Biomed. Eng.* **66**(5), 1297–1308 (2018).

161. Y. Zhao, Q. Dong, S. Zhang, W. Zhang, H. Chen, X. Jiang, L. Guo, X. Hu, J. Han, and T. Liu, Automatic recognition of fMRI-derived functional networks using 3-D convolutional neural networks, *IEEE Trans. Biomed. Eng.* **65**(9), 1975–1984 (2017).

162. L. Zou, J. Zheng, C. Miao, M. J. Mckeown, and Z. J. Wang, 3D CNN based automatic diagnosis of attention deficit hyperactivity disorder using functional and structural MRI, *IEEE Access* **5**, 23626–23636 (2017).

163. M. Agn, P. M. af Rosenschöld, O. Puonti, M. J. Lundemann, L. Mancini, A. Papadaki, S. Thust, J. Ashburner, I. Law, and K. Van Leemput, A modality-adaptive method for segmenting brain tumors and organs-at-risk in radiation therapy planning, *Med. Imag. Anal.* **54**, 220–237 (2019).

164. L. Chen, P. Bentley, K. Mori, K. Misawa, M. Fujiwara, and D. Rueckert, DRINet for medical image segmentation, *IEEE Trans. Med. Imag.* **37**(11), 2453–2462 (2018).

165. A. de Brebisson and G. Montana. Deep neural networks for anatomical brain segmentation. In *Proceedings of the IEEE Conference on Computer Vision and Pattern Recognition Workshops*, pp. 20–28 (2015).

166. Y. Deng, Y. Sun, Y. Zhu, Y. Xu, Q. Yang, S. Zhang, Z. Wang, J. Sun, W. Zhao, X. Zhou, *et al.*, A new framework to reduce doctor's workload for medical image annotation, *IEEE Access* **7**, 107097–107104 (2019).

167. Y. Ding, C. Li, Q. Yang, Z. Qin, and Z. Qin, How to improve the deep residual network to segment multi-modal brain tumor images, *IEEE Access* **7**, 152821–152831 (2019).

168. Y. Ding, F. Chen, Y. Zhao, Z. Wu, C. Zhang, and D. Wu, A stacked multi-connection simple reducing net for brain tumor segmentation, *IEEE Access* **7**, 104011–104024 (2019).

169. J. Dolz, K. Gopinath, J. Yuan, H. Lombaert, C. Desrosiers, and I. B. Ayed, HyperDense-Net: a hyper-densely connected CNN for multi-modal image segmentation, *IEEE Trans. Med. Imag.* **38**(5), 1116–1126 (2018).

170. J. Enguehard, P. O'Halloran, and A. Gholipour, Semi-supervised learning with deep embedded clustering for image classification and segmentation, *IEEE Access* **7**, 11093–11104 (2019).

171. B. Hou, G. Kang, N. Zhang, and C. Hu, Robust 3D convolutional neural network with boundary correction for accurate brain tissue segmentation, *IEEE Access* **6**, 75471–75481 (2018).

172. K. Hu, Q. Gan, Y. Zhang, S. Deng, F. Xiao, W. Huang, C. Cao, and X. Gao, Brain tumor segmentation using multi-cascaded convolutional neural networks and conditional random field, *IEEE Access* **7**, 92615–92629 (2019).

173. W. Li, G. Wang, L. Fidon, S. Ourselin, M. J. Cardoso, and T. Vercauteren. On the compactness, efficiency, and representation of 3D convolutional networks: Brain parcellation as a pretext task. In *International Conference on Information Processing in Medical Imaging*, pp. 348–360 (2017).

174. M. Li, L. Kuang, S. Xu, and Z. Sha, Brain tumor detection based on multimodal information fusion and convolutional neural network, *IEEE Access* **7**, 180134–180146 (2019).

175. H. Li, G. Jiang, J. Zhang, R. Wang, Z. Wang, W.-S. Zheng, and B. Menze, Fully convolutional network ensembles for white matter hyperintensities segmentation in MR images, *NeuroImage* **183**, 650–665 (2018).

176. F. Milletari, S.-A. Ahmadi, C. Kroll, A. Plate, V. Rozanski, J. Maiostre, J. Levin, O. Dietrich, B. Ertl-Wagner, K. Bötzel, *et al.*, Hough-CNN: Deep learning for segmentation of deep brain regions in MRI and ultrasound, *Comput. Vis. Imag. Understand.* **164**, 92–102 (2017).

177. P. Moeskops, J. de Bresser, H. J. Kuijf, A. M. Mendrik, G. J. Biessels, J. P. Pluim, and I. Išgum, Evaluation of a deep learning approach for the segmentation of brain tissues and white matter hyperintensities of presumed vascular origin in MRI, *NeuroImage: Clin.* **17**, 251–262 (2018).

178. M. A. Morrison, S. Payabvash, Y. Chen, S. Avadiappan, M. Shah, X. Zou, C. P. Hess, and J. M. Lupo, A user-guided tool for semi-automated cerebral microbleed detection and volume segmentation: Evaluating vascular injury and data labelling for machine learning, *NeuroImage: Clin.* **20**, 498–505 (2018).

179. T. Nair, D. Precup, D. L. Arnold, and T. Arbel, Exploring uncertainty measures in deep networks for multiple sclerosis lesion detection and segmentation, *Med. Imag. Anal.* **59**, 101557 (2020).

180. D. Nie, L. Wang, E. Adeli, C. Lao, W. Lin, and D. Shen, 3-D fully convolutional networks for multimodal isointense infant brain image segmentation, *IEEE Trans. Cybern.* **49**(3), 1123–1136 (2018).

181. S. Pereira, A. Pinto, J. Amorim, A. Ribeiro, V. Alves, and C. A. Silva, Adaptive feature recombination and recalibration for semantic segmentation with fully convolutional networks, *IEEE Trans. Med. Imag.* **38**(12), 2914–2925 (2019).

182. M. I. Razzak, M. Imran, and G. Xu, Efficient brain tumor segmentation with multiscale two-pathway-group conventional neural networks, *IEEE J. Biomed. Health Informat.* **23**(5), 1911–1919 (2018).

183. A. G. Roy, S. Conjeti, N. Navab, C. Wachinger, Alzheimer's Disease Neuroimaging Initiative, *et al.*, QuickNAT: A fully convolutional network for quick and accurate segmentation of neuroanatomy, *NeuroImage* **186**, 713–727 (2019).

184. S. S. M. Salehi, D. Erdogmus, and A. Gholipour, Auto-context convolutional neural network (auto-net) for brain extraction in magnetic resonance imaging, *IEEE Trans. Med. Imag.* **36**(11), 2319–2330 (2017).

185. M. D. Schirmer, A. V. Dalca, R. Sridharan, A.-K. Giese, K. L. Donahue, M. J. Nardin, S. J. Mocking, E. C. McIntosh, P. Frid, J. Wasselius, *et al.*, White matter hyperintensity quantification in

large-scale clinical acute ischemic stroke cohorts–the MRI-GENIE study, *NeuroImage: Clin.* **23**, 101884 (2019).

186. M. Shao, S. Han, A. Carass, X. Li, A. M. Blitz, J. Shin, J. L. Prince, and L. M. Ellingsen, Brain ventricle parcellation using a deep neural network: Application to patients with ventriculomegaly, *NeuroImage: Clin.* **23**, 101871 (2019).

187. F. Shi, Q. Yang, X. Guo, T. A. Qureshi, Z. Tian, H. Miao, D. Dey, D. Li, and Z. Fan, Intracranial vessel wall segmentation using convolutional neural networks, *IEEE Trans. Biomed. Eng.* **66**(10), 2840–2847 (2019).

188. M. F. Stollenga, W. Byeon, M. Liwicki, and J. Schmidhuber. Parallel multi-dimensional LSTM, with application to fast biomedical volumetric image segmentation. In *Advances in Neural Information Processing Systems*, pp. 2998–3006 (2015).

189. B. Thyreau, K. Sato, H. Fukuda, and Y. Taki, Segmentation of the hippocampus by transferring algorithmic knowledge for large cohort processing, *Med. Imag. Anal.* **43**, 214–228 (2018).

190. L. Wang, C. Xie, and N. Zeng, RP-Net: A 3D convolutional neural network for brain segmentation from magnetic resonance imaging, *IEEE Access* **7**, 39670–39679 (2019).

191. G. Wang, M. A. Zuluaga, W. Li, R. Pratt, P. A. Patel, M. Aertsen, T. Doel, A. L. David, J. Deprest, S. Ourselin, *et al.*, DeepIGeoS: A deep interactive geodesic framework for medical image segmentation, *IEEE Trans. PAMI* **41**(7), 1559–1572 (2018).

192. G. Wang, W. Li, M. A. Zuluaga, R. Pratt, P. A. Patel, M. Aertsen, T. Doel, A. L. David, J. Deprest, S. Ourselin, *et al.*, Interactive medical image segmentation using deep learning with image-specific fine tuning, *IEEE Trans. Med. Imag.* **37**(7), 1562–1573 (2018).

193. L. Chauvin, K. Kumar, C. Wachinger, M. Vangel, J. de Guise, C. Desrosiers, W. Wells, M. Toews, A. D. N. Initiative, *et al.*, Neuroimage signature from salient keypoints is highly specific to individuals and shared by close relatives, *NeuroImage* **204**, 116208 (2020).

194. S. Liu, D. Utriainen, C. Chai, Y. Chen, L. Wang, S. K. Sethi, S. Xia, and E. M. Haacke, Cerebral microbleed detection using susceptibility weighted imaging and deep learning, *NeuroImage* **198**, 271–282 (2019).

195. R. McKinley, R. Wepfer, L. Grunder, F. Aschwanden, T. Fischer, C. Friedli, R. Muri, C. Rummel, R. Verma, C. Weisstanner, *et al.*, Automatic detection of lesion load change in multiple sclerosis using convolutional neural networks with segmentation confidence, *NeuroImage: Clinical* **25**, 102104 (2020).

196. J. Zhang, M. Liu, and D. Shen, Detecting anatomical landmarks from limited medical imaging data using two-stage task-oriented deep neural networks, *IEEE Trans. Imag. Process.* **26**(10), 4753–4764 (2017).

197. S. Bollmann, K. G. B. Rasmussen, M. Kristensen, R. G. Blendal, L. R. Østergaard, M. Plocharski, K. O'Brien, C. Langkammer, A. Janke, and M. Barth, DeepQSM-using deep learning to solve the dipole inversion for quantitative susceptibility mapping, *NeuroImage* **195**, 373–383 (2019).

198. J. H. Cole, R. P. Poudel, D. Tsagkrasoulis, M. W. Caan, C. Steves, T. D. Spector, and G. Montana, Predicting brain age with deep learning from raw imaging data results in a reliable and heritable biomarker, *NeuroImage* **163**, 115–124 (2017).

199. F. Dubost, P. Yilmaz, H. Adams, G. Bortsova, M. A. Ikram, W. Niessen, M. Vernooij, and M. de Bruijne, Enlarged perivascular spaces in brain MRI: Automated quantification in four regions, *NeuroImage* **185**, 534–544 (2019).

200. Z. Li, T. Gong, Z. Lin, H. He, Q. Tong, C. Li, Y. Sun, F. Yu, and J. Zhong, Fast and robust diffusion kurtosis parametric mapping using a three-dimensional convolutional neural network, *IEEE Access* **7**, 71398–71411 (2019).

201. G. Mårtensson, D. Ferreira, L. Cavallin, J.-S. Muehlboeck, L.-O. Wahlund, C. Wang, E. Westman, Alzheimer's Disease Neuroimaging Initiative, *et al.*, AVRA: Automatic visual ratings of atrophy from MRI images using recurrent convolutional neural networks, *NeuroImage: Clinical.* **23**, 101872 (2019).

202. S. S. M. Salehi, S. Khan, D. Erdogmus, and A. Gholipour, Real-time deep pose estimation with geodesic loss for image-to-template rigid registration, *IEEE Trans. Med. Imag.* **38**(2), 470–481 (2018).

203. H. Wei, S. Cao, Y. Zhang, X. Guan, F. Yan, K. W. Yeom, and C. Liu, Learning-based single-step quantitative susceptibility mapping reconstruction without brain extraction, *NeuroImage* **202**, 116064 (2019).

204. J. Yoon, E. Gong, I. Chatnuntawech, B. Bilgic, J. Lee, W. Jung, J. Ko, H. Jung, K. Setsompop, G. Zaharchuk, *et al.*, Quantitative susceptibility mapping using deep neural network: QSMnet, *NeuroImage* **179**, 199–206 (2018).

205. X. Yang, R. Kwitt, M. Styner, and M. Niethammer, Quicksilver: Fast predictive image registration: A deep learning approach, *NeuroImage* **158**, 378–396 (2017).

206. C. Han, L. Rundo, R. Araki, Y. Nagano, Y. Furukawa, G. Mauri, H. Nakayama, and H. Hayashi, Combining noise-to-image and image-to-image GANs: Brain MR image augmentation for tumor detection, *IEEE Access* **7**, 156966–156977 (2019).

207. L. Xiang, Q. Wang, D. Nie, L. Zhang, X. Jin, Y. Qiao, and D. Shen, Deep embedding convolutional neural network for synthesizing CT image from T1-weighted MR image, *Med. Imag. Anal.* **47**, 31–44 (2018).

208. Y. Hong, J. Kim, G. Chen, W. Lin, P.-T. Yap, and D. Shen, Longitudinal prediction of infant diffusion MRI data via graph convolutional adversarial networks, *IEEE Trans. Med. Imag.* **38**(12), 2717–2725 (2019).

209. J. Liu, F. Chen, C. Pan, M. Zhu, X. Zhang, L. Zhang, and H. Liao, A cascaded deep convolutional neural network for joint segmentation and genotype prediction of brainstem gliomas, *IEEE Trans. Biomed. Eng.* **65**(9), 1943–1952 (2018).

210. E. Jung, P. Chikontwe, X. Zong, W. Lin, D. Shen, and S. H. Park, Enhancement of perivascular spaces using densely connected deep convolutional neural network, *IEEE Access* **7**, 18382–18391 (2019).

211. M. Ran, J. Hu, Y. Chen, H. Chen, H. Sun, J. Zhou, and Y. Zhang, Denoising of 3D magnetic resonance images using a residual encoder-decoder Wasserstein generative adversarial network, *Med. Imag. Anal.* **55**, 165–180 (2019).

212. J. Du, L. Wang, Y. Liu, Z. Zhou, Z. He, and Y. Jia, Brain MRI super-resolution using 3D dilated convolutional encoder-decoder network, *IEEE Access* **8**, 18938–18950 (2020).

213. J. Gu, Z. Li, Y. Wang, H. Yang, Z. Qiao, and J. Yu, Deep generative adversarial networks for thin-section infant MR image reconstruction, *IEEE Access* **7**, 68290–68304 (2019).

214. Z. N. K. Swati, Q. Zhao, M. Kabir, F. Ali, Z. Ali, S. Ahmed, and J. Lu, Content-based brain tumor retrieval for MR images using transfer learning, *IEEE Access* **7**, 17809–17822 (2019).

215. H. Gudbjartsson and S. Patz, The Rician distribution of noisy MRI data, *Magnet. Res. Med.* **34**(6), 910–914 (1995).

216. D. Moratal, A. Vallés-Luch, L. Martí-Bonmatí, and M. E. Brummer, K-space tutorial: An MRI educational tool for a better understanding of k-space, *Biomed. Imag. Interv. J.* **4**(1), e15 (2008).

217. M. Zaitsev, J. Maclaren, and M. Herbst, Motion artifacts in MRI: a complex problem with many partial solutions, *J. Magnet. Res. Imag.* **42**(4), 887–901 (2015).

218. R. Shaw, C. H. Sudre, T. Varsavsky, S. Ourselin, and M. J. Cardoso, A k-space model of movement artefacts: Application to segmentation augmentation and artefact removal, *IEEE Trans. Med. Imag.* **39**(9), 2881–2892 (2020).

219. K. Sommer, A. Saalbach, T. Brosch, C. Hall, N. Cross, and J. Andre, Correction of motion artifacts using a multiscale fully convolutional neural network, *Am. J. Neuroradiol.* **41**(3), 416–423 (2020).

220. D. Tamada, M.-L. Kromrey, S. Ichikawa, H. Onishi, and U. Motosugi, Motion artifact reduction using a convolutional neural network for dynamic contrast enhanced MR imaging of the liver, *Magnet. Reson. Med. Sci.* **19**(1), 64–76 (2020).

221. J. V. Manjón and P. Coupe. MRI denoising using deep learning. In *International Workshop on Patch-based Techniques in Medical Imaging*, pp. 12–19 (2018).

222. M. Kidoh, K. Shinoda, M. Kitajima, K. Isogawa, M. Nambu, H. Uetani, K. Morita, T. Nakaura, M. Tateishi, Y. Yamashita, *et al.*, Deep learning based noise reduction for brain MR imaging: Tests on phantoms and healthy volunteers, *Magnet. Reson. Med. Sci.* **19**(3), 195 (2020).

223. Z. Zhang, Y. Xie, F. Xing, M. McGough, and L. Yang. Mdnet: A semantically and visually interpretable medical image diagnosis network. In *Proceedings of the IEEE Conference on Computer Vision and Pattern Recognition*, pp. 6428–6436 (2017).

224. X. Yi and P. Babyn, Sharpness-aware low-dose CT denoising using conditional generative adversarial network, *J. Digit. Imag.* **31**(5), 655–669 (2018).

225. R. Pomponio, G. Erus, M. Habes, J. Doshi, D. Srinivasan, E. Mamourian, V. Bashyam, I. M. Nasrallah, T. D. Satterthwaite, Y. Fan, *et al.*, Harmonization of large MRI datasets for the analysis of brain imaging patterns throughout the lifespan, *NeuroImage* **208**, 116450 (2020).

226. L. Yue, D. Tian, W. Chen, X. Han, and M. Yin, Deep learning for heterogeneous medical data analysis, *World Wide Web*, pp. 1–23 (2020).

227. S.-C. Huang, A. Pareek, S. Seyyedi, I. Banerjee, and M. P. Lungren, Fusion of medical imaging and electronic health records using deep learning: A systematic review and implementation guidelines, *NPJ Digit. Med.* **3**(1), 1–9 (2020).

228. M. Rakić, M. Cabezas, K. Kushibar, A. Oliver, and X. Lladó, Improving the detection of autism spectrum disorder by combining structural and functional MRI information, *NeuroImage: Clin.* **25**, 102181 (2020).

229. M. T. Ribeiro, S. Singh, and C. Guestrin, Model-agnostic interpretability of machine learning, *coRR.* **abs/1606.05386** (2016).

230. N. Xie, G. Ras, M. van Gerven, and D. Doran, Explainable deep learning: A field guide for the uninitiated, *coRR.* **abs/2004.14545** (2020).

231. A. Saxe, S. Nelli, and C. Summerfield, If deep learning is the answer, what is the question? *Nat. Rev. Neurosci.* 1–13 (2020).

232. J. Rieke, F. Eitel, M. Weygandt, J.-D. Haynes, and K. Ritter. Visualizing convolutional networks for MRI-based diagnosis of Alzheimer's disease. In *Understanding and Interpreting Machine Learning in Medical Image Computing Applications*, pp. 24–31. Springer (2018).

233. Y. Gal and Z. Ghahramani. Dropout as a Bayesian approximation: Representing model uncertainty in deep learning. In *International Conference on Machine Learning*, pp. 1050–1059 (2016).

Chapter 3

The Evolution of Mining Electronic Health Records in the Era of Deep Learning

Isotta Landi[*,†,‡], Jessica De Freitas[*,†,§], Brian A. Kidd[†,¶],
Joel T. Dudley[†,‖], Benjamin S. Glicksberg[*,†,**], and
Riccardo Miotto[*,†,††]

*Hasso Plattner Institute for Digital Health at Mount Sinai;
Institute for Next Generation Healthcare;
Department of Genetics and Genomic Sciences,
1 Gustave L. Levy Place, New York, NY 10029, USA
†Icahn School of Medicine at Mount Sinai,
1 Gustave L. Levy Place, New York, NY 10029, USA
‡isotta.landi2@mssm.edu
§jessica.defreitas@icahn.mssm.edu
¶briankidd1@gmail.com
‖joel.dudley@mssm.edu
**benjamin.glicksberg@icahn.mssm.edu
††miotto.r@gmail.com

Electronic health records (EHRs) contain a wealth of biomedical data and offer great promise to improving healthcare for individuals and providing essential data for enhancing population health. During each clinical visit, medical personnel capture a snapshot of a person's health, and these records accumulate in massive storehouses of structured and unstructured data. As the size and scope of these repositories have expanded, opportunities abound to investigate biological and medical questions in new modes and on an unprecedented scale. One powerful tool to this end is deep learning (DL), a subfield of machine learning, which aims to algorithmically represent structure within data using layers of neural networks. Here, we review applications of DL with EHRs, in particular focusing on how the advent of DL changed how we mine EHRs for research.

1. Introduction

Over the past three decades, electronic health records (EHRs) and information technology have revolutionized healthcare and biomedical research. What started as a system to catalog the digital version of a patient's medical history to facilitate administrative processing and improve clinical workflow has gradually migrated to a complex framework that houses massive swaths of digital data and permits new investigations into human health and biomedicine. These digital records provide a snapshot of a patient's state of health, which can augment medical decisions through easier sharing of critical health information. With time, these records accumulate into timelines that can improve the predictive modeling of health trajectories. At the individual level, these trajectories are becoming the basis for personalized medicine. Across multiple people, these records provide a vital resource to understand population health management and make better decisions for healthcare policy.[1]

EHRs represent a collection of data and functions that reflect the often competing needs of the four primary stakeholders these systems have evolved to accommodate. First and foremost, providers want accounting schemes to capture a wide array of events, visits, insurance, diagnoses, treatments, procedures, payments and to monitor healthcare administration. Second, information technology engineers need the latest software and hardware, along with the necessary infrastructure to support the increasing functionality and demands placed on EHRs by providers and healthcare administrators. Third, scientists require applications and data organized for research. Fourth, and often considered as an afterthought, patients desire access to their medical data over time and location. All these different use-cases, in many hospitals, led to large databases consisting of heterogeneous data elements, including patient demographic information, diagnoses, laboratory test results, medication prescriptions, clinical notes, and medical images.

A common approach to mine meaningful information from EHRs is to define a clinical hypothesis and have a domain expert specify the clinical features to use in *ad hoc* manner. However, supervised definition of the feature space scales poorly and misses the opportunities to discover novel patterns, which are one of the major promises of large-scale EHRs. The resulting models also often have limited generalizability across datasets or institutions. Alternatively, machine learning (ML), specifically representation learning, can be used to automatically discover the representations needed for prediction from the raw data.[2] Deep learning (DL) is a form of representation learning with multiple levels of abstractions, obtained by composing simple but nonlinear modules that each transform the representation at one level (starting with the raw input) into a representation at a higher, slightly more abstract level.[3] DL has seen a dramatic resurgence in the recent years, largely driven by increases in computational power and the availability of massive new datasets. The field has witnessed striking advances in the ability of machines to understand and manipulate data, including images,[4] language,[5] and speech.[6] Healthcare and medicine are starting to benefit from DL as well, mostly because of the large volume of data being generated (150 exabytes or 10^{18} bytes in United States alone, growing 48% annually[7]).

In the EHR domain, DL has introduced a shift to a completely data-driven research paradigm where we fully exploit all patient data without requiring manual supervision and feature engineering. Research publications have skyrocketed over the past few years, leading to the first steps towards the next generation of clinical systems that can scale to include many millions to billions of heterogeneous patient records and can effectively support clinicians in their daily activities. In this chapter, we introduce the basic frameworks of EHRs and DL, and we review some of the most effective stories, applying DL in clinical informatics to accelerate translational research. Despite enormous investment, interest, and early successes, however, ML (and DL) has yet to reach its potential in healthcare. Therefore, we also provide commentary on how ML can become more mainstream for clinicians and patients as well as more sustainable for clinical deployment and research moving forward.

2. Data Organization and Structure of EHRs

This section summarizes the origins and evolution of EHRs to their current status in most clinical settings. We highlight the common data types found in an EHR and how they are organized. The development of modern EHRs has led to a number of benefits across the health space. As these systems have grown in complexity, multiple challenges and solutions are presented for bringing them together to work across various domains for different research and clinical needs.

2.1. *Brief history*

EHRs consist of data from patient interactions at a clinic or a hospital. During each visit, medical staff captures a snapshot of a person's health that gets added to their previous information. Originally, digital conversion replaced the analog version of a patient's medical history to facilitate administrative processing and to improve clinical workflow. In particular, the concept of EHR originated in the 1960s to use electronic methods and data processing systems to record patient information (i.e., "problem-oriented" medical record). The Regenstrief Institute developed the first functioning EMR systems in 1972.[8] However, due to high costs, these systems were not appealing to physicians and adopted by government hospitals and larger medical institutions.

It took more than 30 years and two confluent forces to merge modern medical practice with EHRs as they function today.[9] The first was a series of recommendations, which later became regulations, from the Institute of Medicine regarding privacy and confidentiality of medical records. The Health Insurance Portability and Accountability Act (HIPAA) was introduced in 1996 in response to growing issues facing healthcare coverage, privacy, and security in the United States. The second was the rise of the Internet coupled with the decrease in the cost of computing and information technologies. As digital technologies became ubiquitous during the 2000s, EHRs progressively became more prevalent in healthcare facilities, working hand-in-hand with physicians and professionals to provide the best quality care for patients. Today's EHR systems inherit this developmental evolution and focus primarily on facilitating administrative tasks and hospital workflow for patient care — billing, alerts, patient and diagnostic record-keeping, and insurance data. Over the past five-plus years, researchers and physician-scientists have started populating the EHR with additional data, such as imaging, molecular, clinical lab tests (previously kept in ancillary systems), to facilitate new scientific questions and clinical opportunities to improve patient care.

2.2. *Benefits*

The conversion from paper to EHRs brought multiple benefits to patients, providers, and the healthcare industry. The greatest benefit to the patient is that EHRs offer a way to store medical records in a secure format that is now accessible online. This feature gives each person, as well as any designated third party, the ability to view their personal health history at any time and from anywhere. Providers also benefit from the capacity to have a patient's medical information available when needed. This option helps improve medical decisions and ensures that all members of the care team have access to the same information.

2.3. *Data types and organization*

In the United States, as well as several other countries, the information in the EHRs is used primarily for billing and administrative purposes. That said, EHRs provide comprehensive health information about patients, consequently including many different types of information based on input from a variety of providers involved in a patient's care (Table 1).

The array of data types and clinical descriptors available to represent the digital patient create challenges for data analysis and interpretation. These data have a broad range of dimensionality and are subject to various degrees of noise, heterogeneity, sparseness, incompleteness, random errors, and systematic biases.[1,10] For example, some measures are common and result in multiple measurements entered into EHRs (e.g., a comprehensive metabolic panel during regular check-ups). Other lab tests are atypical and ordered under certain conditions (e.g., estimated glomerular filtration rate [eGFR] will be measured if a physician is concerned about a patient's kidney function). Similarly, common diseases like type 2 diabetes mellitus and hypertension are often diagnosed and appear more frequently in EHRs, whereas other less frequent diseases such as multiple myeloma will only be present in a limited number of patients.

In particular, data deficiencies and missingness have risen concerns about the translational efficacy of EHR-based studies in that

Table 1.   Data types commonly found in the electronic health records.

Data category	Description or Example
Patient demographics	Captures personal (e.g., gender, date of birth, race, nationality) and geographical (e.g., address) information.
Clinical notes	Reflects combination of clinical terms and prose written by the clinicians and nurses to summarize a clinical event, such as a patient visit, surgery, and so on.
Vital signs	Blood pressure, temperature, oxygen level, pulse, heartbeat, height, and weight.
Medical histories	Includes both the patient's own medical history — clinical events, allergies, visits, immunization dates — and the patient's family history of disease, such as cancer, diabetes, and hypertension.
Diagnoses	The official disease classification associated to a patient during each encounter. Commonly, these are encoded using the International Classification of Diseases, Ninth (ICD-9) or Tenth revision (ICD-10), codes (https://www.cdc.gov/nchs/icd).
Medications	Record of all the drugs prescribed to the patients during each encounter.
Clinical images	MRI, X-ray, and ultrasound scans, which are usually serialized, stored, and managed in the Digital Imaging and Communications in Medicine (DICOM) standard.
Laboratory and test results	Includes both common tests, such as metabolic panels, as well as more specific tests related to certain conditions. Test results can be reported as a value and unit of measure or as categorical labels against range values (e.g., high, normal, low). Recently, healthcare facilities have started to record lab tests as Logical Observation Identifiers Names and Codes (LOINC) to favor standardization and reduce data dispersion (https://loinc.org).

they may not only introduce unintentional bias but also exacerbate disparities intrinsic to healthcare systems, e.g., racial[11] and sex/gender[12] biases. DL have been applied to EHR with different missing data patterns for direct modeling[13,14] and imputation.[15] Nevertheless, in the context of precision medicine, focus has shifted to model interpretability,[12] bias detection and mitigations,[16,17] and the implementation of guidelines and strategies that could help raise awareness on health disparities and contrast the phenomenon of biased outputs produced by biased inputs.[11]

Other intrinsic EHR challenges include data imbalances and cohort selection. Each patient entry will contain different amounts of information based on the frequency of their visits and their disease status and these data imbalances can confound statistical analyses. Moreover, the same clinical phenotype can be expressed using different codes and terminologies. For example, a patient diagnosed with "type 2 diabetes mellitus" can be identified in multiple ways — a laboratory value of hemoglobin A1C greater than 7.0%, the International Classification of Disease, 10th version (ICD-10) code E11.9, or free text in the clinical notes mentioning "type 2 diabetes mellitus". Each selection procedure can bias the analysis and interpretation of data in the EHRs and it is important to illuminate the potential pitfalls early on in any examination of patient records.

The range of data types used for medicine also creates challenges for how best to store, organize, and format the data for efficient usage from multiple parties. The most common framework for EHRs is a relational database (e.g., Oracle, MySQL) that is updated at every patient clinical event.[18] Recent efforts are underway to aggregate all the data types into formats that facilitate query and large-scale analytics.[19] These new formats aim to handle natural queries that a physician or patient might have and be able to compute on all the clinical records at the scale of millions of patients. Point-and-click dashboards are also ways in which queries for data can be performed without advanced knowledge of computer science or format structure.[20,21]

2.4. *Data standardization and interoperability*

Large healthcare systems must contend with how best to combine multiple sources of data, standardize a variety of data types, and facilitate interoperability among institutions. Data standardization, particularly, is a critical activity for researchers interested in running EHR studies across multiple institutions.[22] Standards play a role in (i) facilitating EHR interoperability, (ii) structuring research databases that house EHR data, and (iii) enabling research reproducibility. All three of these domains are critical for efficient and effective operations on EHRs.

Derivative databases, used primarily for research, also require their own standards for extracting health data from the EHRs. Multiple consortia, committees, and other research collaborations are developing and maintaining standards for the three layers mentioned above as common data models. For example, one group that facilitates standards involved in EHR interoperability is Health-Level 7 (HL-7), which developed a specification called Fast Healthcare Interoperability Resources (FHIR).[23, 24] Their focus is to ensure that healthcare information is transferred appropriately across EHRs and institutions. Another large-scale research project, Integrating Biology and the Bedside (i2b2), was one of the first to design an open-source framework to interface with EHR data for translational research including an interactive dashboard to assist with such tasks as cohort identification.[25] This platform is used widely (as of January 2020, it is used at over 250 locations worldwide[a]) and has countless extensions. The Observational Health Data Sciences and Informatics (OHDSI) consortium recently developed the OMOP Common Data Model[26] that enables researchers to develop code at a single institution and share it across all institutions that conform to the same research-EHR structure. This approach is convenient for researchers who develop at a single institution and look for replicating analyses on a completely independent set of patients.

Standardization also involves algorithm development, which evolves and improves through community engagement and feedback. In fact, clinical algorithms are often derived through an iterative process with medical and informatics experts across multiple institutions. For example, phenotyping algorithms for different diseases have been collected in this way and made available via the Phenotype Knowledge Base (PheKB).[27] The first step in this iterative process is a proposed algorithm contributed by one institution. Other participating institutions then examine the proposed algorithm and make improvements or refinements on the original design. A final algorithm

---

[a]https://community.i2b2.org/wiki/.

is reached through this collaborative coding process that includes a series of tests and validation steps. The finalized algorithm is then treated as a "standard" for future researchers to utilize.[28]

3. A Brief Introduction to Deep Learning

Machine learning (ML) is a general-purpose paradigm that learns relationships from the data without the need to define them *a priori*.[29] ML transforms the inputs of an algorithm into outputs using statistical, data-driven rules that are automatically derived from a large set of examples rather than being explicitly specified by humans.[30] Historically, the typical ML workflow involves four steps: data harmonization, representation learning, model fitting and evaluation.[31] For decades, representation learning has been heavily relying on domain expert and feature engineering to manually define feature extractors.[32] Raw input variables are preprocessed using such feature extractors and transformed into a new space of variables where the desired patterns are easier to detect by the learning subsystem, which is often a classifier.[29]

Deep learning (DL) is a class of representation learning methods, which automatically yields distributed feature representations from raw data for pattern detection and classification. To obtain such representations, DL architectures enable the composition of different layers of simple nonlinear functions, usually based on neural networks, that progressively transform raw data across higher and more abstract levels.[3] The learning procedure aims at deriving distributed representations from training examples. These representations combine many computing elements to represent one entity and favor the generalization to new data unseen during the learning phase.[3] This process is based on stochastic gradient descent, provided that all modules are composed by relatively smooth functions. Specifically, internal weights are updated by computing the gradient of an objective function with respect to the output and working backwards according to the chain rule for derivatives. Known as backpropagation, this approach computes the gradient with respect to the weights of each module.[32]

There are different types of neural networks that shape DL architectures. In particular, among multi-layer networks, we can distinguish between feed-forward neural networks and recurrent neural networks (RNNs). Feed-forward networks learn to map fixed-size inputs to fixed-size outputs. In this category, convolutional neural networks (CNNs) are the standard base for computer vision systems that learn internal hierarchical representations from images to detect and classify objects.[33] Images, expressed as arrays of pixel values, are processed by a stack of layers that first learn to detect edges and then gradually combine edges into motifs, motifs into objects, and objects into scenes.[34] Differently, RNNs learn to process sequential inputs that carry an intrinsic temporal structure (e.g., speech or language) while maintaining in their hidden units relevant information about the past elements of the sequence. Long short-term memory networks (LSTMs) are the most commonly used type of RNNs due to their natural ability of remembering information for long periods of time, limiting the long-term dependency issues that characterized first RNN implementations.[35]

As in ML, DL architectures can be used, and consequently trained, for different tasks. In many applications, DL architectures are trained in a supervised fashion. In this case, training datasets include both input data points (e.g., lab results) and output labels (e.g., "disease-free", "affected") and the models usually aim to provide classification scores. In the absence of known output labels, training is done within an unsupervised framework, where the goal is to reconstruct or model the original input and to discover patterns in the data. Unsupervised learning is commonly done using autoencoders[36] and self-supervised learning (i.e., systems extract and use the naturally available relevant context and embedded metadata as supervisory signals).[37] Alternatively, reinforcement learning (RL), which has recently gained a lot of attention, tries to find the best combination of actions that maximize a reward by trial and error.[38] RL differs from supervised learning because it does not need labeled input/output pairs, nor sub-optimal actions to be explicitly corrected. Instead, the focus is to find a balance between exploration (of uncharted territory) and exploitation (of current knowledge). Originally proposed for unsupervised learning, generative adversarial networks (GANs)[39] have recently been used for reinforcement learning.[40] In GANs, two models are trained simultaneously. A generative model captures the data distribution to produce examples, whereas a discriminator estimates the probability that a sample comes from the training data rather than the generative model. The generator examples are trained, maximizing the probability of the discriminator to make a mistake.

4. Deep Learning with EHRs

This section highlights the successful studies applying DL to EHRs to improve healthcare in a few relevant clinical domains. The main advantage of using DL with EHRs is the natural ability of processing different types of data, leading to effective and efficient heterogeneous learning frameworks that can leverage personalized medicine and next-generation healthcare. When patients come to the hospital, their clinical status is deconstructed into the EHRs (see Figure 1); ML, specifically DL, can help to reconstruct and use for predictive analysis this clinical status by modeling all the different heterogeneous pieces of EHRs. As such, leveraging multi-layer representations, DL methods can implement different fusion strategies to combine heterogeneous data modalities into the same learning process within an EHR, e.g., medical imaging and clinical data.[41]

The literature of this growing field is summarized in different excellent review papers and books.[30,42–50] Here, we cover a few relevant applications, in particular those related to disease prediction,

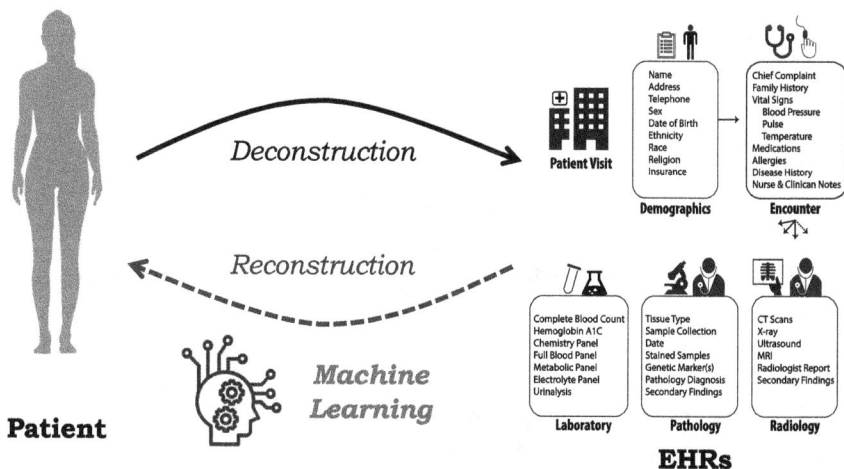

Fig. 1.   The clinical status of a patient visiting a medical facility is deconstructed to be stored in the different tables of the EHRs. ML can help to reconstruct this status and to use it for predictive modeling and medical analysis.

disease phenotyping, patient stratification, and clinical notes understanding. For each one of these, we provide a comprehensive description of at least one study from the literature, briefly overview other relevant works, and highlight the main differences with pre-DL studies.

Incorporating DL models into clinical practice is central to personalized medicine. This translational gap is narrowing in fields such as histopathology, where digital images allow one to leverage machine learning methods across a wide range of diagnostic applications.[51] Moreover, RL has proven to be particularly suited for tasks that require sequential evaluation of trials and errors,[52] such as dynamic treatment regimes in chronic diseases[53] or critical care.[54] Although computational models can already provide useful insights to clinicians, their real-time applications are still complicated by different factors, such as the use of retrospective cohorts and small sample sizes[52] and the need for human-annotated data to provide reliable predictions.[51] Further discussion on this topic would be out of scope here and we point interested readers to other review works.[51,52]

4.1. *Disease prediction*

The large-scale data stored in EHRs can leverage personalized medicine by forecasting the likelihood that an individual will develop particular diseases. These data-driven models create a healthcare platform that learns optimal care pathways from the historical patient data and automatically estimates the risk of new diseases.[55–57] Physicians can monitor their patients, check if any disease is likely to occur in the near future given the current clinical status, and potentially alter the disease course by suggesting an intervention from a selection of possible options based on the evidence.[1] Similarly, these platforms automatically detect patients in the hospital with high probability to develop certain diseases and alert the appropriate care providers.

Early approaches in this domain relied on disease comorbidities and diagnosis to derive predictions.[58,59] Jensen *et al.*, for example, studied temporal disease trajectories over 15 years and 6 million patients to describe how disease diagnoses progress over time.[58] These disease trajectories were defined by analyzing series of consecutive ICD-9 and ICD-10 codes that were observed in the patients. Such trajectories offer tools for personalized medicine as the patient's history of previous diagnoses forms the basis for predicting the most likely next diagnosis.

More recent research trends based on ML included other clinical variables in the analysis, such as medications and lab values. However, a common approach was to have a domain expert to specify clinical variables in an *ad hoc* manner.[60–63] Although appropriate in some situations, defining the feature space in a supervised manner does not scale or generalize well, and does not allow for the discovery of novel patterns and features. DL can mitigate these limitations by reducing the need of manual feature engineering. In particular, methods based on neural networks and deep learning can be used to process aggregated EHRs, including both structured (e.g., diagnoses, medications, laboratory test results, procedures) unstructured (e.g., free-text clinical notes) data, to obtain semantic representations that are used for specific disease prediction.

In one of the first applications of DL to EHRs, Miotto *et al.* presented an unsupervised deep feature learning framework, named "Deep Patient", to derive general-purpose patient representations from EHR data that facilitate clinical predictive modeling.[64] Specifically, they used a deep stack of denoising autoencoders[65] to model EHRs in an unsupervised manner with the goal of capturing structures and patterns in the data, which, grouped together, composed the deep patient representation. The Deep Patient framework is domain-free (i.e., not related to any specific task since learned over a large multi-domain dataset), does not require any additional human effort, and can be easily applied to different predictive applications, both supervised and unsupervised. Figure 2 includes the high-level conceptual architecture to derive the deep patient representations. All EHRs are first extracted from the clinical data warehouse, preprocessed to normalize clinically relevant phenotypes, and grouped in "raw" patient vectors. Each patient can be described by just a single vector or by a sequence of vectors summarizing predefined temporal windows. All the vectors for each patient are fed to the deep unsupervised neural network to discover high-level general descriptors. Every patient in the data warehouse is then represented using these features and such deep representations can be efficiently and effectively applied to different clinical tasks.[66]

To prove the effectiveness of the idea, Deep Patient was used to process the aggregated EHRs of about 700,000 patients from the

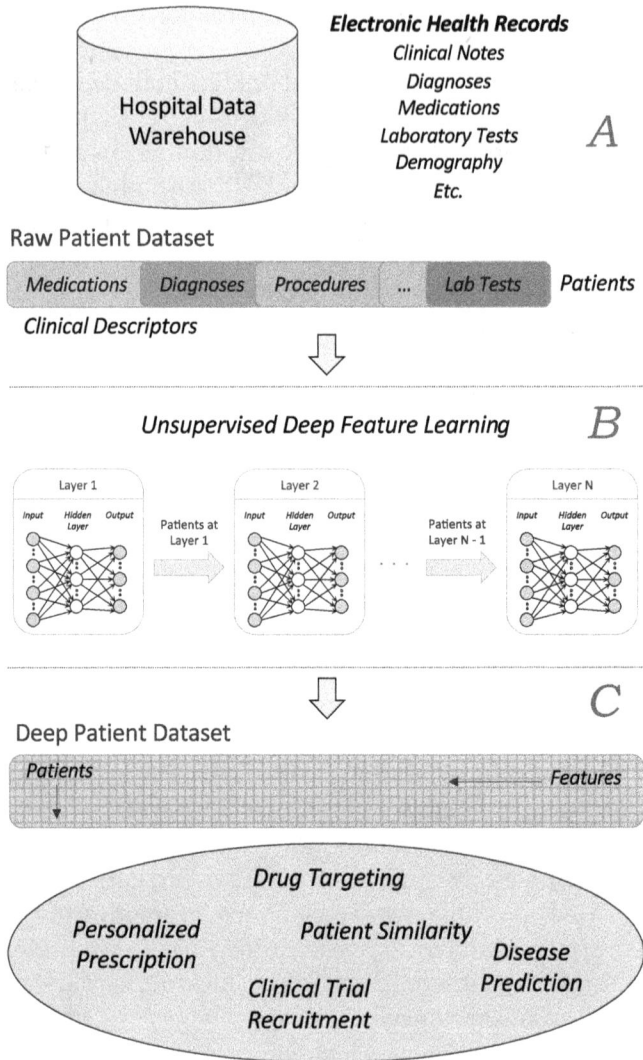

Fig. 2.   Conceptual framework used to derive the Deep Patient representations through unsupervised deep learning of a large EHR data warehouse.[64]

Mount Sinai Hospital in New York City. Patient records included demographic details (e.g., age, gender, and race), common clinical descriptors available in a structured format, such as diagnoses (ICD-9 codes), medications, procedures, and lab tests, and preprocessed clinical notes (summarized using topic modeling[67]). The authors

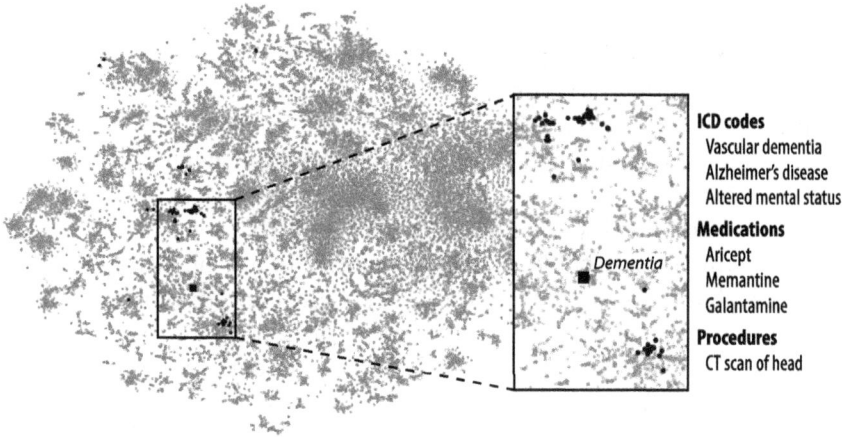

Fig. 3. Disease definition for dementia derived using medical concept embeddings starting from ICD-9 code 294.20 "Dementia".[85]

evaluated this representation as broadly predictive of health states by assessing the probability of patients to develop various diseases within different time windows. The evaluation included 76,214 test patients comprising 78 diseases from diverse clinical domains and temporal windows. Results significantly outperformed those achieved using representations based on raw EHR data and alternative feature learning strategies (see Figure 3). Interestingly, prediction performance for severe diabetes, schizophrenia, and various cancers obtained the largest improvements compared to other algorithms. This is likely related to the chronic nature of these diseases, which lead to a larger and more consistent quantity of data.

These findings showed that deep learning is able to extract features from EHRs that are general and conducive to processing by automated methods in different clinical domains and for different applications, such as disease forecasting. This work represented a first step towards the next generation of clinical systems that can (i) scale to include many millions to billions of patient records and (ii) use a single, distributed patient representation to effectively support clinicians in their daily activities — rather than multiple systems working with different patient representations derived for different tasks.

A large number of studies related to disease prediction built up on this idea and addressed some of the limitations of Deep Patient (e.g., time was not explicitly modeled, predictions are difficult to explain). Doctor AI uses patient history to predict diagnosis and medications for subsequent encounters using RNNs;[68] DeepCare is an end-to-end deep dynamic network based on LSTMs to infer current illness states and predict future medical outcomes, which showed promising performance in the domains of mental health and type 2 diabetes for disease progression modeling, intervention recommendations, and future risk prediction[69]; RETAIN (REverse Time AttentIoN) is an interpretable predictive model based on attention and LSTMs that was evaluated on heart failure prediction[70]; Lipton *et al.* used LSTMs to recognize patterns in multivariate time series of clinical measurements and classify different diagnosis[71]; and Rajkomar *et al.* used deep learning to predict in-hospital mortality, 30-day unplanned readmission, prolonged length of stay, and patient's final discharge diagnosis.[72]

An important consideration to remark is that disease prediction needs to include temporal indications about when a disease is likely to occur. This feature would help physicians to determine the severity of the risk and enable them to prioritize the appropriate intervention strategies. Temporal indication and time risk stratification can be tailored to clinical needs, e.g., in days/months for ordinary patient–physician encounters or in hours/minutes for critical or intensive care situations. For example, Miotto *et al.*[64] evaluated disease predictions over different time windows (i.e., in 30–180 days); Pham *et al.*[69] evaluated their deep architecture by also predicting the time period of disease occurrence; and Lipton *et al.*[71] showed effective temporal disease predictions in ICU.

DL applied to clinical images, such as X-rays and MRI scans, also had several successes in disease prediction and diagnosis.[73] Gulshan *et al.* used deep learning based on CNNs to identify diabetic retinopathy and diabetic macular edema in retinal fundus photographs.[74] Retinal photography with manual interpretation is a widely accepted screening tool for diabetic retinopathy, with performance that usually exceeds that of in-person dilated eye examinations. Automated grading of diabetic retinopathy can increase efficiency, reproducibility, and coverage of screening programs, reduce barriers to access, and improve patient outcomes by providing early detection and treatment. The DL method obtained high sensitivity and specificity over about 10,000 test images with respect to certified ophthalmologist annotations. This study is the first example of an artificial intelligence architecture that performed similar to human experts in a well-defined task routinely done by clinicians while requiring minimum data engineering, when compared to similar efforts based on pre-computed statistics.[75]

DL also obtained accuracy on par with 21 board-certified dermatologists in classifying biopsy-proven clinical images of different types of skin cancers over a large dataset of 130, 000 images.[76] Zech *et al.* built deep neural networks to automatically detect pneumonia in chest radiographs.[77] Their study involved combined images from three different hospitals. One of the major findings, apart from the ability to detect pneumonia, was that models can learn other factors related to healthcare processes that are not relevant to the disease, which resulted in variable performance between sites. For example, the automated methods were able to reliably identify what hospital system the image came from, raising concerns for generalizability.

The actual inclusion of disease prediction models into clinical practice requires efforts in delivering results that can be interpreted in meaningful ways by healthcare workers. Within DL models, the difficult global interpretability and feature selections further complicate the reliability of outcomes, especially for studies that focus on specific disease cohorts or that do not take into account intrinsic biases.[78] Interpretable models and efficient generalizable prediction solutions are fundamental steps to support clinical decision-making and ensure quality and better patient' outcomes. Promising steps towards precision medicine have been made with the development of models which can provide rationales for specific individual predictions (i.e., locally interpretable).[79] Moreover, recent applications to healthcare have proven successful, e.g., in identifying the features that best predict hypoxaemia during surgery.[80] Nevertheless, additional improvements in the model's interpretability and generalizability are still required to enable ML models to effectively support clinical decision-making.

4.2. *Disease phenotyping*

EHR-based research requires accurate case-control definitions for phenotypes (i.e., disease definition) of interest to build robust cohorts similar to how prospective studies implement rigorous selection criteria. However, accurately identifying patients with a certain phenotype in an EHR system can be quite challenging. ICD codes were designed to represent diseases and symptoms but often cannot be relied on as a definitive diagnosis.[81] Depending on the disease, varying data modalities can be best at producing reliable diagnosis. Relevant medication prescriptions may identify patients in a certain disease with high precision, but contribute little to classification in another. Additional challenges come from input errors, coding biases, medical reporting biases, data availability, sparsity and limitations in how the data is structured. The current gold standards for cohort construction are electronic phenotyping algorithms, which are rule-based, manually built, and require validation through expert chart review, before ultimately being deposited in PheKB.[27] Although these algorithms have been successful for biomedical discovery, they are time-consuming, effort-intensive, and domain-specific, restricting broad applicability and scalability. As such, there are only a limited amount of algorithms that exist.

Automated phenotyping methods have been successful in disease classification in a data-driven manner that is more scalable than rule-based methods.[82] Halpern *et al.*, for example, proposed the semi-supervised "learning with anchors" method and applied it to patients in the emergency department.[83] The anchors are observations within the EHRs with high predictive value for a particular phenotype, as manually defined by domain experts. Logistic regression is used to predict the presence or absence of the anchor in the patient's EHR. The final phenotype estimator incorporates all the information in the patient's record as well as the anchor classifier. Compared to a supervised training approach that used gold-standard labels, this method performed better in identifying acute events such as pneumonia, infection, cardiac events, or septic shock, and whether the patient had a history of immunosuppression, anticoagulation therapy, or cancer.

Ho *et al.* developed Limestone, a high-throughput method via non-negative tensor factorization to generate phenotype composed of diagnoses and medications from Geisinger Health System' EHRs.[84] This approach is unsupervised and does not require expert supervision to drive the phenotype learning; however, the study did rely on medical expert annotation when assessing the clinical significance of the derived phenotypes. Specifically looking at heart failure, their method was more interpretable and had increased predictive power compared to the traditional dimensionality reduction approaches, such as principal components analysis and non-negative matrix factorization.

Effort in applying deep learning to EHR-based phenotype definition is limited but promising. Glicksberg *et al.* used a shallow neural network to create unsupervised embeddings of the phenotype space within a large EHR system.[85] Specifically, they used the skip-gram algorithm of word2vec[86] to learn embeddings of the medical concepts found in the structured EHRs of over a million patients. They first divided the patient data in consecutive time intervals of 15 days in length, removing duplicates and random-shuffling the concepts. Each time interval comprising a sequence of unique medical concepts was then considered as a "sentence" which was used to train the word2vec algorithm using stochastic gradient descent. In the trained model, every medical concept was represented as an embedded vector, with all the medical concepts mapped in the same metric space. Concepts adjacent to each other in the original sequence should cluster together in the learned metric space. Figure 3 shows the phenotype space that can be created for dementia, starting from the ICD-9 code 294.20 "Dementia". Of note, most of the concepts in the neighborhood are clinically related to the condition and create a "disease definition" that can be used to better identify cohorts of patients.

In order to create such disease cohorts, the authors summarized the clinical history of patients using a weighted average of these embeddings. For each disease of interest, they selected a single disease-relevant clinical concept as the seed for query, extended it to the nearest concepts in the embedding space, and ranked patients based on their distance from this extended query. Putative cohorts were automatically generated for the disease concept based on patient embeddings with highest similarity, and compared against the gold-standard cohorts derived from PheKB. Results from experiments showed good overlap with manually derived gold-standard phenotypes for five diseases (i.e., ADHD, dementia, herpes zoster, sick cell, and type 2 diabetes mellitus).[87]

This study shows the promise of applying deep learning on EHRs to derive vector-based representations of patients and medical concepts. The hope is that this can be used to efficiently identify meaningful insights for different clinical domains. Specifically, in the disease phenotype applications, deep learning can provide scalable solutions that lead to intuitive definitions of the disease space based on similarity relationships. Advances in self-supervised learning for text modeling, such as GloVE,[88] FastText,[89] Poincarè,[90] BERT (Bidirectional Encoder Representations from Transformers),[91] or XLNet,[92] can potentially be used to extend the work of Glicksberg *et al.* towards more robust and comprehensive understanding of the disease space.

4.3. *Patient stratification*

Heterogeneity among individuals can lead to different disease progression patterns within the same condition and may require different types of interventions. Even seemingly simple diseases can show different degrees of complexity that can create challenges for identification, treatment, and prognosis. For instance, despite being Mendelian disorders, both cystic fibrosis and Huntington's disease exhibit a broad array of symptoms and varying degrees of phenotypic manifestations.[93, 94] This aspect is particularly evident for *complex disorders*, whose etiology is still mostly unknown, possibly due to multiple genetic, environmental, and lifestyle factors. Characteristics of patients with complex disorders may differ on multiple levels of analyses (e.g., comorbid conditions, behavioral aspects, disrupted molecular mechanisms) and in response to treatments throughout the disease trajectory, making these conditions difficult to evaluate. For example, the heterogeneity of neurodevelopmental conditions, such as autism spectrum conditions (ASCs), has been detected at different levels. Coexisting conditions are registered in 70% of individuals with ASC.[95] Genetic studies report hundreds of ASC-linked risk genes and a heritability ranging from 50% to 80%.[96, 97] Moreover, the investigation of developmental trajectories[98] differentiates behavioral growth patterns according to symptom severity and cognitive and language impairments relative to the norm.

Heterogeneous phenotypic manifestations presumably reflect the existence of multiple subgroups of individuals whose conditions are linked to diverse genetic and environmental etiologies and that, although convergent to the diagnostic profile, show a range of clinical characteristics. In the context of personalized medicine, the identification of latent patterns within a cohort of patients can contribute to the development of improved personalized therapies.[99] Moreover, disentangling clinical heterogeneity can lead to the identification of high-impact biomarkers, whose effect may be masked in case-control studies.[100]

The growing interest towards unsupervised deep learning techniques[3] presents a way to examine disease complexity. From a computational perspective, patient stratification is a data-driven, unsupervised learning task that groups patients according to their clinical characteristics.[101] The task of identifying subgroups within a disease cohort from EHRs is usually referred to as "EHR-based patient stratification". Work in this domain aggregates clinical data at a patient level, representing each patient as multi-dimensional vectors, and derives subtypes within a disease-specific population via clustering (e.g., in autism[61]) or topological analysis (e.g., for T2D[62]). Deep learning has been used to model EHRs to derive more robust patient representations to improve disease subtyping.[101, 102] Baytas *et al.* used LSTM networks to leverage stratification of longitudinal data of patients with Parkinson's disease (PD).[101] Similarly, Zhang *et al.* used LSTMs to identify three subgroups of patients with idiopathic PD that differ in disease progression patterns and symptom severity.[102]

Patient stratification studies are mostly focused on a specific disease using *ad hoc* cohorts of patient data.[61, 62, 101, 102, 104, 105] These studies obtained relevant clinically meaningful results, however the computational framework is hard to replicate for different diseases as it is tied to the specific cohorts of patients. Because EHRs tend to be incomplete, using a diverse cohort of patients to derive disease-specific subgroups can adequately capture the features of heterogeneity within the disease of interest.[46] A first approach in this direction is proposed by Landi *et al.* and combines CNNs and autoencoders (ConvAE) to learn patient representations from a large and diverse EHR collection of ~1.6 million patients from the Mount Sinai Health system's data warehouse.[103] These latent representations combine different clinical features, including ICD codes, medications, lab tests, clinical notes, vital signs, and procedures, and aim to enable the identification of disease subgroups from any cohort of patients with complex disorders. The evaluation, firstly, showed that ConvAE performed better than several baselines, including Deep Patient, in clustering patients with different conditions. Secondly, the authors showed that ConvAE leads to effective patient stratification with minimal effort. To this end, they used the encodings learnt from domain-free and heterogeneous EHRs to derive subtypes for different complex disorders and provide a qualitative analysis to determine their clinical relevance. In particular, they evaluated six conditions: T2D, PD, Alzheimer's disease, multiple myeloma, prostate cancer, and breast cancer. Results identified disease progression, symptom severity, and comorbidities as contributing the most to the EHR-based clinical phenotypic variability of complex disorders. For example, T2D patients are divided into three subgroups (see Figure 4) according to comorbidities (i.e., cardiovascular and microvascular problems) and symptom severity (i.e., newly diagnosed with milder symptoms), while individuals with PD showed different disease duration and symptoms (i.e., motor, non-motor). This architecture is

Type 2 diabetes

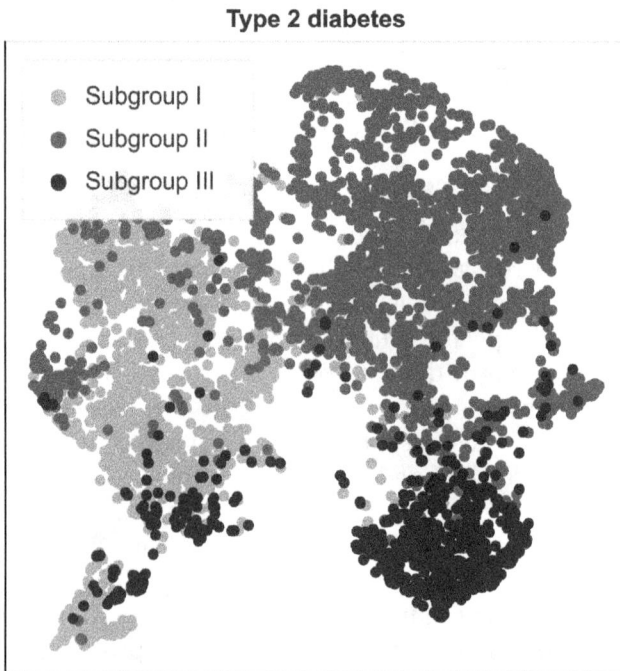

Fig. 4. Disease subgroups identified for type 2 diabetes mellitus (T2D) via EHR-based patient stratification.[103] Patients clustered into three subgroups characterized by the following: common T2D symptoms, e.g., metabolic syndrome, (Subgroup I); microvascular problems (Subgroup II); and cardiovascular problems (Subgroup III).

a first attempt to unlock patient stratification at scale, where we learn multi-purpose EHR-based representations from heterogeneous cohorts of patients without requiring any manual feature engineering and explicit labeling of events.

4.4. *Clinical note understanding*

A large amount of research in machine learning for healthcare focuses on structured EHRs to understand patient clinical trajectories and create opportunities to derive new clinical insights. However, a wealth of relevant clinical information remains locked behind clinical narratives in the free text of notes. Natural language processing (NLP), a branch of computer science that enables machines to process human language for applications such as machine translation,[106] text generation,[107] and image captioning[108] has been used to parse clinical notes to extract relevant insights that can guide clinical decisions.[47]

Before the rise of DL, clinical NLP largely focused on the automatic extraction of clinical concepts, such as diseases, lab tests, medications, and events from the free text (i.e., concept extraction). These concepts were usually identified by matching n-grams (i.e., sequences of adjacent words) to ontologies, such as the Unified Medical Language System (UMLS). The clinical concepts extracted from the text were then used to integrate structured EHRs or to broadly identify/define the clinical status of patients using shallow supervised methods, such as random forest and support vector machine. These approaches were used to, e.g., identify patient eligible for clinical trials,[109] automatically assign diagnosis codes based on discharge summaries,[110] and to identify medical conditions, such as rheumatoid arthritis,[111] obesity[112] and pulmonary disease.[113]

DL applied to clinical NLP has obtained promising results and is receiving growing acceptance in the medical community.[114] In particular, deep learning enables reducing the need of preprocessing, eliminating the step of concept extraction, and using instead all the words in the text. Most of the works rely on techniques such as word embeddings based on word2vec and RNNs (usually implemented as LSTM or GRU networks).[50] Common applications process the information in the free text to explore the automatic assignment of disease codes (i.e., ICD-9/10 codes),[115–117] prediction of disease onset[118] and three-day readmission.[119]

Miotto *et al.* used word embeddings and multi-kernel CNNs to identify the presence of acute low back pain (LBP) episodes in the clinical notes to inform an automated framework that can help front-line primary care providers in the development of targeted strategies for LBP in clinical practice.[120] Acute and chronic low back pain are different conditions with different treatments. However, they are coded in electronic health records with the same ICD-10 code (M54.5) and can be differentiated only by retrospective chart reviews. This prevents an efficient definition of data-driven guidelines for billing and therapy recommendations, such as return-to-work options. This study was the first to explore the use of automated approaches based on machine learning and information retrieval to analyze free-text clinical notes and identify acute LBP episodes. In particular, they used a dataset of $17,409$ clinical notes from different primary care practices, with 891 of them manually annotated as acute LBP and $2,973$ generally associated with LBP via the recorded ICD-10 code. They compared different supervised and unsupervised strategies for automated identification, such as keyword search, topic modeling, logistic regression with bag of n-grams and manual features, and deep learning (based on CNNs). The DL-based architecture obtained the best results and was also robust to the reduction of the number of manually annotated documents used for training. This type of work promises to reduce well-known problems of structured EHRs, such as billing biases and incompleteness, improving the use of patient data for translational research and data-driven analysis.

Advances in NLP based on transformers, specifically BERT,[91] have been recently explored with medical and clinical text as well.[121] In particular, Huang *et al.* developed and evaluated representations of clinical notes using bidirectional transformers (Clinical-BERT).[119] Experiments showed the following: (1) ClinicalBERT was able to uncover high-quality relationships between medical concepts as judged by humans. (2) It outperformed several baselines on 30-day hospital readmission prediction using both discharge summaries and the first few days of notes in the intensive care unit. While this was just the initial studies, techniques based on BERT and extensions, which have the ability to process large amount of data and are more evolved in understanding word semantics from its context, will play a key role in the next year to leverage all the information stored in free-text reports and support clinical decision systems.

5. Discussion

In this chapter, we hope to have illustrated the co-evolution of EHRs and ML methodologies, which hand-in-hand have enabled a new modality of biomedical research. To get to where we are today where ML in healthcare is almost commonplace, there was a tremendous amount of method development and refinement to unlock this source of data for research purposes, as described in previous section. There are a slew of issues that limit the impact such discoveries can make, especially translating findings into the clinic. The first major issue is in regard to the generalizability of models built on healthcare data. In fact, models built using data from one hospital's population does not necessarily generalize to others. In other words, models that may have high AUC-ROC (Area Under the Receiver Operating Characteristic) or specificity/sensitivity on the test set of the data it was trained on might have drastically lower performance on an outside cohort. This discrepancy stems, in part, from the fact that there are biases and system processes that are unique to certain systems, which are independent of the actual features that influence outcome.[122] For instance, in a given hospital, a particular imaging machine may be used for ascertaining certain suspected pathologies, which may be learned by ML algorithms. While it is conceivable that adding the machine details as a feature may prove valuable in some situations, it can lead to learning aspects of a certain hospital system which in essence constitute overfitting and do not translate to other hospitals that use different machines. Another important issue in creating generalizable models, however, is when models are unfair to underrepresented patients. This issue of unfairness in healthcare ML models has already been seen. This could mean that individuals of racial and ethnic populations that are less represented in biomedicine receive sub-optimal recommendations that can lead to real consequences. These unfair models can occur when certain factors are not taken into consideration because they are not available from EHR data. Such facets like socio-economic status, access to care and healthy food options absolutely influence health outcomes, but are not provided to the models to control for. These models, therefore, may improperly assign risk estimates which could further punish those who need assistance the most. Ensuring fairness in healthcare-related ML is an unsolved issue and will be a continued fight.

These aspects represent challenges for the proper use of ML for healthcare. Researchers have developed a set of technical implementations and recommendations that can alleviate some of these issues.[123] To ensure that there is sufficient representation of different populations in training data, there are certain trade-offs of performance that can be enacted to promote equity depending on the situation at hand. Balancing factors, such as equalized odds and predictive power, to ensure fairness will require bespoke reasoning per clinical question. Furthermore, the implementation of explainable models could help interpret the decisional process and hence identify potential pitfalls of algorithms trained on misrepresented data.[12]

In conjunction with the fairness modeling considerations, increasing representation of underserved populations will also improve utility of ML in clinical practice. As we saw, it is traditionally difficult to connect data from various institutions due to data format as well as legal and privacy concerns. Common data models like OMOP have certainly alleviated the burden to connect data and has enabled replication efforts. Here, code can be shared instead of data, which greatly reduces the burden to run such studies. The ability to jointly learn from multiple sources of data is still an issue though. Advances in techniques such as federated learning allow for models to be deployed and refined without the need to share data.[124] Of course, there are still many concerns about how federated learning can work in practice for healthcare-related ML and there are still concerns for attacks, but it represents an effective way forward.

The last key area that will benefit ML in biomedicine is the collection of more refined and continuous data that can fill in gaps in care.[125] When clinicians treat patients they operate on imperfect representations of information and there are a slew of important data that they do not know, such as the patient's diet, sleep, and exercise regimen between visits. These pieces of information can undoubtedly enhance the clinician's ability to treat patients and it is no stretch of the imagination to think that they would also improve the ML performance. Passive data collection modalities, such as sensors,[126] wearables and mobile apps,[127] and smart mirrors,[128] can fill this gap.

With the increased availability of the growing amount of patient-related data, there will be a new set of infrastructural, legal, ethical, and IT-related issues that come with it. With the continued awareness of these problems, particularly regarding fairness, we are encouraged that the field will be able to tackle them, but it will require rigorous standards and continued focus.

Acknowledgments

The authors would like to thank the support from the Hasso Plattner Foundation. R.M. also acknowledges the support from the Alzheimer's Drug Discovery Foundation.

References

1. P. B. Jensen, L. J. Jensen, and S. Brunak, Mining electronic health records: Towards better research applications and clinical care, *Nat. Rev. Genet.* **13**, 395 (2012).
2. Y. Bengio, A. Courville, and P. Vincent, Representation learning: A review and new perspectives, *IEEE Trans. PAMI.* **35**(8), 1798–1828 (2013).
3. Y. LeCun, Y. Bengio, and G. Hinton, Deep learning, *Nature* **521**(7553), 436–444 (2015).
4. O. Russakovsky, J. Deng, H. Su, J. Krause, S. Satheesh, S. Ma, Z. Huang, A. Karpathy, A. Khosla, M. Bernstein, *et al.*, Imagenet large scale visual recognition challenge, *Int. J. Comput. Vis.* **115**(3), 211–252 (2015).
5. J. Hirschberg and C. D. Manning, Advances in natural language processing, *Science* **349**(6245), 261–266 (2015).
6. G. Hinton, L. Deng, D. Yu, G. E. Dahl, A.-R. Mohamed, N. Jaitly, A. Senior, V. Vanhoucke, P. Nguyen, T. N. Sainath, *et al.*, Deep neural networks for acoustic modeling in speech recognition: The shared views of four research groups, *IEEE Signal Process. Mag.* **29**(6), 82–97 (2012).
7. A. Esteva, A. Robicquet, B. Ramsundar, V. Kuleshov, M. DePristo, K. Chou, C. Cui, G. Corrado, S. Thrun, and J. Dean, A guide to deep learning in healthcare, *Nat. Med.* **25**(1), 24–29 (2019). doi: 10.1038/s41591-018-0316-z.
8. C. J. McDonald, J. Overhage, W. M. Tierney, P. R. Dexter, D. K. Martin, J. G. Suico, A. Zafar, G. Schadow, L. Blevins, T. Glazener, J. Meeks-Johnson, L. Lemmon, J. Warvel, B. Porterfield, J. Warvel, P. Cassidy, D. Lindbergh, A. Belsito, M. Tucker, B. Williams, and

C. Wodniak, The regenstrief medical record system: A quarter century experience, *Int. J. Med. Inform.* **54**(3), 225–253 (1999).

9. J. M. Fitzmaurice, K. Adams, and J. M. Eisenberg, Three decades of research on computer applications in health care: Medical informatics support at the agency for healthcare research and quality, *J. Am. Med. Inform. Assoc.* **9**(2), 144–160 (2002).

10. N. G. Weiskopf and C. Weng, Methods and dimensions of electronic health record data quality assessment: Enabling reuse for clinical research, *J. Am. Med. Inform. Assoc.* **20**(1), 144–151 (2013).

11. E. M. Cahan, T. Hernandez-Boussard, S. Thadaney-Israni, and D. L. Rubin, Putting the data before the algorithm in big data addressing personalized healthcare, *NPJ Digit. Med.* **2**(1), 1–6 (2019).

12. D. Cirillo, S. Catuara-Solarz, C. Morey, E. Guney, L. Subirats, S. Mellino, A. Gigante, A. Valencia, M. J. Rementeria, A. S. Chadha, *et al.*, Sex and gender differences and biases in artificial intelligence for biomedicine and healthcare, *NPJ Digit. Med.* **3**(1), 1–11 (2020).

13. Z. C. Lipton, D. Kale, and R. Wetzel. Directly modeling missing data in sequences with rnns: Improved classification of clinical time series. In *Machine Learning for Healthcare Conference*, pp. 253–270, PMLR (2016).

14. Z. Che, S. Purushotham, K. Cho, D. Sontag, and Y. Liu, Recurrent neural networks for multivariate time series with missing values, *Sci. Rep.* **8**(1), 1–12 (2018).

15. B. K. Beaulieu-Jones and J. H. Moore. Missing data imputation in the electronic health record using deeply learned autoencoders. In *Pacific Symposium on Biocomputing*, pp. 207–218, World Scientific (2017).

16. B. H. Zhang, B. Lemoine, and M. Mitchell. Mitigating unwanted biases with adversarial learning. In *Proceedings of the 2018 AAAI/ACM Conference on AI, Ethics, and Society*, pp. 335–340, Association for Computing Machinery (2018).

17. A. Amini, A. P. Soleimany, W. Schwarting, S. N. Bhatia, and D. Rus. Uncovering and mitigating algorithmic bias through learned latent structure. In *Proceedings of the 2019 AAAI/ACM Conference on AI, Ethics, and Society*, pp. 289–295, Association for Computing Machinery (2019).

18. A. Boonstra, A. Versluis, and J. F. J. Vos, Implementing electronic health records in hospitals: A systematic literature review, *BMC Health Serv. Res.* **14**(1), 370 (2014).

19. J. Pathak, A. N. Kho, and J. C. Denny, Electronic health records-driven phenotyping: Challenges, recent advances, and perspectives, *J. Am. Med. Inform. Assoc.* **20**(e2), e206–e211 (2013).

20. M. A. Badgeley, M. Liu, B. S. Glicksberg, M. Shervey, J. Zech, K. Shameer, J. Lehar, E. K. Oermann, M. V. McConnell, T. M. Snyder, and J. T. Dudley, CANDI: An R package and Shiny app for annotating radiographs and evaluating computer-aided diagnosis, *Bioinformatics* **35**(9), 1610–1612 (2018).

21. B. S. Glicksberg, B. Oskotsky, P. M. Thangaraj, N. Giangreco, M. A. Badgeley, K. W. Johnson, D. Datta, V. A. Rudrapatna, N. Rappoport, M. M. Shervey, R. Miotto, T. C. Goldstein, E. Rutenberg, R. Frazier, N. Lee, S. Israni, R. Larsen, B. Percha, L. Li, J. T. Dudley, N. P. Tatonetti, and A. J. Butte, PatientExploreR: An extensible application for dynamic visualization of patient clinical history from electronic health records in the OMOP common data model, *Bioinformatics* **35**(21), 4515–4518 (2019).

22. M. R. Boland, K. J. Karczewski, and N. P. Tatonetti, Ten simple rules to enable multi-site collaborations through data sharing, *PLoS Comput. Biol.* **13**(1), e1005278–e1005278 (2017).

23. D. Bender and K. Sartipi. Hl7 fhir: An agile and restful approach to healthcare information exchange. In *Proceedings of the 26th IEEE International Symposium on Computer-based Medical Systems*, pp. 326–331, IEEE (2013).

24. G. Alterovitz, J. Warner, P. Zhang, Y. Chen, M. Ullman-Cullere, D. Kreda, and I. S. Kohane, SMART on FHIR genomics: Facilitating standardized clinico-genomic apps, *J. Am. Med. Inform. Assoc.* **22**(6), 1173–1178 (2015).

25. S. Murphy and A. Wilcox, Mission and sustainability of informatics for integrating biology and the bedside (i2b2), *eGEMs* **2**(2) (2014).

26. G. Hripcsak, J. D. Duke, N. H. Shah, C. G. Reich, V. Huser, M. J. Schuemie, M. A. Suchard, R. W. Park, I. C. K. Wong, P. R. Rijnbeek, *et al.*, Observational health data sciences and informatics (ohdsi): Opportunities for observational researchers, *Stud. Health Technol. Inform.* **216**, 574 (2015).

27. J. Kirby, P. Speltz, L. Rasmussen, M. Basford, O. Gottesman, P. Peissig, J. Pacheco, G. Tromp, J. Pathak, D. Carrell, S. Ellis, T. Lingren, W. Thompson, G. Savova, J. Haines, D. M. Roden, P. Harris, and J. Denny, PheKB: A catalog and workflow for creating electronic phenotype algorithms for transportability, *J. Am. Med. Inform. Assoc.* **23**(6), 1046–1052 (2016).

28. H. Mo, W. K. Thompson, L. V. Rasmussen, J. A. Pacheco, G. Jiang, R. Kiefer, Q. Zhu, J. Xu, E. Montague, D. S. Carrell, *et al.*, Desiderata for computable representations of electronic health records-driven phenotype algorithms, *J. Am. Med. Inform. Assoc.* **22**(6), 1220–1230 (2015).

29. C. M. Bishop, *Pattern Recognition and Machine Learning*. Springer, New York (2006).
30. A. Esteva, A. Robicquet, B. Ramsundar, V. Kuleshov, M. DePristo, K. Chou, C. Cui, G. Corrado, S. Thrun, and J. Dean, A guide to deep learning in healthcare, *Nat. Med.* **25**(1), 24–29 (2019).
31. M. I. Jordan and T. M. Mitchell, Machine learning: Trends, perspectives, and prospects, *Science* **349**(6245), 255–260 (2015).
32. I. Goodfellow, Y. Bengio, and A. Courville, *Deep Learning*. MIT press, Cambridge, Massachusetts (2016).
33. Y. LeCun *et al.*, Generalization and network design strategies, *Connectionism in Perspective* **19**, 143–155 (1989).
34. Y. LeCun, K. Kavukcuoglu, and C. Farabet. Convolutional networks and applications in vision. In *Proceedings of 2010 IEEE International Symposium on Circuits and Systems*, pp. 253–256, IEEE (2010).
35. S. Hochreiter and J. Schmidhuber, Long short-term memory, *Neural Comput.* **9**(8), 1735–1780 (1997). doi: 10.1162/neco.1997.9.8.1735.
36. D. E. Rumelhart, G. E. Hinton, and R. J. Williams. Learning internal representations by error propagation. Technical report, California Univ. San Diego La Jolla Inst for Cognitive Science (1985).
37. T. Mikolov, I. Sutskever, K. Chen, G. S. Corrado, and J. Dean. Distributed representations of words and phrases and their compositionality. In *Advances in Neural Information Processing systems*, pp. 3111–3119, NeurIPS (2013).
38. Y. Li, Deep reinforcement learning: An overview, *arXiv preprint arXiv:1701.07274* (2017).
39. I. J. Goodfellow, J. Pouget-Abadie, M. Mirza, B. Xu, D. Warde-Farley, S. Ozair, A. Courville, and Y. Bengio. Generative adversarial nets. In *Proceedings of the 27th International Conference on Neural Information Processing Systems*, vol. 2, pp. 2672–2680, MIT Press, Cambridge, MA, USA (2014).
40. J. Ho and S. Ermon, Generative adversarial imitation learning, *arxiv preprint 1606.03476* (2016).
41. S.-C. Huang, A. Pareek, S. Seyyedi, I. Banerjee, and M. P. Lungren, Fusion of medical imaging and electronic health records using deep learning: A systematic review and implementation guidelines, *NPJ Digit. Med.* **3**(1), 1–9 (2020).
42. R. Miotto, F. Wang, S. Wang, X. Jiang, and J. T. Dudley, Deep learning for healthcare: Review, opportunities and challenges, *Brief. Bioinform.* **19**(6), 1236–1246 (2017).
43. K. W. Johnson, J. T. Soto, B. S. Glicksberg, K. Shameer, R. Miotto, M. Ali, E. Ashley, and J. T. Dudley, Artificial intelligence in cardiology, *J. Am. Coll. Cardiol.* **71**(23), 2668–2679 (2018).

44. C. Xiao, E. Choi, and J. Sun, Opportunities and challenges in developing deep learning models using electronic health records data: A systematic review, *J. Am. Med. Inform. Assoc.* **25**(10), 1419–1428 (2018).
45. K.-H. Yu, A. L. Beam, and I. S. Kohane, Artificial intelligence in healthcare, *Nat. Biomed. Eng.* **2**(10), 719–731 (2018).
46. D. Chen, S. Liu, P. Kingsbury, S. Sohn, C. B. Storlie, E. B. Habermann, J. M. Naessens, D. W. Larson, and H. Liu, Deep learning and alternative learning strategies for retrospective real-world clinical data, *NPJ Digit. Med.* **2**(1), 1–5 (2019).
47. S. Sheikhalishahi, R. Miotto, J. T. Dudley, A. Lavelli, F. Rinaldi, and V. Osmani, Natural language processing of clinical notes on chronic diseases: Systematic review, *JMIR Med. Informat.* **7**(2), e12239 (2019).
48. E. Topol, *Deep Medicine: How Artificial Intelligence can Make Healthcare Human Again.* Hachette UK (2019).
49. A. Rajkomar, J. Dean, and I. Kohane, Machine learning in medicine, *New Engl. J. Med.* **380**(14), 1347–1358 (2019).
50. S. Wu, K. Roberts, S. Datta, J. Du, Z. Ji, Y. Si, S. Soni, Q. Wang, Q. Wei, Y. Xiang, *et al.*, Deep learning in clinical natural language processing: A methodical review, *J. Am. Med. Inform. Assoc.* **27**(3), 457–470 (2020).
51. D. F. Steiner, P.-H. C. Chen, and C. H. Mermel, Closing the translation gap: AI applications in digital pathology, *Biochimica et Biophysica Acta (BBA)-Reviews on Cancer* p. 188452 (2020).
52. C. Yu, J. Liu, and S. Nemati, Reinforcement learning in healthcare: A survey, *arXiv preprint arXiv:1908.08796* (2019).
53. J. D. Martín-Guerrero, F. Gomez, E. Soria-Olivas, J. Schmidhuber, M. Climente-Martí, and N. V. Jiménez-Torres, A reinforcement learning approach for individualizing erythropoietin dosages in hemodialysis patients, *Expert Syst. Appl.* **36**(6), 9737–9742 (2009).
54. M. Komorowski, L. A. Celi, O. Badawi, A. C. Gordon, and A. A. Faisal, The artificial intelligence clinician learns optimal treatment strategies for sepsis in intensive care, *Nat. Med.* **24**(11), 1716–1720 (2018).
55. R. Bellazzi and B. Zupan, Predictive data mining in clinical medicine: Current issues and guidelines, *Int. J. Med. Inform.* **77**(2), 81–97 (2008).
56. J. Wu, J. Roy, and W. F. Stewart, Prediction modeling using ehr data: Challenges, strategies, and a comparison of machine learning approaches, *Med. Care.* **48**(6 Suppl), S106–S113 (2010).

57. M. R. Boland, P. Parhi, L. Li, R. Miotto, R. Carroll, U. Iqbal, P.-A. Nguyen, M. Schuemie, S. C. You, D. Smith, *et al.*, Uncovering exposures responsible for birth season–disease effects: A global study, *J. Am. Med. Inform. Assoc.* **25**(3), 275–288 (2018).

58. A. B. Jensen, P. L. Moseley, T. I. Oprea, S. G. Ellesøe, R. Eriksson, H. Schmock, P. B. Jensen, L. J. Jensen, and S. Brunak, Temporal disease trajectories condensed from population-wide registry data covering 6.2 million patients, *Nat. Commun.* **5**(1), 4022 (2014). doi: 10.1038/ncomms5022. https://doi.org/10.1038/ncomms5022.

59. J. Hu, C. Thomas, and S. Brunak, Network biology concepts in complex disease comorbidities, *Nat. Rev. Genet.* **17**(10), 615–629 (2016).

60. N. P. Tatonetti, P. Y. Patrick, R. Daneshjou, and R. B. Altman, Data-driven prediction of drug effects and interactions, *Sci. Transl. Med.* **4** (125), 125ra31–125ra31 (2012).

61. F. Doshi-Velez, Y. Ge, and I. Kohane, Comorbidity clusters in autism spectrum disorders: An electronic health record time-series analysis, *Pediatrics* **133**(1), e54–e63 (2013). doi: 10.1542/peds.2013-0819.

62. L. Li, W. Y. Cheng, B. S. Glicksberg, O. Gottesman, R. Tamler, R. Chen, E. P. Bottinger, and J. T. Dudley, Identification of type 2 diabetes subgroups through topological analysis of patient similarity, *Sci. Transl. Med.* **7**(311), 311ra174 (2015).

63. K. Shameer, K. W. Johnson, A. Yahi, R. Miotto, L. Li, D. Ricks, J. Jebakaran, P. Kovatch, P. P. Sengupta, S. Gelijns, *et al.* Predictive modeling of hospital readmission rates using electronic medical record-wide machine learning: A case-study using mount sinai heart failure cohort. In *Pacific Symposium on Biocomputing*, pp. 276–287, World Scientific (2017).

64. R. Miotto, L. Li, B. A. Kidd, and J. T. Dudley, Deep patient: An unsupervised representation to predict the future of patients from the electronic health records, *Sci. Rep.* **6**, 26094 (2016). doi: 10.1038/srep26094.

65. P. Vincent, H. Larochelle, I. Lajoie, Y. Bengio, and P.-A. Manzagol, Stacked denoising autoencoders: Learning useful representations in a deep network with a local denoising criterion, *J Mach Learn. Res.* **11**(Dec), 3371–3408 (2010).

66. R. Miotto, L. Li, and J. T. Dudley. Deep learning to predict patient future diseases from the electronic health records. In *European Conference on Information Retrieval*, pp. 768–774, Springer, Cham (2016).

67. D. M. Blei, Probabilistic topic models, *Commun. ACM* **55**(4), 77–84 (2012).

68. E. Choi, M. Bahadori, and J. Sun, Doctor AI: Predicting clinical events via recurrent neural networks, *CoRR.* **abs/1511.05942** (2015). http://arxiv.org/abs/1511.05942.

69. T. Pham, T. Tran, D. Phung, and S. Venkatesh. Deepcare: A deep dynamic memory model for predictive medicine. In *Advances in Knowledge Discovery and Data Mining*, pp. 30–41, Springer International Publishing (2016).

70. E. Choi, M. T. Bahadori, J. Sun, J. Kulas, A. Schuetz, and W. Stewart. Retain: An interpretable predictive model for healthcare using reverse time attention mechanism. In *Advances in Neural Information Processing Systems*, pp. 3504–3512, NeurIPS (2016).

71. Z. C. Lipton, D. C. Kale, C. Elkan, and R. Wetzel, Learning to diagnose with lstm recurrent neural networks, *arXiv preprint arXiv:1511.03677* (2015).

72. A. Rajkomar, E. Oren, K. Chen, A. Dai, N. Hajaj, M. Hardt, P. Liu, X. Liu, J. Marcus, M. Sun, P. Sundberg, H. Yee, K. Zhang, Y. Zhang, G. Flores, G. Duggan, J. Irvine, Q. Le, K. Litsch, A. Mossin, J. Tansuwan, D. Wang, J. Wexler, J. Wilson, D. Ludwig, S. Volchenboum, K. Chou, M. Pearson, S. Madabushi, N. Shah, A. Butte, M. Howell, C. Cui, G. Corrado, and J. Dean, Scalable and accurate deep learning with electronic health records, *NPJ Digit. Med.* **1**(1), 18 (2018). doi: 10.1038/s41746-018-0029-1. https://doi.org/10.1038/s41746-018-0029-1.

73. G. Litjens, T. Kooi, B. E. Bejnordi, A. A. A. Setio, F. Ciompi, M. Ghafoorian, J. A. Van Der Laak, B. Van Ginneken, and C. I. Sánchez, A survey on deep learning in medical image analysis, *Med. Imag. Anal.* **42**, 60–88 (2017).

74. V. Gulshan, L. Peng, M. Coram, M. C. Stumpe, D. Wu, A. Narayanaswamy, S. Venugopalan, K. Widner, T. Madams, J. Cuadros, *et al.*, Development and validation of a deep learning algorithm for detection of diabetic retinopathy in retinal fundus photographs, *JAMA* **316**(22), 2402–2410 (2016).

75. I. J. MacCormick, B. M. Williams, Y. Zheng, K. Li, B. Al-Bander, S. Czanner, R. Cheeseman, C. E. Willoughby, E. N. Brown, G. L. Spaeth, *et al.*, Accurate, fast, data efficient and interpretable glaucoma diagnosis with automated spatial analysis of the whole cup to disc profile, *PLOS One* **14**(1), e0209409 (2019).

76. A. Esteva, B. Kuprel, R. A. Novoa, J. Ko, S. M. Swetter, H. M. Blau, and S. Thrun, Dermatologist-level classification of skin cancer with deep neural networks, *Nature* **542**(7639), 115–118 (2017).

77. J. R. Zech, M. A. Badgeley, M. Liu, A. B. Costa, J. J. Titano, and E. K. Oermann, Variable generalization performance of a deep learning model to detect pneumonia in chest radiographs: A cross-sectional study, *PLoS Med.* **15**(11) (2018).

78. G. Stiglic, P. Kocbek, N. Fijacko, M. Zitnik, K. Verbert, and L. Cilar, Interpretability of machine learning-based prediction models in healthcare, *WIREs Data Min. Knowl. Discov.* **10**(5), e1379 (2020). doi: https://doi.org/10.1002/widm.1379.

79. M. Du, N. Liu, and X. Hu, Techniques for interpretable machine learning, *Commun. ACM* **63**(1), 68–77 (2019).

80. S. M. Lundberg, B. Nair, M. S. Vavilala, M. Horibe, M. J. Eisses, T. Adams, D. E. Liston, D. K.-W. Low, S.-F. Newman, J. Kim, *et al.*, Explainable machine-learning predictions for the prevention of hypoxaemia during surgery, *Nat. Biomed. Eng.* **2**(10), 749–760 (2018).

81. W. Wei, P. Teixeira, H. Mo, R. Cronin, J. Warner, and J. Denny, Combining billing codes, clinical notes, and medications from electronic health records provides superior phenotyping performance, *J. Am. Med. Inform. Assoc.* **23**(e1), e20–e27 (09, 2015).

82. J. Banda, M. Seneviratne, T. Hernandez-Boussard, and N. Shah, Advances in electronic phenotyping: From rule-based definitions to machine learning models, *Annu. Rev. Biomed. Data Sci.* **1**(1), 53–68 (2018).

83. Y. Halpern, S. Horng, Y. Choi, and D. Sontag, Electronic medical record phenotyping using the anchor and learn framework, *J. Am. Med. Inform. Assoc.* **23**(4), 731–740 (2016).

84. J. C. Ho, J. Ghosh, S. R. Steinhubl, W. F. Stewart, J. C. Denny, B. A. Malin, and J. Sun, Limestone: High-throughput candidate phenotype generation via tensor factorization, *J. Biomed. Inform.* **52**, 199–211 (2014).

85. B. S. Glicksberg, R. Miotto, K. W. Johnson, K. Shameer, L. Li, R. Chen, and J. T. Dudley. Automated disease cohort selection using word embeddings from Electronic Health Records. In *Biocomputing 2018*, pp. 145–156, World Scientific (2017). doi: 10.1142/9789813235533_0014.

86. T. Mikolov, K. Chen, G. Corrado, and J. Dean. Efficient Estimation of Word Representations in Vector Space, *arXiv preprint arXiv*:1301.3781 (2013).

87. J. K. De Freitas, K. W. Johnson, E. Golden, G. N. Nadkarni, J. T. Dudley, E. P. Bottinger, B. S. Glicksberg, and R. Miotto, Phe2vec: Automated disease phenotyping based on unsupervised embeddings from electronic health records, *medRxiv* (2020). doi: 10.1101/2020.11.14.20231894.

88. J. Pennington, R. Socher, and C. D. Manning. Glove: Global vectors for word representation. In *Conference on Empirical Methods in Natural Language Processing (EMNLP)*, pp. 1532–1543, ACL (2014).

89. P. Bojanowski, E. Grave, A. Joulin, and T. Mikolov, Enriching word vectors with subword information, *Trans. Assoc. Comput. Linguist.* **5**, 135–146 (2017).

90. B. K. Beaulieu-Jones, I. S. Kohane, and A. L. Beam. Learning contextual hierarchical structure of medical concepts with poincairé embeddings to clarify phenotypes. In *PSB*, pp. 8–17, World Scientific (2019).

91. J. Devlin, M.-W. Chang, K. Lee, and K. Toutanova, Bert: Pre-training of deep bidirectional transformers for language understanding, *arXiv preprint arXiv:1810.04805* (2018).

92. Z. Yang, Z. Dai, Y. Yang, J. Carbonell, R. R. Salakhutdinov, and Q. V. Le. Xlnet: Generalized autoregressive pretraining for language understanding. In *Advances in Neural Information Processing Systems*, pp. 5754–5764, NeurIPS (2019).

93. V. Alexandrov, D. Brunner, L. B. Menalled, A. Kudwa, J. Watson-Johnson, M. Mazzella, I. Russell, M. C. Ruiz, J. Torello, E. Sabath, A. Sanchez, M. Gomez, I. Filipov, K. Cox, M. Kwan, A. Ghavami, S. Ramboz, B. Lager, V. C. Wheeler, J. Aaronson, J. Rosinski, J. F. Gusella, M. E. MacDonald, D. Howland, and S. Kwak, Large-scale phenome analysis defines a behavioral signature for Huntington's disease genotype in mice, *Nat. Biotechnol.* **34**(8), 838–844 (2016).

94. G. R. Cutting, Cystic fibrosis genetics: From molecular understanding to clinical application, *Nat. Rev. Genet.* **16**(1), 45–56 (2014).

95. M. C. Lai, M. V. Lombardo, and S. Baron-Cohen, Autism, *Lancet.* **383**, 896–910 (2014). doi: 10.1016/S0140-6736(13)61539-1.

96. D. Bai, B. H. K. Yip, G. C. Windham, A. Sourander, R. Francis, R. Yoffe, E. Glasson, B. Mahjani, A. Suominen, H. Leonard, M. Gissler, J. D. Buxbaum, K. Wong, D. Schendel, A. Kodesh, M. Breshnahan, S. Z. Levine, E. T. Parner, S. N. Hansen, C. Hultman, A. Reichenberg, and S. Sandin, Association of genetic and environmental factors with autism in a 5-country cohort, *JAMA Psychiatry* **76**(10), 1035–1043 (2019). doi: 10.1001/jamapsychiatry.2019.1411.

97. M. Quesnel-Vallières, R. J. Weatheritt, S. P. Cordes, and B. J. Blencowe, Autism spectrum disorder: Insights into convergent mechanisms from transcriptomics, *Nat. Rev. Genet.* **20**(1), 51–63 (2018). doi: 10.1038/s41576-018-0066-2.

98. C. Lord, S. Bishop, and D. Anderson, Developmental trajectories as autism phenotypes, *AAm. J. Med. Genet. Part A: Semin. Med. Genet.* **169**(2), 198–208 (2015). doi: 10.1002/ajmg.c.31440.

99. S. A. Dugger, A. Platt, and D. B. Goldstein, Drug development in the era of precision medicine, *Nat. Rev. Drug Discov.* **17**(3), 183–196 (2017). doi: 10.1038/nrd.2017.226.

100. M. Manchia, J. Cullis, G. Turecki, G. A. Rouleau, R. Uher, and M. Alda, The impact of phenotypic and genetic heterogeneity on results of genome wide association studies of complex diseases, *PLoS ONE*. **8**(10), e76295 (2013). doi: 10.1371/journal.pone.0076295.

101. I. M. Baytas, C. Xiao, X. Zhang, F. Wang, A. K. Jain, and J. Zhou. Patient Subtyping via Time-Aware LSTM Networks. In *Proceedings of the 23rd ACM SIGKDD International Conference on Knowledge Discovery and Data Mining*, pp. 65–74, ACM, New York, NY, USA (2017). doi: 10.1145/3097983.3097997. http://doi.acm.org/10.1145/3097983.3097997.

102. X. Zhang, J. Chou, J. Liang, C. Xiao, Y. Zhao, H. Sarva, C. Henchcliffe, and F. Wang, Data-driven subtyping of parkinson's disease using longitudinal clinical records: A cohort Study, *Sci. Rep.* **9**(1), 797 (2019).

103. I. Landi, B. S. Glicksberg, H.-C. Lee, S. Cherng, G. Landi, M. Danieletto, J. T. Dudley, C. Furlanello, and R. Miotto, Deep representation learning of electronic health records to unlock patient stratification at scale, *NPJ Digit. Med.* **3**(96) (2020).

104. M. V. Lombardo, M.-C. Lai, B. Auyeung, R. J. Holt, C. Allison, P. Smith, B. Chakrabarti, A. N. Ruigrok, J. Suckling, E. T. Bullmore, *et al.*, Unsupervised data-driven stratification of mentalizing heterogeneity in autism, *Sci. Rep.* **6**(1), 1–15 (2016).

105. E. Stevens, D. R. Dixon, M. N. Novack, D. Granpeesheh, T. Smith, and E. Linstead, Identification and analysis of behavioral phenotypes in autism spectrum disorder via unsupervised machine learning, *Int. J. Med. Inform.* **129**, 29–36 (2019). doi: 10.1016/j.ijmedinf.2019.05.006.

106. Y. Wu, M. Schuster, Z. Chen, Q. V. Le, M. Norouzi, W. Macherey, M. Krikun, Y. Cao, Q. Gao, K. Macherey, *et al.*, Google's neural machine translation system: Bridging the gap between human and machine translation, *arXiv preprint arXiv:1609.08144* (2016).

107. A. Kannan, K. Kurach, S. Ravi, T. Kaufmann, A. Tomkins, B. Miklos, G. Corrado, L. Lukacs, M. Ganea, P. Young, *et al.* Smart reply: Automated response suggestion for email. In *ACM International Conference on Knowledge Discovery and Data Mining*, pp. 955–964, ACM (2016).

108. O. Vinyals, A. Toshev, S. Bengio, and D. Erhan. Show and tell: A neural image caption generator. In *IEEE Conference on Computer Vision and Pattern Recognition*, pp. 3156–3164, IEEE (2015).

109. R. Miotto and C. Weng, Case-based reasoning using electronic health records efficiently identifies eligible patients for clinical trials, *J. Am. Med. Inform. Assoc.* **22**(e1), e141–e150 (2015).

110. A. Perotte, R. Pivovarov, K. Natarajan, N. Weiskopf, F. Wood, and N. Elhadad, Diagnosis code assignment: Models and evaluation metrics, *J. Am. Med. Inform. Assoc.* **21**(2), 231–237 (2014).

111. R. J. Carroll, W. K. Thompson, A. E. Eyler, A. M. Mandelin, T. Cai, R. M. Zink, J. A. Pacheco, C. S. Boomershine, T. A. Lasko, H. Xu, *et al.*, Portability of an algorithm to identify rheumatoid arthritis in electronic health records, *J. Am. Med. Inform. Assoc.* **19**(e1), e162–e169 (2012).

112. R. L. Figueroa and C. A. Flores, Extracting information from electronic medical records to identify the obesity status of a patient based on comorbidities and bodyweight measures, *J. Med. Syst.* **40**(8), 191 (2016).

113. M. R. Ananda-Rajah, D. Martinez, M. A. Slavin, L. Cavedon, M. Dooley, A. Cheng, and K. A. Thursky, Facilitating surveillance of pulmonary invasive mold diseases in patients with haematological malignancies by screening computed tomography reports using natural language processing, *PLoS One* **9**(9) (2014).

114. Y. Goldberg, A primer on neural network models for natural language processing, *J. Artif. Intell. Res.* **57**, 345–420 (2016).

115. H. Shi, P. Xie, Z. Hu, M. Zhang, and E. P. Xing, Towards automated icd coding using deep learning, *arXiv preprint arXiv:1711.04075* (2017).

116. T. Baumel, J. Nassour-Kassis, R. Cohen, M. Elhadad, and N. Elhadad. Multi-label classification of patient notes: Case study on icd code assignment. In *Workshops at the AAAI Conference on Artificial Intelligence*, AAAI (2018).

117. J. Mullenbach, S. Wiegreffe, J. Duke, J. Sun, and J. Eisenstein, Explainable prediction of medical codes from clinical text, *arXiv preprint arXiv:1802.05695* (2018).

118. J. Liu, Z. Zhang, and N. Razavian, Deep ehr: Chronic disease prediction using medical notes, *arXiv preprint arXiv:1808.04928* (2018).

119. K. Huang, J. Altosaar, and R. Ranganath, Clinicalbert: Modeling clinical notes and predicting hospital readmission, *arXiv preprint arXiv:1904.05342* (2019).

120. R. Miotto, B. L. Percha, B. S. Glicksberg, H.-C. Lee, L. Cruz, J. T. Dudley, and I. Nabeel, Identifying acute low back pain episodes in primary care practice from clinical notes: Observational study, *JMIR Med. Inform.* **8**(2), e16878 (2020).

121. J. Lee, W. Yoon, S. Kim, D. Kim, S. Kim, C. H. So, and J. Kang, Biobert: A pre-trained biomedical language representation model for biomedical text mining, *Bioinformatics* **36**(4), 1234–1240 (2020).

122. M. A. Badgeley, J. R. Zech, L. Oakden-Rayner, B. S. Glicksberg, M. Liu, W. Gale, M. V. McConnell, B. Percha, T. M. Snyder, and

J. T. Dudley, Deep learning predicts hip fracture using confounding patient and healthcare variables, *NPJ Digit. Med.* **2**(1), 31 (2019).

123. A. Rajkomar, M. Hardt, M. D. Howell, G. Corrado, and M. H. Chin, Ensuring fairness in machine learning to advance health equity, *Ann. Intern. Med.* **169**(12), 866–872 (2018).

124. J. Xu and F. Wang, Federated learning for healthcare informatics, *arXiv preprint arXiv:1911.06270* (2019).

125. B. S. Glicksberg, K. W. Johnson, and J. T. Dudley, The next generation of precision medicine: Observational studies, electronic health records, biobanks and continuous monitoring, *Hum. Mol. Genet.* **27** (R1), R56–R62 (2018).

126. S. Xu, A. Jayaraman, and J. A. Rogers. Skin sensors are the future of health care, *Nature* **571**, 319–321 (2019).

127. F. F. Chaudhry, M. Danieletto, E. Golden, J. Scelza, G. Botwin, M. Shervey, J. K. De Freitas, I. Paranjpe, G. N. Nadkarni, R. Miotto, *et al.*, Sleep in the natural environment: A pilot study, *Sensors* **20**(5), 1378 (2020).

128. R. Miotto, M. Danieletto, J. R. Scelza, B. A. Kidd, and J. T. Dudley, Reflecting health: Smart mirrors for personalized medicine, *NPJ Digit. Med.* **1**(1), 1–7 (2018).

https://doi.org/10.1142/9781800610941_0004

Chapter 4

Natural Language Technologies in the Biomedical Domain

Horacio Rodríguez

Computer Science Department, Universitat Politècnica de Catalunya, Campus Nord, Carrer de Jordi Girona, 1, 3, 08034 Barcelona, Spain

horacio@cs.upc.edu

In this chapter, we face the problems associated with natural language processing in the biomedical domain. We strive to provide enough technical background to allow the reader to develop real applications in this area while also providing the needed theoretical basis for supporting practical techniques. For the sake of self-containment, we organize the chapter as a general to specific tour following two orthogonal dimensions: the dimension of the techniques and the dimension of the domains. In the first dimension, we begin by presenting the generalities of natural language processing, i.e. linguistic units, tasks, applications, resources. After superficially discussing the symbolic approaches, we move into empirical methods, machine learning, shallow neural models and, finally, deep learning. In parallel, we start with open domain scenarios to further move into domain-restricted ones and, finally, into the biomedical domain.

1. Introduction to Natural Language Processing

Natural Language Processing (NLP) is an old discipline evolving from the origin of the commercial use of computers under the umbrella of Artificial Intelligence (AI).[a] Both disciplines follow

---

[a] Although frequently NLP does not use AI techniques.

parallel itineraries, littered with periods of exaggerated expectations followed by long periods of skepticism as a result of the discredit after the hypes and lack of public funding. NLP is in a sweet spot for the time being. NLP is useful because it seeks solutions to language-related problems in situations where manual processing is not technically or economically feasible. The utility of NLP is manifested in the multiple applications that have reached commercial level, far beyond research status, as discussed in Section 1.2. NLP is, however, difficult due to a number of reasons:

- **Multilingualism:** The term "language" refers to any human language. According to *Ethnologue*,[b] there are currently 7,117 languages spoken in the world although the 23 most spoken cover half of the world's population. NLP focuses on languages with enough resources for supporting some degree of processing. For instance, Wikipedia covers 314 languages, DBPedia 125, MultiWordNet 75, BabelNet 271, *MUSE* 110, LASER 93, and Spacy 61.
- **Multi-modality:** Although most NLP applications use text as an input mode, other modes, such as voice (as in phone interaction) and image (radiological reports), could be used as well.
- **Multi-domain:** Some applications of NLP are open domain while others are domain-dependent. The health and biomedical domains are by far the most important.
- **Multi-genre:** Input documents for NLP belong to a variety of genres, frequently using sub-languages, jargons, abbreviations, etc. In Section 4.1, we discuss this issue in the medical domain.
- **Comprehension vs. Generation:** NL can be used both as input and output in NLP.
- **Ambiguity:** Present at any level of language, i.e., lexical (e.g., "Washington" can be a state, a city, or a person), morphological (e.g., "building" can be a noun or a verb), syntactic, semantic, etc.

1.1. *NLP tasks*

The processes involved in NLP over a document include locating, extracting, and representing pieces of linguistic information from the

---

[b]https://www.ethnologue.com/.

text. These pieces are usually organized into a layered structure. Different tasks are assigned to each layer and different processors face each task. A common structure is as follows:

- **Textual layer:** Over the original document, some tasks could be performed: encoding and script guessing, locating of textual fragments, language identification, paragraph and sentence splitting, and, the basic one, tokenizing, i.e., decomposing the text into the minimal units owning a meaning (lexemes).
- **Morphological layer:** Over the tokenized text, the basic task is the morphological analysis, i.e., assigning to each token the set of their morpho-syntactic categories (part of speech (POS)). Other tasks are POS tagging, Named Entities Recognition and Classification (NERC), co-reference resolution, Word Sense Disambiguation (WSD).
- **Syntactic layer:** Over each sentence, syntactic analysis could be carried out. Parsers can be full, including constituency and dependency parsers, shallow parsers, spotters, chunkers, etc.
- **Semantic layer:** For each parsed sentence, a semantic parser should obtain the representation of its meaning. Full semantic parsing is only feasible in very narrow domains; in other cases, simpler processes could be performed, such as lexical tagging or Semantic Role Labelling.
- **Pragmatic layer:** Pragmatics means the intended use of language. The basic task here is the Discourse Analysis.

1.2. *NLP applications*

NLP applications can be classified into two large fields (without exclusion):

- **Human–machine interaction,** including different modes of dialog, Question Answering (QA), Linguistic Inference (LI), among others.
- **Massive textual information processes,** including Information Retrieval, Extraction, Filtering, Routing, etc. Automatic Summarization (AS), Machine Translation (MT), Machine Comprehension (MC), Opinion Mining, Sentiment Analysis (SA), terminology extraction, text classification, or concept linking, among others.

1.3. *NLP approaches*

Many different approaches can be followed for NLP. At the first level, they can be classified into two categories, the rationalist and the empiricist approaches:

- The rationalist approach proposed by Noam Chomsky sets that a considerable part of the knowledge to be used in NLP tasks can be fixed in advance and has to be prescribed, codified and incorporated explicitly to any NLP process. The usually named symbolic or knowledge-based systems follow this approach.
- The empiricist approach proposed by Zellig Harris sets, in turn, that linguistic knowledge can be inferred from experience and collected through textual corpora by using a few simple mechanisms, such as association or generalization. This way corresponds to Firth's Distributional Hypothesis: "We can know a word by the company it owns".

All the tasks presented in Section 1.1 could be faced with different processors belonging to one (or both) of these approaches. While morphology and syntax are usually faced by symbolic approaches, the empirical approach is usually applied to semantics. We focus on the latter, presented in Section 2, because this chapter is devoted to Deep Learning (DL). For the sake of completeness, however, we propose some general references. Studies in Refs. [1] and [2] cover both approaches, while Refs. [3] and [4] focus on DL, Ref. [5] focuses on statistical approaches, including conventional machine learning systems, and Ref. 6 goes into implementation details using Python.

2. Empirical Methods in NLP

Besides the use of stochastic context-free grammars at syntactic level, the empirical methods focus on semantics. Within the paradigm of distributional semantics, the base is the vector space model (VSM), where linguistic units are represented as vectors in high-dimensional vectorial spaces. In symbolic models, these vector spaces are of an enormous dimension, although the tendency to contract vector spaces to sub-symbolic representations of much smaller dimension (of the order of hundreds) is growing. When using *NN*, these dense representations are named embeddings, as described in Section 5.1. In

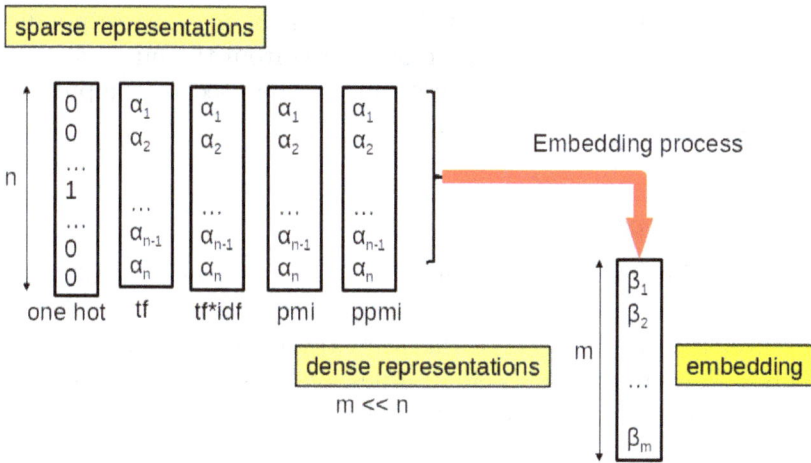

Fig. 1. Examples of vector representations of words.

Figure 1, some of the possible representations of words in a VSM model are presented. On the left, we find sparse representations in a vector space of dimension n, where n is the size of the vocabulary. In the *one-hot* representation, only one of the components of the vector takes the value 1, as there is no context here. The next columns correspond to different weighting schemata of the words in the context. A dense representation (an embedding) is shown on the right; the dimension m is several orders of magnitude below n.

Once the words or other linguistic units are represented by sparse or dense vectors, we can use on these vectors all the paraphernalia of instruments that linear algebra provides, such as addition, distance, projection, dimension reduction, and change of base.

Not only can words be represented in VSM, but we can also represent sub-word units as characters and complex units such as sentences. Documents and collections of linguistic units can be represented as matrices. For example, given a collection of D documents $d_1, d_2, \ldots, d_D$, in which N different words occur: $w_1, w_2, \ldots, w_N$, we can construct the word/document matrix of dimension $N \times D$ in which the rows are the words and the columns the documents, so that the element of row p and column d will contain the count of the occurrences of p in d. Word/document matrices are used to detect which documents are relevant to a user's query, represented as a set of keywords. The words of the query are represented in the rows of the matrix and each document is represented in its corresponding column. Documents containing more words from the query are proposed as a result. These matrices can also be used to compute the similarity between two documents.

2.1. *Resources*

The key point for the development of DL techniques for NLP is the availability of huge datasets for learning deep models. Consider, for instance, the case of QA. In the past, the richest dataset, "CuratedTREC",[7] contained only 2,180 (question, answer) pairs; obviously not enough for learning even a shallow NN. The dataset "Quora Q Pairs"[c] contains 404,302 pairs and allows learning accurate NN models.

Similarly, for the LI task, we can compare the old 5,800 pairs of Microsoft Research Paraphrase Corpus[d] with the 570,000 pairs of SNLI.[e] Other datasets for these and other tasks are described in Ref. 8. Besides these NLP resources (and many others), we have to mention generic resources, such as the Wikipedia(s), the DBPedia(s), WordNet, MultiWN, BabelNet, ConceptNet, and others, which are often used by NLP processors.

3.   Statistical Methods in NLP

Basically, VSM represents linguistic units as vectors in a high-dimensional vectorial space. Three basic problems have to be faced in this setting: (1) composition of vectors representing words for getting vector representations of more complex units; (2) computation of distances between vectors; and (3) dimensionality reduction. We present them in the following.

Let x be a complex unit, consisting on a sequence of tokens $x_1, x_2, \ldots, x_n$. Let $\vec{x_i}$ be the vector representing the token x_i. The vector representing x could be computed applying a composition

---

[c]https://www.kaggle.com/quora/question-pairs-dataset/.
[d]https://www.wikidata.org/wiki/Q47463175.
[e]https://nlp.stanford.edu/projects/snli/.

function ϕ over the components of x: $\overrightarrow{x} = \phi([\overrightarrow{x_1}, \ldots, \overrightarrow{x_n}])$. Different formulas have been used for ϕ. The most popular is a simple summation of the components of the sequence, i.e., $\overrightarrow{x} = \sum_{i=1}^{n} \overrightarrow{x_i}$. This function does not take into account the order of the components and assumes that all are equally important. These assumptions are clearly false. Consider, for instance, the nominal phrase x = "black cat", so $\overrightarrow{black\ cat} = \phi([\overrightarrow{black}, \overrightarrow{cat}])$. The vector $\overrightarrow{black\ cat}$ should be closer to $\overrightarrow{cat}$ than to $\overrightarrow{black}$ and this effect cannot be obtained using the simple summation. Another possibility is a linear combination of the components such as $\overrightarrow{x} = \sum_{i=1}^{n} \alpha^i \times \overrightarrow{x_i}$, with the weights α^i manually set according to the POS of the components, or learned for minimizing the distance between the complex unit and its head. For instance, in the case of noun phrases composed by an adjective and a noun, we can weight the adjective with 0.1 and the noun with 0.9, or learn α^i for minimizing the distance between the vector representing the nominal phrase <ADJ, NOUN> and the vector representing the head (<NOUN>).

For defining a distance (or similarity[f]) measure, our space, χ, should be a metric space. So, a distance d has to be defined. Such d is a function $\chi \times \chi \rightarrow \mathbb{R}$ satisfying the following properties, being $\overrightarrow{x}$, $\overrightarrow{y}$, and $\overrightarrow{z} \in \chi$:

(1) $d(\overrightarrow{x}, \overrightarrow{y}) \geq 0$,
(2) $d(\overrightarrow{x}, \overrightarrow{y}) = 0$ if and only if $\overrightarrow{x} = \overrightarrow{y}$,
(3) $d(\overrightarrow{x}, \overrightarrow{y}) = d(\overrightarrow{y}, \overrightarrow{x})$,
(4) $d(\overrightarrow{x}, \overrightarrow{z}) \leq d(\overrightarrow{x}, \overrightarrow{y}) + d(\overrightarrow{y}, \overrightarrow{z})$.[g]

Two popular distances are the L_1 norm, or the Manhattan distance, $d_{\text{man}}(\overrightarrow{x}, \overrightarrow{y}) = \sum_{i=1}^{d} |x_i - y_i|$, and the L_2 norm, or the Euclidean distance, $d_{\text{euc}}(\overrightarrow{x}, \overrightarrow{y}) = \sqrt{\sum_{i=1}^{d} |x_i - y_i|^2}$. L_1 and L_2 can be generalized into L_p, named the Minkowski distance. If we need normalized distances (in the interval [0,1]), we can normalize the vectors $\overrightarrow{x}$ in χ; this is equivalent to project $\overrightarrow{x}$ into a hyper-sphere of radius 1 and then compute the cosine distance (cosine of the

---

[f]Conversion between these two measures is straightforward.
[g]This property, the triangular inequality, is frequently not needed.

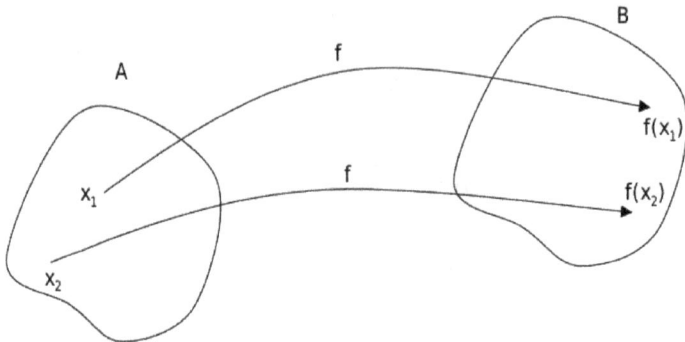

Fig. 2.   Mapping a vectorial space into a semantic space.

angle between the two vectors) or the geodesic distance. Other popular metrics are Dice and Jaccard. See Ref. [9] for details of all these metrics and many others and Ref. 10 for a Python library of implementations.[h]

An important issue of all these measures is that all the components of the vectors are equally important. Weighting the dimensions is an effective way of facing this issue. Mahalanobis proposes the following metric: $d_M(\overrightarrow{x}, \overrightarrow{y}) = \sqrt{\sum_{i=1}^{d}(\overrightarrow{x} - \overrightarrow{y})^T M(\overrightarrow{x} - \overrightarrow{y})}$, where $M = \Sigma^{-1}$ is the covariance matrix of the input vectors. A generalization of d_M allows M to be whatever semidefinite positive matrix.[i] Matrix M has a dimension $n \times n$ and has to be learned. If M is the identity matrix I, d_M reduces to d_{euc}. If M is a diagonal matrix, e.g., containing the eigenvalues, each dimension in the space is weighted by the value of the corresponding diagonal row. Also tri-diagonal matrices are used.

Sometimes, we have a semantic space where the distances own a clearer semantic interpretation: consider Figure 2. A is a vectorial space where vectors x_1 and x_2 are represented, B is a semantic space and f maps x_1 and x_2 into their semantic representations. We define our semantic distance in A of x_1 and x_2 as the semantic distance in B of the images of the application of f to x_1 and x_2: $d_{\text{sem}}^A(\overrightarrow{x_1}, \overrightarrow{x_2}) = d_{\text{sem}}^B(f(\overrightarrow{x_1}), f(\overrightarrow{x_2}))$. Different measures can be used in B. If B has

---

[h]https://pypi.python.org/pypi/metric-learn.
[i]That is, all the eigenvalues are non-negative.

a taxonomic structure, the most popular methods are path-based, i.e., the distance between two elements in B is the length of the shortest path between them following taxonomic links. The original path-based metrics were applied using WordNet as semantic space. NLTK provides[j] a library of path-based measures. This approach has been later applied to other semantic spaces, such as Wikipedia in the open domain and UMLS and DrugBank[k] in the medical domain, see Ref. [11].

The third topic we have to face is dimensionality reduction. The task is important for reducing the cost of computation and for improving the generalization process. Basically, what is done is approximating an n-dimensional space by a k-dimensional one with $k \ll n$. The most popular approach is Latent Semantic Indexing (LSI) based on Singular Value Decomposition. Others are Probabilistic LSI and Latent Dirichlet Allocation. Both models are generative and based on topic distributions. Note that while in LSI, reduction is obtained by selecting only the highest k eigenvalues, in the other approaches, it is done by selecting the k most relevant topics.

4. NLP in the Biomedical Domain

4.1. *Characteristics of biomedical language*

According to Refs. [12] and [13], the biomedical domain has specific characteristics that, in some aspects, make the process more complicated (noted in the following list as "–") although, fortunately, there are also positive aspects (noted as "+"):

- Many genres exist with different wording: electronic health reports (EHR), discharge reports, radiological reports, medical articles, drug leaflets, medical fora (for expert and lay users), clinical trials, etc.
- Complex terminology, including extremely ambiguous acronyms.
+ Domain-specific lexical, terminological, and ontological resources, including large-sized corpora.
+ Tools and methods for exploiting the semantic information.

---

[j]https://www.nltk.org/howto/wordnet.html.
[k]See Ref. [1].

– The gap between non-expert users and target documents may be larger than in other restricted domains. For instance, the "Creutzfeldt–Jakob disease" also named "subacute spongiform encephalopathy" or "vCJD" is known at the lay level as the "mad cow disease".

4.2. *Resources available in the biomedical domain*

Table 1[1] presents some datasets (first three rows) and ontologies belonging to the medical domain. Most of the ontologies can be accessed through BioPortal.[m] Although most of these resources are for English language, some of them, such as Snomed-CT, ICD-10, and Orphanet, provide resources for other languages.

4.3. *Approaches for facing NLP tasks in the biomedical domain*

The tasks and the applications of NLP in the biomedical domain are basically the same as those in the other domains or in the domain-free settings,[16] including some specific tasks such as diagnosis support, outcome and risk prediction, patient phenotyping, among others. Various types of EHR have been used in addressing these tasks, such as lab measurements, clinical narratives, and medical images. Requirement constraints used to be more severe with respect to robustness, efficiency, reliability, and explainability.

With some limitations, so, the same generic approaches and tools can be used here. There are, however, two points where specific processes have to be done. The first is the preprocessing step, detailed in Section 4.4. The latter, detailed in Section 5.1, is the use of biomedical models, such as embeddings, when following *DL* approaches. As discussed in Section 4.1, the biomedical language presents characteristics that complicate the process. The tasks needing specific processors are the tokenizers and the NERCs (semantic taggers). Consider, for instance, the question $z =$ "Can I go home when I have

---

[1]Legends for size: w: words, p: pairs of sentences, d: documents, c: concepts.
[m]https://bioportal.bioontology.org/ provides access to 909 ontologies in the biomedical domain.

Table 1. Some relevant resources in the medical domain.

Resource	Ref.	Content	Size
Clinical-QE(2016)	Ref. [14]	QA	8,588 p
MedQuAD	Ref. [15]	QA	47,457 p
CORD-19	https://registry.opendata.aws/cord-19/	Various	200,000 d
FMA	http://si.washington.edu/projects/fma	Anatomy	174,329 c
Snomed-CT	https://www.snomed.org/	Various	665,940 c
Galen	https://www.opengalen.org/	Various	39,264 c
MeSH	https://www.ncbi.nlm.nih.gov/mesh/	Various	205,522 c
DrugBank	https://go.drugbank.com/	Drugs	15,867 w
Orphanet	https://www.orpha.net/	Rare diseases	2,206 w
DO	https://disease-ontology.org/	Diseases	21,273 w
ICD-10	https://www.cdc.gov/nchs/icd/icd10cm.htm	Diseases	142,000 w
RadLex	https://www.rsna.org/	Radiology	2,626 w
MIMIC-III	https://mimic.physionet.org/	EHR	40,000 d
UMLS	https://www.nlm.nih.gov/research/umls/	Various	1M c
Medline	https://www.nlm.nih.gov/bsd/medline.html	Links to journals	26M d
PubMed	https://pubmed.ncbi.nlm.nih.gov/	Medline citations	30M d
PMC	https://www.ncbi.nlm.nih.gov/pmc/	Medline full texts	6M d

COVID-19 and pneumonia?". Applying a conventional spacy processor for getting the entities occurring in z, we have the following:

```
import spacy; import en_core_web_lg
nlp = en_core_web_lg.load()
doc = nlp(z); doc.ents → ()
```

We obtain deceiving 0 entities. If we use, instead, the scientific domain-restricted scispacy,[n] four entities (only two correct) are recognized:

---

[n]Health and medicine have the highest representation in the scientific domain.

```
import scispacy; import en_core_sci_md
nlp = spacy.load("en_core_sci_md")
doc = nlp(z); doc.ents → (home, I, COVID-19, pneumonia)
```

If we use the NCBO accessor to Bioportal, using 'SNOMEDCT' and 'ICD10PCS' as source ontologies, we obtain three entities (only 2 correct):

ontologies = ['SNOMEDCT', 'ICD10PCS']; NCBO = BioPortal()
$NCBO.semantic\_tagging\_text(z)$ → 'home', 'pneumonia', 'covid-19'

It is clear from these examples that domain-specific processors result in an improvement of the results on these basic tasks.

4.4. *Linguistic preprocessing for NN models in the biomedical domain*

Although some NN models use raw text as input, linguistic preprocessing is sometimes needed. Fortunately, there are currently many publicly accessible toolkits that provide most of the processors needed, at least for English (although the multilingual offer is growing). The most popular within those following symbolic approaches are as follows: Natural Language Toolkit (NLTK),[o,71] Stanford CoreNLP,[p,17] OpenNLP,[q] LingPipe,[r] and Freeling.[s,72] Within those following empirical approaches, we can find the following: AllenNLP,[t,18] SpaCy,[u,19] Pythia,[v] PyTorch-NLP,[w] or Jack the Reader.[x] *Transformers* provides easy access to its models,

---

[o]https://www.nltk.org/.
[p]https://stanfordnlp.github.io/CoreNLP/.
[q]https://opennlp.apache.org/.
[r]http://alias-i.com/lingpipe/.
[s]http://nlp.lsi.upc.edu/freeling/node/1.
[t]https://www.linuxlinks.com/allennlp-apache-nlp-research-library/.
[u]https://spacy.io/.
[v]https://github.com/facebookresearch/pythia.
[w]https://github.com/PetrochukM/PyTorch-NLP.
[x]https://github.com/uclnlp/jack.

but there exist more comfortable and fast frameworks built upon it, such as FARM[y] (Framework for Adapting Representation Models).

Most of these resources are domain-free, although some of them have developed (Bio-)Medical-specific tools.

LingMed[z] is the biomedical domain version of LingPipe, basically designed for accessing Biomedical resources, such as MED-LINE, Entrez-Gene, and the Gene Ontology. Scispacy[aa] is a full spaCy pipeline for biomedical data. MedaCy[bb] is a text processing and learning framework built over spaCy to support medical NLP models. Pythia Predict[cc] focuses on the prediction of the interaction of medical devices. FreeLing-Med[dd] allows one to analyze clinical documents written in Spanish.

Besides these systems, derived from existing domain-free ones, there exist processors built specifically for the (Bio-)Medical domain. Some of them are MedLEE, BioMedLEE, cTAKES,[ee] HITEX,[ff] and Metamap.[gg] BioPortal offers a rest API[hh] with facilities for accessing its ontologies, such as the NCBO annotator that allows annotating a text with mentions of terms of one or more of the ontologies.

5. Neural Models for NLP: General Issues

Along the history of AI, neural systems appear and disappear intermittently. Periods of euphoria with exaggerated expectations are followed by periods of deception, lack of funding, and abandonment of this line of research. In 1956, Rosenblatt presented the Perceptron, the first neuronal model. The proposal aroused great expectations. The Perceptron managed to solve some theoretical or toy problems, but failed to scale up to real dimensions. In 1995, LeCun applied

---

[y]https://farm.deepset.ai/.
[z]http://www.alias-i.com/lingpipe-3.9.3/web/sandbox.html.
[aa]https://allenai.github.io/scispacy/.
[bb]https://github.com/NLPatVCU/medaCy.
[cc]http://ehealthanalytics.net/new-pythia-predict/.
[dd]http://ixa2.si.ehu.eus/prosamed/resources.html.
[ee]https://ctakes.apache.org/.
[ff]https://www.i2b2.org/software/projects/hitex/hitex_manual.html.
[gg]https://metamap.nlm.nih.gov/.
[hh]http://data.bioontology.org/documentation.

the "back-propagation" algorithm to carry out the learning of NN. Again, excellent results were obtained in tasks, such as the classification of handwritten figures. Scaling up to more complex cases in the state of hardware technology of the time proved impossible and the model was again abandoned. However, in 2005, "Deep Learning" was *launched*. The development of much more powerful processors (such as GPU and later TPU[ii]), the production of parallelizable and task-specific software for the implementation of the models led to spectacular results, first in image recognition and later in NLP. Can we consider that this time NN are here to stay?

The starting point in the application of NN to NLP was probably SENNA,[jj] a multi-task system created by Collobert and Weston.[20] SENNA annotates a text with POS tags, chunks, NE tags, semantic roles, semantically similar words and a language model. The entire network is trained jointly on all these tasks in a semi-supervised setting. The language models are learned from unannotated texts, while for the other tasks, the learning is supervised. SENNA was built using a simple two-layer CNN architecture without pooling and reaches state-of-the-art (SOTA) scores in all the tasks (97.29% in POS tagging, 94.32% in Chunking, 89.59% in NER, 75.49% in Semantic Role Labeling, 87.92% in Syntactic Parsing).

Most of the existing NN architectures have been applied to NLP. Especially important are Convolutional NN (CNN), Recurrent NN (RNN), Recursive NN (RecNN), Autoencoders, Attention-based NN, and the encoder–decoder NN, among others. Excellent surveys of the use of these models for NLP have been provided[3, 21] (see also Chapter 2).

CNN is probably the best method for extracting features from images, video and text data. The basic idea in a convolutional layer is to use a nonlinear convolution operation (filter) to sample on the layer for getting a feature map. NLP uses one-dimensional CNN (Conv-1), where the filter is implemented as a vector. Although the values of the filter are learned, sometimes a good initialization improves the learning process. Reference [22] has built a repository

---

[ii]https://iq.opengenus.org/cpu-vs-gpu-vs-tpu.
[jj]https://ronan.collobert.com/senna/.

of learned filters (Bank of Weight Filters for Deep CNNs) that could be used without the need of learning.

CNNs have been applied with success to many NLP tasks, such as the SENNA system, cited before. The first proposal was due to Yoon Kim,[23] who applied CNN to sentence classification. See Ref. [21] for some other interesting references.

RNNs introduce time on NN models and, as a result, are useful for processing sequential information. These models perform the same task over each instance of the sequence such that the output is dependent on the previous computations. RNNs are deep in both space and time in the sense that information flows either vertically (through the different layers) or horizontally (through the different time steps). This model is naturally suited for many NLP tasks showing a sequential structure of the language, where units are characters, words, or sentences as presented by Alex Graves in Ref. [24]. Simple RNN can be stacked for improving its representational power.

Contrary to CNNs that can be computed in parallel, RNNs must be computed sequentially. But contrary to the local features of CNNs, RNNs capture much of the previous units. As in the case of CNN, this model has been successfully applied to many NLP tasks at word and sentence levels. References [21] and [24] and provide interesting references of some of these applications.

The hidden state of the RNN accumulates information from other time steps and can thus be used for semantic matching between texts. A problem of these simple RNN nets (the vanishing gradient problem) is that the action of previous information decreases asymptotically with the distance. To face this important problem, variants of RNNs such as long short-term memories (LSTM) or gated recurrent units (GRU) have been introduced.

RNN and CNN represent a natural way to model sequences. However, language exhibits a natural recursive structure, which can be represented by a parsing tree. RecNNs use these tree structures as input. In fact, RecNNs can be seen as generalizations of RNN from sequences to binary trees. An important issue of RecNN is that a preprocessing step of the texts including parsing and binarization is mandatory. Parsing is costly and not error-free. Richard Socher[25–27] has proposed several RecNN models and applied them to several NLP tasks.

Autoencoders are a family of NN models, by themselves a subclass of the encoder–decoder model, that learn to transform the input into a compressed representation that generates a reconstruction of the input, minimizing reconstruction loss, i.e., the difference between the input and its reconstruction.

The encoder–decoder framework is a generalization of autoencoders when the input and output spaces are different, as in the case of sequence-to-sequence models, applied, for instance, to tasks such as MT (input and output are texts in different languages), AS (output is a reduced version of input), or human dialogs. For instance, in Ref. [28], in an MT task, an LSTM is used to encode the input sequence as a fixed-size vector, which is used as the initial state of another LSTM, used as decoder.

A problem existing in the encoder–decoder framework is that the encoder sometimes is forced to encode information which might not be relevant to the task at hand. In tasks such as AS and MT, certain alignment exists between the input and output texts. This is the base of the attention mechanism. This mechanism allows the decoder to refer back to the input sequence. During decoding, in addition to the last hidden state and generated token, the decoder is also conditioned on an attention (or context) vector calculated based on the input hidden state sequence.

Attention-based models have been applied to many NLP tasks. Some examples are as follows: Ref. [29], which introduced the Bi-Directional Attention Flow (BIDAF) network, a multi-stage hierarchical process that represents the context at different levels of granularity and uses a bi-directional attention flow mechanism; Ref. [8], which introduced a dynamic attention model applied to QA; and Ref. [30], which, in their attention-over-attention model, used a 2D similarity matrix between the query and context words.

Evolving from these attention-based models, Ref. [31] has recently proposed the transformers model, which is basic for the extraordinary development of DL for NLP. We will describe the transformers model in Section 6.1.

5.1. *Embeddings*

As shown in Section 2.1, words and other linguistic units can be represented as vectors in a vectorial space. Dense representations were obtained through dimensionality reduction techniques. The name "embedding" usually refers to these dense representations when produced by NN models. An embedding is simply a mapping of a linguistic unit (a word, a phrase, a sentence, an entity, a relation, a predicate with or without arguments, an RDF triple, an image, a node of a graph, etc.) into an element of a low-dimensional vectorial space. Within the scope of NLP, initial embedding models were first applied to words, basically for building accurate language models. Lexical embeddings can serve as useful representations for words for a variety of NLP tasks and are not difficult to learn, but learning embeddings for more complex units can be challenging. While separate embeddings are learned for each word, doing the same is unfeasible for every sentence.

Embeddings can be used directly for some NLP tasks involving operations on the embedding space (distances, similarities, projections, etc.), although in most cases embeddings are used as input layer in more complex models. In these cases, the embedding layer can be frozen or allow a retraining in the overall model. The simpler word embedding system consists in mapping a word token w into a vector of reals $\overrightarrow{x}$: $w \xrightarrow{\text{one\_hot}} \overrightarrow{w} \xrightarrow{\text{emb}} \overrightarrow{x}$ with $\overrightarrow{w} \in X^n$ and $\overrightarrow{x} \in X^d$, $d \ll n$ where n is the dimension of the input space and d that of the embedding space. Tomas Mikolov in his seminal paper[32] proposed two model architectures, CBOW and *Skip-Gram*, for computing embeddings of words from very large datasets. CBOW computes the conditional probability of a target word given the context while *skip-gram* does the opposite. Both models form the Word2Vec[kk] system, which has been, until the recent apparition of contextualized word representations (*CWR*), the most widely used word embeddings model. A popular software for using Word2Vec models or learning new models from specific corpora is Gensim.[ll] An alternative to Word2Vec is Glove,[mm,33] also widely used. In the biomedical domain, Sampo Pyysalo[34] has made public an embedding[nn] learned from Medline[oo] datasets.

[kk]https://code.google.com/archive/p/word2vec/.

[ll]https://rare-technologies.com/word2vec-tutorial/.

[mm]https://nlp.stanford.edu/projects/glove/.

[nn]http://bio.nlplab.org/.

[oo]https://medlineplus.gov/.

All these embeddings have been built for English language. A notable contribution to build embeddings in other languages (usually less resourced) is the Multilingual Unsupervised and Supervised Embeddings[pp] (MUSE)[35] using FastText,[qq] a library for learning word representations and sentence classification.[36] MUSE has produced embeddings in more than 100 languages and LASER[rr] in 93 languages. The Nordic Language Processing Laboratory maintains a repository of embeddings[ss] for numerous languages along with algorithms for their learning and use. All these embedding models belong to the class of static embeddings.

A serious limitation of traditional static word embeddings is the polisemy of words. In these models, a word has a unique vector representation regardless of its different senses, i.e., its context in the distributional semantics setting. Reference [37] creates *Sense2Vec* setting the problem as WSD. Going further, this limitation has been recently faced by the CWR. Replacing static embeddings by CWR has lead to significant improvements in many NLP tasks. CWR will be described in Section 6.2.

Embedding words is only the first step of the application of NN for obtaining dense vectorial representations of linguistic units. For subword units (characters, stems, character n-grams), the techniques are basically the same as explained above. For complex, units the techniques mimic those described in Section 3. A popular software for building these embeddings is *FastText* quoted above.

6. Deep Learning Models for NLP

The development of deep models for NLP has always gone one step behind those applied to image recognition. While AlexNet[38] success in the ImageNet Large Scale Visual Recognition Challenge in 2012, attributed to the depth of a conventional CNN model, is considered the kickoff of DL on image recognition, the year 2018, with the

---

[pp] https://github. com/facebookresearch/MUSE.
[qq] https://github.com/facebookresearch/fastText.
[rr] https://github.com/facebookresearch/LASER.
[ss] http://vectors.nlpl.eu/repository/.

apparition of deep CWR, was an inflection point in transfer learning for NLP models. Starting with the CWR and OpenAI's Transformers model,[31] many systems including Allen AI2's ELMo, Google's BERT, fast.ai's ULMFiT, OpenAI's GPT, GPT-2 and GPT-3, CMU, Google's XLNet and Microsoft's MT-DNN have emerged and compete for the supremacy in NLP tasks. A nice introduction to this topic can be found in Ref. [39].

CWR has been used in unsupervised approaches applying two layers biLSTM (ELMo), three layers AWD-LSTM[40] (ULMFIT) and, more recently, Transformers (BERT, GPT, GPT-2 and GPT-3). These systems are deep neural language models that are fine-tuned to create models for a wide range of downstream NLP tasks. ELMo and ULMFIT use sentences consisting of sequences of words as input, while BERT and GPT versions deal with sub-word units. While ELMo and ULMFIT are rather shallow NNs (two and three layers), the simplest configurations of BERT and GPT have 12 layers. ELMo uses two-layer biLSTM for training. In contrast, GPT-2 and BERT are transformer-based language models: the former uni-directional and the latter bi-directional (using Masked LM).

Each transformer layer of 12-layer BERT (base, cased) and 12-layer GPT-2 creates a contextualized representation of each token by attending to different parts of the input sentence. Reference [41] analyses how contextual are the CWRs produced by these models, i.e., are there infinitely many context-specific representations for each word? Or are words essentially assigned one of a finite number of senses? The conclusion is that the contextualized models do not simply assign one vector to each sense of each word, as, for instance, *Sense2Vec*, but to each context. Upper layers of contextualizing models produce more context-specific representations, much like how upper layers of LSTMs produce more task-specific representations.

A study in Ref. [42] analyses the factors that influence the performance of the models. These factors include the number of model parameters, the size of the dataset, and the amount of computer power used for training. The conclusion is that the performance depends strongly on scale and weakly on model shape. Performance has a power-law relationship with each of the three-scale factors. In brief, big models may be more important than big data.

6.1. *Transformers*

We present in this section the Transformers model and the Transformers library[tt] that implements the model in PyTorch and TensorFlow. The Transformers library provides thousands of pre-trained models to perform NLP tasks. Transformers is the first transduction model relying entirely on self-attention to compute representations of its input and output without using sequence-aligned RNNs or convolution. The model follows this overall architecture using stacked self-attention and pointwise, fully connected layers for both the encoder and the decoder.

The encoder is composed of a stack of $N = 6$ identical layers. Each layer has two sub-layers. The first is a multi-head self-attention mechanism and the second is a simple, positionwise fully connected FFN. All sub-layers in the model, as well as the embedding layers, produce outputs of dimension 512. The decoder is also composed of a stack of $N = 6$ identical layers. In addition to the two sub-layers in each encoder layer, it inserts a third sub-layer, which performs multi-head attention over the output of the encoder stack. Transformers use multi-head attention in the "encoder–decoder attention" layers, in the encoder layers and in the decoder layers.

Once the Transformer is pre-trained, we can start using it for downstream tasks. A number of input transformations to handle the inputs for different types of tasks is outlined in Ref. [43]. Basically, what is done is building a dummy sentence, including what is needed for the task, which is used as input to the transformer. The output of the transformer is usually sent to a final net for completing the task. In the case of classification, this net is reduced to a simple layer, such as a softmax classifier. For classification tasks, the transformations are straightforward:

$$< Start > < Text > < End > < Class >$$

For QA or LI, as two sentences are involved, the transformation is a bit more complex:

$$< Start > < Sentence\ 1 > < Delim > < Sentence\ 2 > < Result >$$

[tt]https://github.com/huggingface/transformers, included into the *huggingface* repository.

In the case of building a language model, we do not need an entire Transformer; the task can be performed with just the decoder of the Transformer.

6.2. *Models*

We present in this section the most widely used CWR models.

Universal Language Model FIne-Tuning (ULMFIT)[44] introduces a language model and a process to effectively fine-tune it for various tasks, achieving SOTA results. ULMFiT incorporates several fine-tuning techniques which are broadly applicable to other methods as well. The training process has three steps: LM pre-training, LM fine-tuning and task-specific fine-tuning. LM pre-training was done using 103M words from Wikipedia. As texts in the specific task/domain have a different distribution with respect to the Wikipedia corpus, an LM fine-tuning step is mandatory. This is accomplished in two steps: one depending on the domain and the other on the task. The LM fine-tuning involves the use of discriminative fine-tuning and slanted triangular learning rates (a learning rate schedule that first linearly increases the learning rate and then linearly makes it decay). The task-specific fine-tuning uses a gradual unfreezing mechanism for preventing overfit.

Embeddings from Language Models (ELMo)[73] creates word embeddings by a task-specific combination (a linear function) of the internal states of a two-layer biLSTM. The training dataset was the 1B WordBenchmark.[uu]

Generative Pretraining Transformer (GPT)[43] has a sequence-to-sequence encoder–decoder architecture and has been implemented using the Transformers framework described above. GPT uses only a 12-layer decoder of the Transformer NN with 117M parameters. Note that while BERT uses only the encoder part of the Transformers, GPT uses the decoder part. Each layer contains 12 independent self-attention heads, totalling 144 distinct attention patterns, each one likely corresponding to a linguistic property captured by the model. As other CWR models, GPT uses a two-stage training procedure, following a semi-supervised setting. First, in an unsupervised mode, an initial generic LM is learned from a huge dataset. The goal is to learn a universal representation that transfers with little adaptation

---

[uu]https://opensource.google/projects/lm-benchmark.

to a wide range of specific tasks. So, the universal LM is fine-tuned to a target domain/task using the corresponding supervised objectives, a small set manually annotated. Pre-training has been carried out using as input dataset the Toronto Book Corpus,[vv] containing 11,308 books totalling about 1B words.

Generative Pretraining Transformer-2 (GPT-2)[45] is just a larger version of its predecessor with a light scaling up of the model size, dataset size and diversity, and length of training, using 1.5B parameters. GPT-2 has been trained on a dataset of 8M web pages, called "WebText". The work in Ref. [45] focuses on fine-tuning, i.e., updating the weights of a pre-trained generic model by training on thousands of supervised labels specific to the desired task. Fine-tuning improves performance on many benchmarks at a cost of annotating huge datasets for every task. GPT-2 is only partially open source. The training dataset is proprietary and not published, the pre-trained models are, however, freely available.

Generative Pre-training Transformer-3 (GPT-3)[46] scales up heavily from GPT-2 (from 1.5B to 175B parameters) maintaining a similar architecture. Training GPT-3 models for a specific task involves two steps: pre-training and fine-tuning. It is possible, however, to use only the first step in what is named a task-agnostic setting. This setting is useful because fine-tuning to a given task is costly due to the supervision of big datasets. In the task-agnostic setting, three learning scenarios are devised: Few-shot (FS), One-shot (1S) and Zero-shot (0S). In FS, the model is given a few (from 10 to 100) K demonstrations of the task (examples of context and completion) at inference time. The model has a extremely light supervision. For 1S, $K = 1$, and for 0S, $K = 0$ and only a natural language description of the task is provided instead of any examples.

Broadly, on NLP tasks, GPT-3 achieves promising results in the 0S and 1S settings and in the FS setting is sometimes competitive with the SOTA. For example, GPT-3 achieves 81.5 F1 on CoQA in the 0S setting, 84.0 F1 on CoQA in the 1S setting, 85.0 F1 in the FS setting and 90.7 of SOTA. Similarly, GPT-3 achieves 64.3% accuracy on TriviaQA in the 0S setting, 68.0% in the 1S setting, 71.2% in the FS setting and 68.0 of SOTA.

[vv] https://huggingface.co/datasets/bookcorpus.

Bidirectional Encoder Representations from Transformers (BERT)[47] is without doubt the most popular CWR and probably the overall best one. BERT consists of L stacked Transformer layers to encode each sentence. Although the standard Transformer is unidirectional (causal), BERT reaches some bidirectional representations of the words by using a Masked Language Model (MLM) and a Next Sentence Prediction in the pre-training step. The model was pre-trained on 2,500M internet words and 800M words of Toronto Book Corpus, totalling 16 GB.

In MLM, about 15% of the input tokens are masked (80% of the time with [MASK] tokens, 10% with random tokens, and 10% with the unchanged input tokens) at random and the model tries to predict these masked tokens and not the entire input sequence.

BERT provides four versions: the base and the larger models cased or uncased with different variants. Let H be the hidden size, A the number of attention heads, and P the number of hyperparameters. The figures of both models are the following:

- BERT-Base, Uncased: $L = 12$, $H = 768$, $A = 12$, $P = 110M$.
- BERT Large, Uncased: $L = 24$, $H = 1024$, $A = 16$, $P = 340M$.
- BERT-Base, Cased: $L = 12$, $H = 768$, $A = 12$, $P = 110M$.
- BERT Large, Cased: $L = 24$, $H = 1024$, $A = 16$, $P = 340M$.
- BERT-Base, Multilingual Cased: $L = 12$, $H = 768$, $A = 12$, $P = 110M$.

The pre-trained model can then be fine-tuned to NLP tasks, resulting in substantial accuracy improvements. The authors claim that fine-tuning the pre-trained model on a new task can be done in at most 1 hour on a single Cloud TPU or a few hours on a GPU. Some of the models are integrated in HuggingFace's Python library Transformers.

For evaluating NLP systems, the most frequently used benchmarks are *GLUE*[ww][48] and its improved version SuperGLUE. A study in Ref. 49 performed an evaluation of most of the CWRs presented so far. This evaluation covers eight NLP tasks. GLUE also provides a global GLUE score and SOTA scores for each task. BERT outperforms SOTA in all the tasks and globally (80.5 vs. 74 of SOTA), ELMo fails in all the tasks but one and globally (71 vs. 74) and GPT

[ww] https://gluebenchmark.com/.

obtains results in the middle range, although the global score is positive (75.1 vs. 74). It is worth noting that this evaluation does not include GPT-2 and GPT-3 that improve the figures of GPT and, in some cases, those of BERT.

Based on BERT and on its pre-trained models, many projects and models have emerged in what has been named Bertology. Some popular models are as follows:

- ALBERT (A Lite BERT for Self-supervised Learning of Language Representations) is similar to BERT with a few changes, the most significant being replacing the next sentence prediction by a sentence ordering prediction.
- RoBERTa (Robustly Optimized BERT Pre-training Approach) is a larger model, with 160GB of text for training (144GB additional data over BERT) and use of dynamic masking, i.e., tokens are masked differently at each epoch; Next sentence prediction is used. It results in an improvement of 2–20% on the performance.
- ERNIE (Enhanced Representation through Knowledge Integration) learns language representation enhanced by knowledge-masking strategies, which include entity-level and phrase-level masking. Knowledge information is provided by knowledge graphs.
- DistilBERT is — smaller (half-size) than BERT using model distillation (approximation). It improves on the inference speed at a cost of 3% of loss in performance.
- BART is a sequence-to-sequence model with an encoder and a decoder. The pre-training process follows the BERT strategy with some transformations on the tokens for input on the encoder. These transformations include mask or delete random tokens, mask a span of k tokens with a single mask token, permute sentences, start at a specific token. For the decoder, BART proceeds left-to-right (like GPT). BART is particularly effective when fine-tuned for text generation, QA, and AS.
- XLM is a cross-lingual model. It applies two methods to learn language models: one unsupervised relying on monolingual data and one supervised that leverages parallel data. XLM obtains SOTA results on cross-lingual classification and MT.
- XLNet is an extension of the Transformer-XLM model, pre-trained to learn bidirectional contexts by considering all permutations of the input sequence. XLNet outperforms BERT on several NLP tasks.

- Sentence Transformer[50] is a library that provides sentence embeddings based on transformer networks. The models are tuned such that sentences with similar meanings are close in vector space.

Many other models have been defined, such as CamemBERT, BARThez, FlauBERT, and others. See the "supported models" list in https://huggingface.co/models[xx] leaving the biomedical variants to Section 6.3.

As previously said, BERT is by far the most popular CWR, but GPT-3 achieves the best results in many NLP tasks, so a comparison of both models could be useful:

- GPT-3 is 470 times bigger in size than BERT-Large. The cost of training increases exponentially. Simply loading the model would use 300GB of VRAM.
- BERT is fully open source, while GPT-3 only partially fits this category.
- BERT only uses the encoder of transformers, while GPT-3 uses both the encoder and the decoder.
- BERT fine-tuning process is more complex and costly.
- Contrary to GPT-3, BERT has models for various languages: both monolingual and multilingual models.
- Many of the BERT models are available from the Transformers library.
- A frequent criticism against GPT-3 is that it has been trained on low-quality internet data.
- GPT-3 can be tuned by providing instructions in plain English, whereas BERT requires task-specific data.
- GPT-3 performs better on language modeling tasks (such as MT or AS) and less well on reasoning tasks (QA, LI, paraphrase).

6.3. *Deep learning models for NLP in the biomedical domain*

Models trained on the general domain do not perform well when applied to domain-specific texts. This is specially true in highly

---

[xx]It is amazing to note the capability of bertologists in locating terms containing the infix "BERT" to become meaningful acronyms of their models.

specialized domains like biomedicine, which present a word distribution drastically different from the general domain. This is why many domain-specific models have been developed, most by fine-tuning general domain pre-trained models. The Transformers library is an excellent source of such models. From BERT, the most popular biomedical variants are SciBERT, BioBERT, ClinicalBERT, Bio_ClinicalBERT, BlueBERT and PubMedBERT. We next briefly describe these models, leaving the reader to seek further details from Ref. 51.

- SciBERT[52] is a model pre-trained on BERT datasets and fine-tuned on the full text of 1.14M biomedical (82%) and computer science (18%) papers from the Semantic Scholar corpus.[yy]
- BioBERT[53] is pre-trained with BERT training datasets complemented with PubMed abstracts (4.5B words) and PMC full text articles (13.5B words). BioBERT performs well on biomedical NERC, relation extraction, and QA tasks, obtaining 0.51–9.61% improvements.
- ClinicalBERT[54] is a BERT variant for clinical notes. It has been fine-tuned with 2M clinical notes in the MIMIC-III database. MIMIC-III is a publicly available EHR database comprising deidentified health data associated with 40,000 critical care patients. The database contains clinical notes, laboratory test results, diagnoses, procedures, and medications. Two variants have been built by using on top of BERT and BioBERT models either all the data in MIMIC-III or just the discharge summaries. ClinicalBERT models outperform others in clinical NLP.
- Bio_ClinicalBERT[54] is similar to ClinicalBERT, but using not BERT but BioBERT as pre-trained model. Depending on the data used from MIMIC-III, two models can be built: Bio+clinical BERT and Bio+Discharge Summary BERT. In Ref. [54], these models are evaluated on tasks included in the i2/b2 benchmark.[zz] BioBERT is the winner in the deidentification task, Bio_ClinicalBERT in temporal relation extraction, and Bio+Discharge Summary BERT in clinical relation extraction.

[yy] https://allenai.org/data/s2orc.
[zz] https://portal.dbmi.hms.harvard.edu/projects/n2c2-nlp/.

- PubMedBERT is pre-trained on biomedical texts from scratch. The pre-training corpus comprises 14M PubMed abstracts with 3B words (21GB). An enriched version is learned by adding full text articles from PMC, with the pre-training corpus increased substantially to 16.8B words (107GB). PubMedBERT outperforms all prior language models across biomedical NLP applications.

The Biomedical Language Understanding and Reasoning Benchmark (BLURB[aaa]) is an evaluation benchmark, similar to GLUE but adapted to PubMed-based biomedical NLP applications. BLURB consists of 13 datasets in six diverse tasks. All these variants have been evaluated in Ref. [55]. There is no variant offering the best performance for all tasks. Using the BLURB score as measure and the BERT results as baseline, the relative improvements in percentage are as follows: RoBERTa: 0.45%, ClinicalBERT: 1.58%, SciBERT (Uncased): 3.7%, BioBERT: 5.66%, and PubMedBERT: 6.72%.

6.4. *Some examples of application of deep learning models in the biomedical domain*

We present in this section several examples of application of DL techniques on NLP tasks.

Open information extraction: Reference [56] performs some experiments of domain adaptation between the news and the biomedical domains. For the news domain, 1,959 sentences from WikiNews are used. For the biomedical domain, the DDI corpus, built from 792 DrugBank definitions and 233 Medline abstracts (used in the DDI Extraction 2013 task[bbb]), is used. Reference [57] addressed the recognition of drugs and extraction of drug–drug interactions; the best scored system (FBK IRST) in this challenge obtained an F1 value of 0.651 in the NERC task. We will consider this score as our baseline. Three transfer approaches were compared in Ref. [56]: (i) transductive, i.e., transferring knowledge learnt from the news domain to the biomedical domain, (ii) inductive, i.e., a small amount of biomedical data from DDI is fed to the NN, and (iii) traditional,

---

[aaa]https://microsoft.github.io/BLURB/.
[bbb]https://www.cs.york.ac.uk/semeval-2013/task9.html.

i.e., both training and testing on biomedical data. Four embeddings were compared: Glove, BERT, XLNet, and XLM-RoBERTa. For the Traditional transfer approach all the embeddings outperformed the baseline with F1 from Glove: 0.71 to BERT and XLM-RoBERTa: 0.79. Also, in the inductive setting, the embeddings outperformed the baseline with F1 from Glove: 0.74 to XLM-RoBERTa: 0.78. Only in the transductive setting, the baseline was the winner with small margin over XLM-RoBERTa: 0.64.

Machine comprehension: Reference [58] has released BioMRC, a dataset for Biomedical Machine Reading Comprehension. The dataset is provided in three versions: large (812,707 instances), lite (100,000 instances), and tiny (60 instances, answered by humans). The authors also introduce a new BERT-based MRC model.

Summarization: Reference [59] has released PreSum,[ccc] which consists of a BERT-based general framework for both extractive and abstractive models. Based on this model, Ref. [60] released MatchSum.[ddd] The authors formulate the AS task as a semantic text matching problem, in which a source document and candidate summaries extracted from the original text will be matched in a semantic space.

Drug mention detection in tweets: Reference [61] applies transfer learning for the automatic classification of tweets mentioning a drug. The problem is set as a binary classification and experiment on using BERT, BioBERT, ClinicalBERT, SciBERT, BioMed-RoBERTa, ELECTRA, and ERNIE. BioMed-RoBERTa achieves the highest F1 score.

Building embeddings of medical units: Several efforts have been made to build static representations of medical entities. Reference [62] proposed the *med2vec*[eee] system that learns embeddings for medical NE from a big set of EHR (1,381,549 patients, 6.3 visits/patient)

[ccc] https://github.com/nlpyang/PreSumm.
[ddd] https://github.com/maszhongming/MatchSum.
[eee] thttps://github.com/mp2893/med2vec.

taking profit of the sequential structure of visits of each patient over time, where each visit includes multiple medical concepts, such as diagnosis, procedure, and medication (often with codes) in the EHR dataset. Reference [63] proposed the *cui2vec*[fff] system that identifies CUI (Concept Unique Identifier of UMLS metathesaurus) codes in medical documents. The system works by first mapping all medical terms occurring in the documents into their corresponding CUI. Next, a CUI–CUI co-occurrence matrix is constructed. The matrix can be directly factored by GloVe to create the embeddings. The input data include a database of claims from health insurance plans, full-text journal articles from PMC, and a dataset of concept co-occurrences in clinical notes.

ICD Coding of EHR: Coding occurrences of medical entities in EHR is a difficult task, as justified in Section 4.1. In the case of diseases, the problem is even more challenging due to the high polysemy of terms, the frequent use of acronyms and abbreviations, the different profiles of the authors of clinical notes, the use of idiosyncratic jargon, etc. The habitual coding is ICD (International Classification of Diseases). The most frequently used version is the 10th, i.e. ICD-10, although some resources are codified with ICD-9, and ICD-11 is increasingly used. A problem is that the mapping between versions is far from easy. ICD-10 codes are presented in two code sets: ICD-10-CM for diseases[ggg] and ICD-10-PCS[hhh] for procedures.

Annotating EHR with ICD-10 codes has attracted the attention of many researchers; A comparison of DL approaches to the task can be found in Ref. [64]. Reference [65] presents the participation of FHDO Biomedical Computer Science Group (BCSG) in the CLEF eHealth 2020 Task 1, Subtask 1 on Multilingual Information Extraction, which focuses on ICD-10 coding for clinical texts in Spanish. The problem is challenging and the approach shows several interesting novelties: Due to the scarcity of the training material, additional data from MIMIC-III is used, but this material is coded in ICD-9

[fff] https://github.com/beamandrew/cui2vec.
[ggg] https://www.cdc.gov/nchs/icd/icd10cm.htm.
[hhh] https://www.icd10data.com/ICD10PCS/Codes.

and the clinical notes are in English, so translation and mapping between ICD versions were needed. BioBERT, ClinicalBERT, and XLNet were tried. An ensemble of BioBERT and XLNet achieved the best results.

Predicting clinical events from EHR: Predicting clinical events, sometimes tied to time constraints, such as suicide, death, aggravation or recovery from an illness, among others, from EHR is an important task both from economic and health points of view. Reference [66] has applied ClinicalBERT for modeling clinical notes and predicting hospital readmission. They use the clinical notes from MIMIC-III associated with the admissions (2,083,180 deidentified notes) for training and compare the performance of a biLSTM model, BERT and ClinicalBERT for the task. As patients are often associated with many notes, and having ClinicalBERT a fixed length of input sequence (512), the sequence of temporally sorted notes is split to this maximum length. On each sub-sequence, the probability of readmission is computed independently. The overall probability of readmission is computed by a weighted combination of the partial probabilities. ClinicalBERT achieves the best results, surprisingly followed by biLSTM.

COVID-19 related applications: Related to COVID-19, many efforts have been put on facing different aspects of the pandemic. Reference [67] released COVID-Twitter-BERT (CT-BERT), a transformer-based model, pre-trained on a large corpus of tweets on the topic of COVID-19. First, a corpus of 97M tweets about COVID-19 was collected. After cleaning and preprocessing, 22.5M tweets (containing 40.7M sentences and 633M tokens) were selected for training. CT-BERT has been applied to five datasets including a subset of its training material, SST-2, an open dataset from SemEval-2016 Task 4, and two datasets related to vaccines. As a baseline, BERT-large was used. CT-BERT outperforms BERT-large in all the datasets from 9% to 26%. Manuel Tonneau has released[iii] two BERT versions pre-trained on a preprocessed version of the

---

[iii]Unpublished.

CORD-19 dataset, see Table 1, namely, ClinicalCovidBERT and Bio-CovidBERT. Reference 68 has built and released COVID-QA,[jjj] a QA dataset consisting of 2,019 question/answer pairs extracted from scientific articles related to COVID-19. Trained on COVID-QA, deepset has built a QA model.[kkk]

Sentence transformers applications: The SentenceTransformers library[lll50] includes the code of NLP applications built using the library.

7. Conclusions

In this chapter, we have presented the application of DL techniques to NLP in the context of the biomedical domain. A *zooming* approach in two dimensions has been followed. In the *methodological dimension*, we have first presented the topic of NLP, linguistics, tasks, applications, approaches, etc. Next, we have focused on empirical methods, then on NN methods, and finally on DL. In the *topic dimension*, we have followed the general-to-biomedical domain route.

Where are we now? We have shown that DL is currently the most accurate paradigm for facing many NLP tasks (many but not all). We count with domain-specific linguistic processors and also domain-specific resources, including datasets, ontologies, terminologies, and embeddings. Furthermore, we count with solid techniques for addressing most NLP tasks, as shown in Section 6.4.

What could be the future of this field? Have we arrived at the end of the road? Is it our task now to just add new items to the huge list of BERT followers? Or, perhaps, we just have to wait for the delivery of GPT-4, or GFPT-10, or GPT-∞? Should we forget the grammars, the grammatical rules, the logical forms, the symbolic approaches, the non-neural empirical approaches?

We first need to note that the CWR are good in many NLP tasks, but not in all the tasks. If we consider the BLURB benchmark, the two best scored models, BioBERT and PubMedBERT, surpass the

---

[jjj]https://github.com/deepset-ai/COVID-QA.
[kkk]deepset/roberta-base-squad2-covid.
[lll]https://github.com/UKPLab/sentence-transformers.

score of 80.0 in 9 (69%) and 10 (77%) out of 13 tasks. So, there is still space for improvement.

Recently, there has been some debate about what is really captured by the Contextual Word Representation or by the static embeddings: just the context? the syntax? the meaning? Are the word embeddings capturing the commonsense knowledge? Reference [69] points out that *DL* models perform poorly on tasks that require commonsense reasoning. They propose the Commonsense Auto-Generated Explanation (CAGE) framework for facing this problem. Reference [70] argues that a system trained only on word forms has no way to learn meaning *a priori*. We can extend their argument to commonsense that in most cases does not occur explicitly into the texts; can a model capture what does not occur in the training text? Without including commonsense knowledge into the models, I think that the upper limit of accuracy in tasks needing meaning representation and management would not be surpassed. Where could such commonsense knowledge be found? In the Wikipedia? In the Linked Open Data Cloud? In children's textbooks? How could this knowledge be integrated into the models? I reckon this is the key point to address in the near future.

References

1. R. Mitkov, *The Oxford Handbook of Computational Linguistics 2nd edn.* Oxford University Press (2014).
2. D. Jurafsky and J. H. Martin, *Speech and Language Processing: An Introduction to Natural Language Processing, Computational Linguistics, and Speech Recognition 3rd edn.* Prentice Hall (2017).
3. Y. Goldberg, *Neural Network Methods in Natural Language Processing, Synthesis Lectures on Human Language Technologies.* Morgan and Claypool Publishers (2017).
4. U. Kamath, J. Liu, and J. Whitaker, *Deep Learning for NLP and Speech Recognition.* Springer (2019).
5. C. Manning and H. Schütze, *Foundations of Statistical Natural Language Processing.* MIT Press (1999).
6. H. Lane, H. Hapke, and C. Howard, *Natural Language Processing in Action: Understanding, Analyzing, and Generating Text with Python 1st edn.* Manning Publications (2019).

7. P. Baudiš and J. Šedivý. Modeling of the question answering task in the yodaqa system. In *Experimental IR Meets Multilinguality, Multimodality, and Interaction,* (eds.) J. Mothe, J. Savoy, J. Kamps, K. Pinel-Sauvagnat, G. Jones, E. San Juan, L. Capellato, and N. Ferro, pp. 222–228, Springer International Publishing (2015).

8. K. M. Hermann, T. Kociský, E. Grefenstette, L. Espeholt, W. Kay, M. Suleyman, and P. Blunsom, Teaching machines to read and comprehend, *Advances in Neural Information Processing Systems 28 (NIPS 2015)* (2015).

9. A. Bellet, A. Habrard, and M. Sebban, *Metric Learning.* Morgan & Claypool Publishers (2015).

10. W. de Vazelhes, C. Carey, Y. Tang, N. Vauquier, and A. Bellet, metric-learn: Metric Learning Algorithms in Python, *J. Mach. Learn. Res.* **21** (138), 1–6 (2020).

11. A. Olivares, I. Stankovic, H. González, and H. Rodriguez. Measuring distances between medical entities. step 1: Drugbank. In *Proceedings of the International Conference of the Catalan Association for Artificial Intelligence,* pp. 106–115 (2018).

12. S. J. Athenikos and H. Han, Biomedical question answering: A survey, *Comput. Methods Programs Biomed.* **99**(1), 1–24 (2010).

13. P. Zweigenbaum. Knowledge and reasoning for medical question-answering. In *Proceedings of the 2009 Workshop on Knowledge and Reasoning for Answering Questions,* KRAQ '09, pp. 1–2 (2009).

14. A. Ben Abacha and D. Demner-Fushman. Recognizing question entailment for medical question answering. In *AMIA 2016, American Medical Informatics Association Annual Symposium, Chicago, IL, USA, November 12-16, 2016* (2016).

15. A. Ben Abacha and D. Demner-Fushman, A question-entailment approach to question answering, *arXiv e-prints* (2019).

16. S. K. P. and R. M. Smart healthcare analytics solutions using deep learning ai. In *Proceedings of International Conference on Recent Trends in Machine Learning, IoT, Smart Cities and Applications. Advances in Intelligent Systems and Computing,* (eds.) Gunjan V.K. and Zurada J.M. Vol 1245, Springer, Singapore (2021).

17. C. D. Manning, M. Surdeanu, J. Bauer, J. Finkel, S. J. Bethard, and D. McClosky. The Stanford CoreNLP natural language processing toolkit. In *Association for Computational Linguistics (ACL) System Demonstrations,* pp. 55–60 (2014).

18. M. Gardner, J. Grus, M. Neumann, O. Tafjord, P. Dasigi, N. Liu, M. Peters, M. Schmitz, and L. Zettlemoyer, Allennlp: A deep semantic natural language processing platform, *arXiv e-prints* (2018).

19. M. Honnibal and I. Montani, spacy 2: Natural language understanding with bloom embeddings, convolutional neural networks and incremental parsing, *Explosion* (2017).
20. R. Collobert, J. Weston, L. Bottou, M. Karlen, K. Kavukcuoglu, and P. Kuksa, Natural language processing (almost) from scratch, *J. Mach. Learn. Res.* **12**, 2493—2537 (2011).
21. T. Young, D. Hazarika, S. Poria, and E. Cambria, Recent trends in deep learning based natural language processing [review article], *IEEE Comput. Intell. Mag.* **13**, 55–75 (2018).
22. S. K. Kumaraswamy, P. Sastry, and K. Ramakrishnan. Bank of weight filters for deep cnns. In eds. R. J. Durrant and K.-E. Kim, *Proceedings of The 8th Asian Conference on Machine Learning*, Vol. 63, *Proceedings of Machine Learning Research*, pp. 334–349, PMLR, The University of Waikato, Hamilton, New Zealand (2016).
23. Y. Kim. Convolutional neural networks for sentence classification. In *Proceedings of EMNLP 2014*, pp. 1746–1751, Doha, Qatar.
24. A. Graves, Generating sequences with recurrent neural networks, *arXiv e-prints* (2013).
25. R. Socher, A. Perelygin, J. Wu, J. Chuang, C. D. Manning, A. Ng, and C. Potts. Recursive deep models for semantic compositionality over a sentiment treebank. In *Proceedings of EMNLP 2013*, pp. 1631–1642, Seattle, Washington, USA.
26. R. Socher, C. C. Lin, A. Y. Ng, and C. D. Manning. Parsing natural scenes and natural language with recursive neural networks. In eds. L. Getoor and T. Scheffer, *Proceedings of the 28th International Conference on Machine Learning, ICML 2011, Bellevue, Washington, USA*, pp. 129–136 (2011).
27. R. Socher, B. Huval, C. D. Manning, and A. Y. Ng. Semantic compositionality through recursive matrix-vector spaces. In eds. J. Tsujii, J. Henderson, and M. Pasca, *Proceedings of EMNLP-CoNLL 2012*, Jeju Island, Korea, pp. 1201–1211.
28. I. Sutskever, O. Vinyals, and Q. V. Le. Sequence to sequence learning with neural networks. In eds. Z. Ghahramani, M. Welling, C. Cortes, N. Lawrence, and K. Q. Weinberger, *Advances in Neural Information Processing Systems*, Vol. 27, pp. 3104–3112, Curran Associates (2014).
29. M. Seo, A. Kembhavi, A. Farhadi, and H. Hajishirzi. Bidirectional attention flow for machine comprehension. In *Proceedings of the International Conference on Learning Representations (ICLR 2017)*, Toulon, France (2017).
30. Y. Cui, Z. Chen, S. Wei, S. Wang, T. Liu, and G. Hu. Attention-over-attention neural networks for reading comprehension. In *Proceedings of the 55th Annual Meeting of the ACL (Volume 1: Long Papers)*, pp. 593–602, Vancouver, Canada (2017).

31. A. Vaswani, N. Shazeer, N. Parmar, J. Uszkoreit, L. Jones, A. N. Gomez, u. Kaiser, and I. Polosukhin. Attention is all you need. In *Proceedings of the 31st International Conference on Neural Information Processing Systems*, NIPS '17, pp. 6000–6010, Curran Associates (2017).

32. T. Mikolov, K. Chen, G. Corrado, and J. Dean. Efficient estimation of word representations in vector space. In *Proceedings of the International Conference on Learning Representations (ICLR 2013)* (2013).

33. J. Pennington, R. Socher, and C. Manning. GloVe: Global vectors for word representation. In *Proceedings of EMNLP 2014*, pp. 1532–1543, Doha, Qatar.

34. S. Pyysalo, F. Ginter, H. Moen, T. Salakoski, and S. Ananiadou, Distributional semantics resources for biomedical text processing, *Proceedings of Languages in Biology and Medicine* (2013).

35. G. Lample, A. Conneau, M. Ranzato, L. Denoyer, and H. Jégou. Word translation without parallel data. In *International Conference on Learning Representations* (2018).

36. P. Bojanowski, E. Grave, A. Joulin, and T. Mikolov, Enriching word vectors with subword information, *Trans. Assoc. Comput. Linguist.* **5**, 135–146 (2017).

37. A. Trask, P. Michalak, and J. Liu. In *sense2vec - A Fast and Accurate Method for Word Sense Disambiguation in Neural Word Embeddings*, arXiv (2015).

38. A. Krizhevsky, I. Sutskever, and G. E. Hinton, Imagenet classification with deep convolutional neural networks, *Commun. ACM* **60**(6), 84–90 (2017).

39. W. Weng and P. Szolovits, Representation learning for electronic health records, *CoRR.* **abs/1909.09248** (2019).

40. S. Merity, N. S. Keskar, and R. Socher. Regularizing and optimizing LSTM language models. In *ICLR* (2018).

41. K. Ethayarajh. How contextual are contextualized word representations? comparing the geometry of BERT, ELMo, and GPT-2 embeddings. In *Proceedings of EMNLP-IJCNLP 2019*, pp. 55–65, Hong Kong, China.

42. J. Kaplan, S. McCandlish, T. Henighan, T. Brown, B. Chess, R. Child, S. Gray, A. Radford, J. Wu, and D. Amodei, Scaling laws for neural language models, *ArXiv* (2020).

43. A. Radford, K. Narasimhan, T. Salimans, and I. Sutskever. Improving language under-standing with unsupervised learning. In *Technical Report, OpenAI* (2018).

44. J. Howard and S. Ruder. Universal language model fine-tuning for text classification. In *Proceedings of the 56th Annual Meeting of the ACL (Volume 1: Long Papers)*, pp. 328–339, Melbourne, Australia (2018).

45. A. Radford, J. Wu, R. Child, D. Luan, D. Amodei, and I. Sutskever. Language models are unsupervised multitask learners. In *Technical Report, OpenAI* (2019).
46. T. Brown, B. Mann, N. Ryder, M. Subbiah, J. Kaplan, P. Dhariwal, A. Neelakantan, P. Shyam, G. Sastry, A. Askell, S. Agarwal, A. Herbert-Voss, G. Krueger, T. Henighan, R. Child, A. Ramesh, D. Ziegler, J. Wu, C. Winter, and D. Amodei. Language models are few-shot learners. In *Proceedings of Advances in Neural Information Processing Systems 33, (NeurIPS 2020)* (2020).
47. J. Devlin, M.-W. Chang, K. Lee, and K. Toutanova. BERT: Pre-training of deep bidirectional transformers for language understanding. In *Proceedings of the 2019 Conference of the North American Chapter of the ACL: Human Language Technologies, Volume 1 (Long and Short Papers)*, pp. 4171–4186, Minneapolis, Minnesota (2019).
48. A. Wang, A. Singh, J. Michael, F. Hill, O. Levy, and S. Bowman. GLUE: A multi-task benchmark and analysis platform for natural language understanding. In *Proceedings of the 2018 EMNLP Workshop BlackboxNLP: Analyzing and Interpreting Neural Networks for NLP*, pp. 353–355, Brussels, Belgium (2018).
49. X. Liu, P. He, W. Chen, and J. Gao. Multi-task deep neural networks for natural language understanding. In *Proceedings of the 57th Annual Meeting of the ACL*, pp. 4487–4496, Florence, Italy (2019).
50. N. Reimers and I. Gurevych. Sentence-bert: Sentence embeddings using siamese bert-networks. In *Proceedings of EMNLP 2019*.
51. F. K. Khattak, S. Jeblee, C. Pou-Prom, M. Abdalla, C. Meaney, and F. Rudzicz, A survey of word embeddings for clinical text, *J. Biomed. Informat.* **4** (2019).
52. I. Beltagy, K. Lo, and A. Cohan. SciBERT: A pretrained language model for scientific text. In *Proceedings of EMNLP-IJCNLP 2019*, pp. 3615–3620, Hong Kong, China.
53. J. Lee, W. Yoon, S. Kim, D. Kim, S. Kim, C. H. So, and J. Kang, BioBERT: A pre-trained biomedical language representation model for biomedical text mining, *Bioinformatics* (2019).
54. E. Alsentzer, J. Murphy, W. Boag, W.-H. Weng, D. Jin, T. Naumann, and M. McDermott. Publicly available clinical BERT embeddings. In *Proceedings of the 2nd Clinical Natural Language Processing Workshop*, pp. 72–78, Minneapolis, Minnesota, USA (2019).
55. Y. Gu, R. Tinn, H. Cheng, M. Lucas, N. Usuyama, X. Liu, T. Naumann, J. Gao, and H. Poon, Domain-specific language model pretraining for biomedical natural language processing, *arXiv e-prints* (2020).
56. I. Sarhan and M. Spruit, Can we survive without labelled data in nlp? transfer learning for open information extraction, *Appl. Sci.* **10**(17) (2020).

57. I. Segura-Bedmar, P. Martínez, and M. Herrero-Zazo, Lessons learnt from the ddi-extraction-2013 shared task, *J. Biomed. Informat.* **51**, 152–164 (2014).

58. D. Pappas, P. Stavropoulos, I. Androutsopoulos, and R. McDonald. BioMRC: A dataset for biomedical machine reading comprehension. In *Proceedings of the 19th SIGBioMed Workshop on Biomedical Language Processing*, pp. 140–149, Online (2020).

59. Y. Liu and M. Lapata. Text summarization with pretrained encoders. In *Proceedings of EMNLP-IJCNLP 2019*, pp. 3730–3740, Hong Kong, China.

60. M. Zhong, P. Liu, Y. Chen, D. Wang, X. Qiu, and X. Huang. Extractive summarization as text matching. In *Proceedings of the 58th Annual Meeting of the ACL* (2020).

61. M. L. and J. R. Using transfer learning for detecting drug mentions in tweets. In *ICT Systems and Sustainability. Advances in Intelligent Systems and Computing*, (eds.) M. Tuba, S. Akashe, A. Joshi, Vol. 1270, Springer, Singapore. (2021).

62. E. Choi, M. T. Bahadori, E. Searles, C. Coffey, M. Thompson, J. Bost, J. Tejedor-Sojo, and J. Sun. Multi-layer representation learning for medical concepts. In *Proceedings of the 22nd ACM SIGKDD International Conference on Knowledge Discovery and Data Mining*, KDD '16, pp. 1495–1504, New York, NY, USA (2016).

63. A. L. Beam, B. Kompa, I. Fried, N. P. Palmer, X. Shi, T. Cai, and I. S. Kohane, Clinical concept embeddings learned from massive sources of medical data, *CoRR* (2018).

64. E. Moons, A. Khanna, A. Akkasi, and M.-F. Moens, A comparison of deep learning methods for icd coding of clinical records, *Appl. Sci.* **10**(5), 152–164 (2020).

65. H. Schäfer and C. Friedrich. Multilingual icd-10 code assignment with transformer architectures using mimic-iii discharge summaries. In *Working Notes of CLEF 2020 — Conference and Labs of the Evaluation Forum, Thessaloniki, Greece, September 22-25, 2020* (2020).

66. K. Huang, J. Altosaar, and R. Ranganath, Clinicalbert: Modeling clinical notes and predicting hospital readmission, *CoRR* (2019).

67. M. Müller, M. Salathé, and P. E. Kummervold, COVID-twitter-bert: A natural language processing model to analyse COVID-19 content on twitter, *arXiv e-prints* (2020).

68. T. Möller, A. Reina, R. Jayakumar, and M. Pietsch. COVID-QA: A question answering dataset for COVID-19. In *ACL 2020 Workshop NLP-COVID* (2020).

69. N. F. Rajani, B. McCann, C. Xiong, and R. Socher. Explain yourself! leveraging language models for commonsense reasoning. In *Proceedings*

of the 57th Annual Meeting of the ACL, pp. 4932–4942, Florence, Italy (2019).

70. E. M. Bender and A. Koller. Climbing towards NLU: On meaning, form, and understanding in the age of data. In *Proceedings of the 58th Annual Meeting of the ACL*, pp. 5185–5198 (2020).

71. S. Bird, E. Klein, and E. Loper. *Natural Language Processing with Python*. O'Reilly Media Inc. (2009).

72. L. Padró and E. Stanilovsky. Freeling 3.0: Towards wider multilinguality. In *Proceedings of the Language Resources and Evaluation Conference (LREC 2012)*, Istanbul, Turkey (May, 2012).

73. M. E. Peters, M. Neumann, M. Iyyer, M. Gardner, C. Clark, K. Lee, and L. Zettlemoyer. Deep contextualized word representations. In *Proceedings of the 2018 Conference of the North American Chapter of the Association for Computational Linguistics: Human Language Technologies, Volume 1 (Long Papers)* (2018).

Chapter 5

Metabolically Driven Latent Space Learning for Gene Expression Data

Marco Barsacchi[*,†,‡,§], Helena Andrés-Terré[‡,¶], and Pietro Lió[‡,‖]

*Department of Information Engineering,
University of Florence, 50000 Florence, Italy
†Department of Information Engineering,
University of Pisa, 56122 Pisa, Italy
‡Computer Laboratory,
University of Cambridge, Cambridge, UK
§barsacchimarco@gmail.com
¶ha376@cam.ac.uk
‖pl219@cam.ac.uk

Gene expression microarrays provide a characterisation of the transcriptional activity of a particular biological sample. Their high-dimensionality hampers the process of pattern recognition and extraction. Several approaches have been proposed for gleaning information about the hidden structure of the data. Among these approaches, deep generative models provide a powerful way for approximating the manifold on which the data reside. Here, we develop GEESE, a deep learning-based framework that provides novel insight into the manifold learning for gene expression data, employing a metabolic model to constrain the learned representation. We evaluated the proposed framework, showing its ability to capture biologically relevant features and encoding these features in a much simpler latent space. We showed how using a metabolic model to drive the autoencoder learning process helps in achieving better generalisation to unseen data. GEESE provides a novel perspective on the problem of unsupervised learning for biological data.

1. Introduction

Metabolism comprises the complex network of chemical reactions allowing an organism to transform nutrients into energy and base components necessary for growth, replication, defence and other cellular tasks. Metabolic reactions are mediated by enzymes which, in turn, are produced through gene expression. Nevertheless, despite this close association, the problem of predicting a metabolic phenotype from gene expression levels is anything but solved.[1]

Gene expression microarrays provide a snapshot of all the transcriptional activity in a biological sample, which, in turn, is the result of the complex interactions among genes and environmental factors. Gene expression profiling aims at capturing gene expression patterns in cellular responses to diseases, genetic perturbations and drug treatments. Nevertheless, while more than two decades have passed since the inception of the transcriptomic era, it is still easier to collect data than to understand it.[2] As a sample is typically characterised by large quantities of variables with unknown correlation structures, it is thus extremely challenging to analyse and make sense of the data. Dimensionality reduction techniques have been widely used to unravel the patterns hidden in the gene expression data.[3] As the difficulty of a learning task depends on how the information is represented, it is of paramount importance to find a good representation for the data.

The *manifold hypothesis* states that high-dimensional data tend to lie in the vicinity of a low-dimensional manifold and represents the foundation of manifold learning.[4] Deep generative models, such as variational autoencoders (VAEs)[5] and generative adversarial networks (GANs),[6] involve learning a mapping (via a generator or decoder network) from a lower-dimensional latent space to the high-dimensional space of observed data;[7] in other words, they approximate the original manifold.

In this paper, we propose an approach for learning structure in gene expression data; advancing the current state of the art, we employ the metabolic knowledge we possess in the form of a genome-scale metabolic model (GSMM),[8] constraining the learnt representation to convey the genotype–phenotype relationship. Furthermore, we endeavour to yield a disentangled representation, in which different latent units are sensible to changes in a single generative factor and approximately invariant with respect to changes of the other factors.[9] To do so, we employ a deep generative model (β-VAE)[10] combined with a genome-scale metabolic model. To the best of our knowledge, even if approaches aimed at extracting latent spaces from transcriptomic data[11] have been proposed before, none of them has integrated the metabolic model to constrain the learnt representation. We dubbed our framework GEESE (Gene Expression latEnt Space Encoder).

The rest of the work is organised as follows. In Section 2, we thoroughly describe the proposed framework as well as the theory and computational methods required; we then proceed to a detailed evaluation in Section 3. Conclusions are drawn in Section 4.

2.   Methods

In this section, we describe the proposed framework. Its schematic diagram is provided in Figure 1. The general idea is introduced here; a detailed description is given in the following sections.

Suppose we have a dataset $\mathcal{D}$ of gene expression data, from which we aim at extracting a (low-dimensional) latent space representation. The dataset of gene expression data is provided as input to the FBA

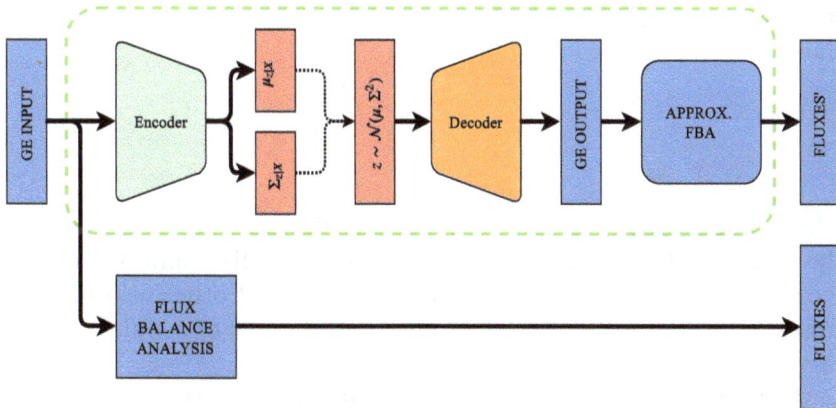

Fig. 1.   Global scheme of the proposed framework. The gene expression data is inputted both to the VAE and FBA models. The VAE is trained in minimizing the loss between the fluxes obtained by passing the reconstructed gene expression through the approximated FBA and the fluxes outputted by the real FBA.

model, which produces a set of reaction fluxes F. We then train the FBA approximator, providing g.e. data as input and minimising the MSE between the fluxes F and the predicted fluxes F'. The VAE is then trained, with g.e. data as input, aiming at minimising the loss between the fluxes F' obtained by passing the reconstructed gene expression through the approximated FBA and the fluxes F, keeping the weights of the FBA approximator fixed.

2.1. *Genome-scale metabolic models*

Metabolic models are based on a well-curated genome-scale metabolic network. A metabolic model comprises both the metabolic reactions and the genes encoding enzymes involved in mediating these reactions.[12] The metabolic network is topologically represented as $\mathbf{S}$, an $M \times N$ stoichiometric matrix, where the M rows represent the stoichiometric coefficients of the corresponding metabolites in all the N reactions. Under the mass balance constraint, the system behaves according to a set of differential equations: $\frac{dx_i}{dt} = \sum_{j=1}^{N} S_{ij} v_j$, $i = 1, \ldots, M$, x_i being the concentration of the ith metabolite and v_j the flux through reaction j.[13] The value of S_{ij} is negative, positive or zero if the ith metabolite acts as reactant, product or does not participate in the jth reaction, respectively. Under the hypothesis of pseudo-steady-state $\frac{dx_i}{dt} = 0$, $\forall i$, the amount of compound being produced equals the total amount being consumed, thus

$$\sum_{j=1}^{N} S_{ij} v_j = 0 \ \forall i. \tag{5.1}$$

The pseudo-steady-state hypothesis holds under the assumption that the time constants for metabolic reactions (milliseconds to tens of seconds) are typically much smaller than those of other cellular processes, such as transcriptional regulation (minutes) or cellular growth (several minutes or hours).[14]

As there are more unknown variables than equations ($N \geq M$), the system is undetermined and there are an infinite number of flux vectors that satisfy Eq. (5.1); that set of vectors represent the *null space* of $\mathbf{S}$. In order to constrain the set of allowable metabolic phenotypes of the systems, thermodynamic and capacity constraints can be introduced into the system as lower and upper bounds on the reaction fluxes: $\mathbf{v}^{\text{inf}} \leq \mathbf{v} \leq \mathbf{v}^{\text{sup}}$. The mass-balance constraints, along with the flux inequalities, define a convex-bounded polytope, in which all feasible solutions lie. The maximisation of a postulate objective function can be used to select the most physiologically relevant metabolic phenotype, leading to the classic FBA optimisation formulation:[15]

$$\max Z = \mathbf{c}^T \mathbf{v}$$
$$\text{s.t.} \quad \mathbf{Sv} = \mathbf{b} \qquad (5.2)$$
$$\mathbf{v}^{\text{inf}} \leq \mathbf{v} \leq \mathbf{v}^{\text{sup}}.$$

The most widely used objective function is the biomass function; it is a fictitious reaction used as a sink for biomass precursors (e.g., DNA, RNA, proteins, lipids) that together define the biomass composition of the cell.[16] The biomass objective relies on the assumption that the cell is striving to maximise its growth, given a fixed amount of resources.

Nonetheless, the usage biomass as the objective imposes a strong limitation, as an organism is often simultaneously optimising multiple and competing objectives.[17] Furthermore, it has been shown that biomass maximising flux states are usually degenerate, in that exist multiple flux distributions that yield the same maximal biomass value.[18]

The limitation can be tackled using a multi-objective optimisation scheme; in this context, the results of the optimisation process is a set of non-dominated points called the Pareto front. As shown by Ref. 19, the multi-objective optimisation problem can be tackled using bilevel linear programming coupled with evolutionary algorithms. In this work, we choose the following bilayer formulation, as proposed before[20]:

$$\max \mathbf{g}^T \mathbf{v}$$
$$\text{s.t.} \quad \max \mathbf{f}^T \mathbf{v}$$
$$\text{s.t.} \quad \mathbf{Sv} = \mathbf{b} \qquad (5.3)$$
$$\mathbf{v}^{\text{inf}} h(\mathbf{y}) \leq \mathbf{v} \leq \mathbf{v}^{\text{sup}} h(\mathbf{y})$$
$$\mathbf{v} \in \mathbb{R}^N,$$

where f and g are arrays of weights associated with the first and second objectives, respectively, and $h(\mathbf{y})$ is a multiplicative function of gene expression vector $\mathbf{y}$ introduced in the following.

In order to exploit multiple sources of information, we use a multi-omic model, integrating gene expression data into the model. Each metabolic reaction in the model depends on a set of genes through gene to protein to reaction (GPR) associations.[21] Each GPR is described as a string of genes linked by AND/OR operators; if a gene set is made up of two genes connected by an AND, both genes are necessary to carry out the reactions, thus they made up an enzymatic complex. Conversely, if two genes are connected by an OR operator, they independently catalyse the same reaction, making up an isozyme. In order to deal with continuous expression values, instead of binary (zero or one) activations, we borrow the standard operators from fuzzy logic.[22] The expression of two genes connected through an AND operator is the minimum of the expression of the individual genes making up the gene set. The gene set expression for two genes connected by an OR operator is the max of expression of the individual genes.

The expression of a gene set can then be applied to the corresponding reaction flux boundaries using the following piecewise multiplicative function:

$$h(y_i) = \begin{cases} (1 + |\log(y_i)|)^{\mathrm{sgn}(y_i - 1)} & \text{if } y_i \in \mathbb{R}^+ \setminus \{1\}, \\ 1 & \text{if } y_i = 1, \end{cases} \tag{5.4}$$

where y_i is the expression of the gene set responsible for the ith reaction.[23] The function approximates the relationship between mRNA abundance and protein synthesis rate.[24] A discussion of the appropriateness of using mRNA levels as a proxy for protein abundance is given elsewhere.[20]

2.2. *Approximating FBA*

In order to be able to train a VAE to reconstruct a GE vector that produces the same fluxes as the input one, we decided to use the mean square loss between the fluxes of the reconstructed GE, let's say F' and the fluxes of the original GE vector, F; nevertheless, doing so requires the FBA layer in Figure 1 to be differentiable with respect to the GE. To the best of our knowledge, no differentiable formulation of linear programming with respect to a non-differentiable function

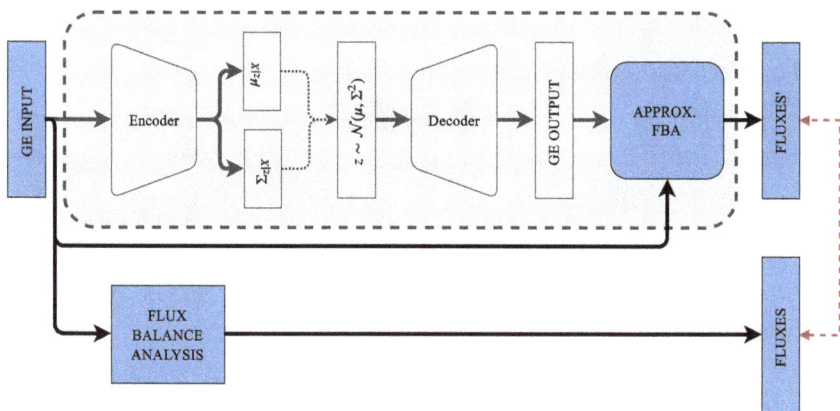

Fig. 2. Schematic diagram of the training process for the FBA approximator. We provide a GE vector as well as the concentration of relevant metabolites in the media (oxygen and glucose) as inputs to the FBA approximator; the approximator is trained to approximate the fluxes obtained via FBA.

of the constraints has been proposed before. Thus, we approximated the FBA using an MLP (APPROX. FBA in Figure 1).

The training is schematised in Figure 2; we provided the GE vector as well as the concentration of relevant metabolites (glucose and oxygen) in the media as inputs. It is worth underlining that the learnt model is limited to particular organisms and to variations of metabolite concentrations for which it has been trained; notably, the model provides a sound approximation only for GE vectors that reside in the convex hull of the training data. Nevertheless, this aspect does not represent a limitation for the current purpose of the model (see Section 3.1). The FBA approximator is trained independently from the remaining architecture, and its weights are kept fixed when training the VAE.

The FBA approximator is five-layered MPL; its architecture is shown in Figure S1. The total number of trainable parameters is 24,337,944. We used *relu* as activation functions for all but the last layer; the last layer uses a linear activation function. We used an adagrad optimizer and mean square error (MSE) between the reconstructed and FBA-produced layer as loss function. We trained the network on a NVIDIA TESLA K80 GPU; we trained for 300 epochs using a batch size of 128.

2.3. Dataset

2.3.1. Real dataset

As a real dataset, we use a compendium of 466 *E. coli* Affymetrix Antisense2 microarray expression profiles.[25] The dataset includes gene expression microarrays collected in different experimental conditions, such as varying oxygen and glucose concentrations, pH changes, heat shock and antibiotics. When running the FBA, we consider oxygen and glucose intake rate depending on the particular media condition.

2.3.2. Generating GE data

In order to construct a dataset, we used a multi-objective optimisation algorithm, generating a set gene expression vectors defining Pareto fronts for different experimental conditions (aerobic/anaerobic, varying concentrations of glucose in the medium). We generated, for a set of 12 experimental conditions, Pareto fronts using the METRADE multi-objective scheme,[20] with 450 iterations and a population of 300 individuals. METRADE couples a bilayer FBA formulation with an NSGA-II algorithm.[26] We followed a previously proposed approach,[23] selecting biomass maximisation and total intracellular flux minimisation as conflicting objectives.

We selected various experimental conditions, anaerobic and aerobic for different glucose concentrations (5.5, 5.6, 6 10, 11, 20, 22 and 44 mmol h^{-1} gDW^{-1}) in order to provide a sufficient number of Pareto fronts. The experimental conditions span the set of glucose and oxygen concentrations found in the dataset of 466 *E. coli* Affymetrix Antisense2 microarray expression profiles described before. The objective space for a sub-sample of the dataset is shown in Figure S4. The resulting dataset is composed of 6'440 gene expression vectors.

2.4. VAEs

Variational autoencoders (VAEs)[5] are a class of deep generative models trained via variational inference methods, hence the name. Given a dataset $\mathcal{D} = \{x^1, \ldots, x^N\}$, a probabilistic encoder and decoder are trained. The generative process considers a set of latent variables

$\mathbf{z} \in \mathbb{R}^k$ and a set of observed variables $\mathbf{x} \in \mathcal{X}$, thus defining a joint probability distribution $p(\mathbf{x}, \mathbf{z}) = p(\mathbf{x}|\mathbf{z})p(\mathbf{z})$.

We want to maximise the marginal probability of each $\mathbf{x}$ in the training set under the generative process $p(\mathbf{x}) = \int p_\theta(\mathbf{x}|\mathbf{z})p(\mathbf{z})d\mathbf{z}$; nevertheless, being the integral intractable, VAEs are generally trained by maximising the evidence lower bound (ELBO) instead:

$$
\begin{aligned}
\log p(\mathbf{x}) = \text{ELBO}(\theta, \phi; \mathbf{x}, \mathbf{z}) + D_{KL}(q_\phi(\mathbf{z}|\mathbf{x})||p(\mathbf{z}|\mathbf{x})) \geq \\
\text{ELBO}(\theta, \phi; \mathbf{x}, \mathbf{z}) = \\
\mathbb{E}_{q_\phi(\mathbf{z}|\mathbf{x})}\left[\log p_\theta(\mathbf{x}|\mathbf{z})\right] - D_{KL}(q_\phi(\mathbf{z}|\mathbf{x})||p(\mathbf{z})),
\end{aligned}
\tag{5.5}
$$

where $q_\phi(\mathbf{z}|\mathbf{x})$ is an approximate (posterior) distribution parametrised via ϕ. Here, $D_{\text{KL}}(q_\phi(\mathbf{z}|\mathbf{x})||p(\mathbf{z}))$ is the Kullback Leiber divergence between q_ϕ and p.

The optimisation is achieved by simultaneously performing gradient descent on both ϕ and θ; to do so, the *reparametrisation trick* is used, i.e. each random variable $z_i \sim q_\phi(z_i|\mathbf{x}) = \mathcal{N}(\mu_i, \sigma_i)$ is rewritten as a differentiable transformation of a noise variable $\epsilon \sim \mathcal{N}(0, 1) : z_i = \mu_i + \sigma_i\epsilon$. In the VAE model, we generally assume $\mathbf{z} \sim p(\mathbf{z}) = \mathcal{N}(\mathbf{0}, \mathbf{I})$ and $\mathbf{x} \sim p_\theta(\mathbf{x}|\mathbf{z})$; furthermore, both p and q are parametrised by *neural networks*.

In this work, we use a particular evolution of the VAE framework, which modifies the original objective function introducing an adjustable hyperparameter β,[10] hence the name:

$$
\begin{aligned}
\mathcal{L}(\theta, \phi; \mathbf{x}, \mathbf{z}, \beta) = \\
\mathbb{E}_{q_\phi(\mathbf{z}|\mathbf{x})}\left[\log p_\theta(\mathbf{x}|\mathbf{z})\right] - \beta D_{KL}(q_\phi(\mathbf{z}|\mathbf{x})||p(\mathbf{z})).
\end{aligned}
\tag{5.6}
$$

The parameter β determines the amount of pressure applied to the latent information channel. Imposing $\beta > 1$, we strongly constrain the latent bottleneck, thus pushing $q_\phi(\mathbf{z}|\mathbf{x})$ towards the isotropic unit Gaussian prior $p(\mathbf{z})$. It has been shown that reconstruction under this bottleneck helps in producing a disentangled representation,[27] in which different latent units are sensible to changes in a single generative factor and approximately invariant with respect to changes of the other factors.

Here, we briefly justify the choice of the model, providing the rationale behind the choice of the VAE instead of a more common AE; although the VAE has an AE-like structure, i.e. it is made of a decoder and an encoder network, it serves a much larger purpose;

still it can be used fruitfully to learn latent representations. Since we are interested in having a probabilistic generative model of the data, a VAE is a better choice. Among the advantages offered by a generative model, it is that of sampling new elements from the distribution, e.g., sampling fake gene expression data for a particular condition.

The overall VAE model is made of an encoder q and a decoder p. The decoder, $p_\theta(\mathbf{x}|\mathbf{z})$, is a three-layered MLP, as shown in Figure S2; the input to the model is the sampled latent state $\mathbf{z}$. The encoder $q_\phi(\mathbf{z}|\mathbf{x})$ is a three-layered MLP, as shown in Figure S3. We train the VAE network on a NVIDIA TESLA K80 GPU for 300 epochs, using a batch size of 128 and keeping the approximated FBA weights fixed.

3.   Experimental Results

In this section, we fit our framework on the dataset we have generated, evaluating its ability to learn a compact and disentangled representation of the gene expression data. We first characterise the FBA approximator (Section 3.1) and later on evaluate the GEESE model (Section 3.2). Then we compare GEESE with a baseline VAE on a real dataset (Section 3.3).

3.1.   *FBA approximation*

We first trained the FBA approximator. Then, we evaluated the approximator on both the train and test sets; we show the results in Figure 3. The MSEs are 0.671 and 1.048 on the train and test sets, respectively.

In Figure 3, we plotted the two objectives for both FBA-generated fluxes (orange circles) and approximated FBA (green + symbols); corresponding points are connected by a black line. According to the experimental results, the approximator learns a property we dubbed *Pareto-preservation*, i.e. it generally learns to map g.e. data in the nearest (true) Pareto Front.

Furthermore, in order to assess the deviation with respect to the steady-state assumption $\mathbf{Sv} = \mathbf{0}$, we measured $D = \frac{||\mathbf{Sv}^{(a)}||_1}{||\mathbf{v}^{(t)}||_1}$, where $\mathbf{v}^{(a)}$ and $\mathbf{v}^{(t)}$ are the approximated and exact flux vectors, respectively; we will refer to D as the deviation index hereafter. The mean

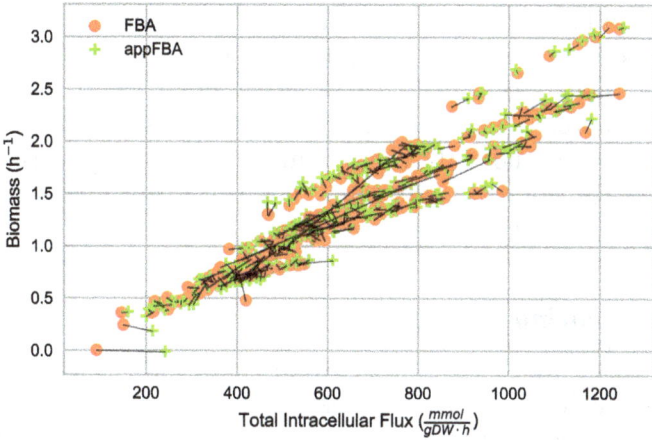

(a) Train

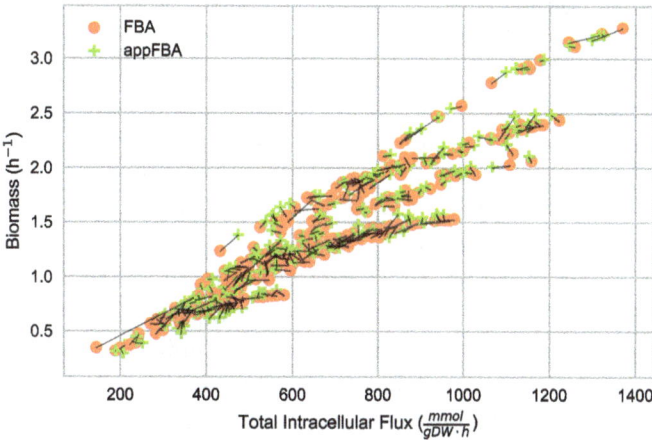

(b) Test

Fig. 3. Pareto preserving properties of the FBA approximator; for sake of clarity we show only 300 random samples from both the train (upper panel) and test (lower panel) sets. The FBA predictions are represented as orange circles, while the approximated FBA ones are marked with green + symbols. Each pair of prediction is connected by a black line.

deviation indexes on the train and test sets are 0.119 and 0.115, respectively.

It is worth noticing that, while the FBA approximator shows promising results, we are not interested in obtaining a perfect approximation of the FBA; as long as the approximator drives the latent space learning in the direction of a better feature extraction, the approximation is good enough. Whether or not this property is fulfilled is the subject of the following sections.

Furthermore, we expect the model to generalise as long as the data on which it is used lie in the convex hull of the training distribution;[28] since the FBA approximator is only used to train the VAE, we can be reasonably confident of its behaviour.

3.2. *Evaluating the VAE*

We trained the variational autoencoder shown in Figure 1. We then evaluated the learnt FBA on a hold-out test set.

We first inspected the output gene expression reconstructed by the autoencoder; interestingly, the reconstructed gene expression data show greater compactness: as shown in Figure S6, the standard deviation of the reconstructed gene expression (right panel) is, for the majority of genes, lower than the original one (left panel). This behaviour suggests that the VAE is denoising the data, discarding all the variations in gene expression that is not strictly useful in terms of reconstructing a particular metabolic phenotype.

We then evaluated the learnt latent space in terms of the original experimental conditions (see Section 2.3.2). In the left panel Figure 4, we show a scatterplot of the encoded latent dimensions for a sample of $n = 2000$ gene expression vectors. As expected, the encoding maps different experimental conditions along different curves in the latent space. The closeness between curves reflects similarities/dissimilarities between experimental conditions. For example, the experimental conditions (Anaerobic, –20) and (Anaerobic, –22) are encoded on partially overlapping curves as are their Pareto fronts in Figure S4. More interesting, each curve is directed in the sense that moving across a specific curve, we span the corresponding Pareto front (see the following and the left panel of Figure 4).

We then compared the latent space generated by GEESE with the one induced by a baseline VAE (without the FBA module); even if the experimental conditions are nicely separated in the latent space, the Pareto front structure is not preserved (Figure S5). Indeed, even if the Pareto front structure is an inherent property of the dataset, it is only captured adding the metabolic constraints imposed by GEESE.

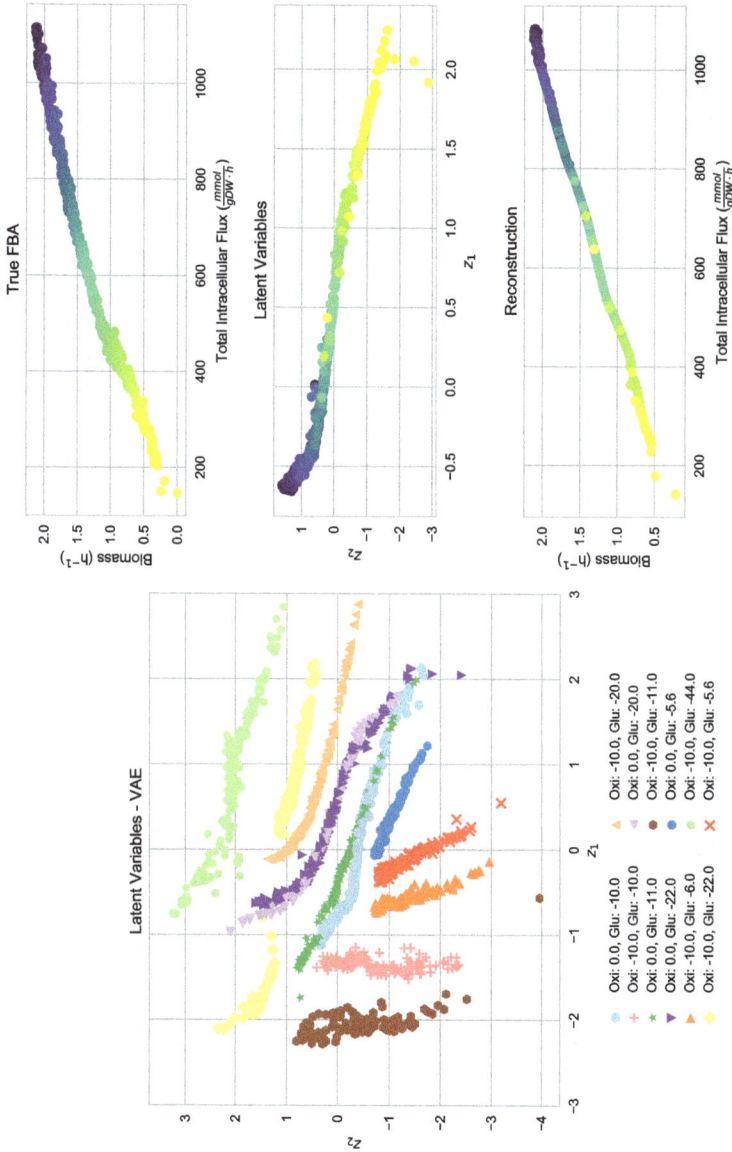

Fig. 4. Left Panel: The (bidimensional) latent space for a sample of $n = 2000$ GE data is reported. The VAE encodes different experimental conditions in different regions (more properly paths) of the latent space. See also Figure S4 in the supplementary material. Right Panel: For a given Pareto Front (Anaerobic, max glucose intake $22 \frac{mmol}{gDW \cdot h}$), dark purple in Figure 4), we plot the two objectives for the true FBA (upper right panel) and the two objectives of the reconstructed FBA, obtained passing the gene expression data through the autoencoder (lower right panel). The colour, shifting from yellow to dark purple, encodes the movement along the Pareto front (middle right panel).

Furthermore, we analysed the capability of the proposed framework with respect to the reconstruction of a given Pareto front. We selected gene expression data from a particular Pareto front (obtained in anaerobic setting with max glucose intake $22\frac{mmol}{gDW \cdot h}$)), and we used our VAE trained with a latent space dimension of 2. In the right panel of Figure 4, we report the objective space produced by the true FBA (upper right panel), the encoding of the gene expression data into the latent space (dark purple curve in the left panel), and the two objectives of the reconstructed FBA, obtained passing the gene expression data through the autoencoder (lower left panel).

Then, we analysed the capability of the proposed framework by locally exploring the adjacent latent space of the given Pareto fronts. New data points were generated in the proximity of a particular Pareto front (obtained in anaerobic setting with max glucose intake $22\frac{mmol}{gDW \cdot h}$)) followed by the reconstruction of their gene expression using our GEESE (see the left panel in Figure 5). The distribution of each gene was used to identify a set of particularly stable and unstable genes along that region of the latent space. We performed the sensitivity analysis to obtain the robustness value of each gene for two different objectives. The genes classified as stable in the local latent space around the Pareto front show high values of robustness, meaning that their role in the optimisation under those specific experimental conditions is replaceable (see the right panel in Figure 5). Instead, the unstable genes show mixed robustness values, which can be understood as having a more critical influence over the optimisation under these experimental conditions. In both groups, the GEESE manages to identify genes that have almost binary optimisation values (either completely breaking or maximising the results). Therefore, GEEESE succeeds in identifying a set of specific genes that are characteristic to each of the experimental conditions, with minimal overlap among Pareto fronts and clear effect over optimisation.

3.3. *Is GEESE helping in reconstructing the latent space?*

In order to inspect how the model generalises in a real-case scenario, we devised the following experiment: we selected a compendium of

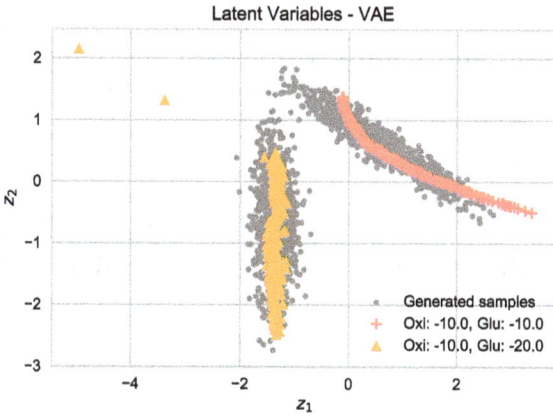

(a) Generated samples

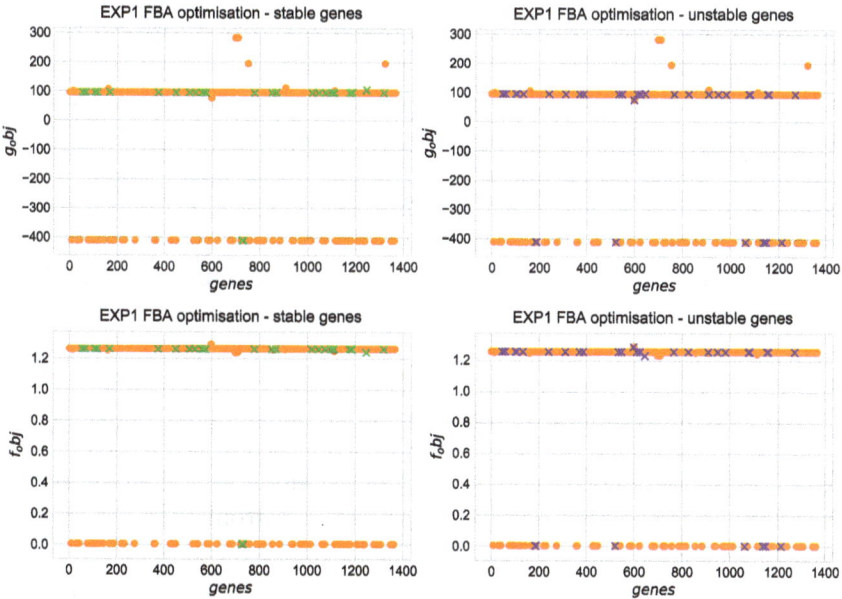

(b) Sensitivity analysis

Fig. 5. New data points were generated in the proximity of a particular Pareto front (left panel) followed by the reconstruction of their gene expression using our VAE. Stable and unstable genes have been identified, and sensitivity analysis for each gene for two different objectives have been performed (right panel). In both groups, the VAE manage to identify genes that have almost binary optimisation values.

466 *E. coli* Affymetrix Antisense2 microarray expression profiles.[25] As described in the following, this dataset collects gene expression microarrays from different experimental conditions, such as varying oxygen and glucose concentrations, pH changes, heat shock and antibiotics. We then generated a dataset, using only the knowledge of glucose and oxygen in the media, using Paretos from the multi-objective evolutionary approach. We trained both a baseline Variational Autoencoder, without the FBA module, and our architecture (GEESE), on this dataset. Both GEESE (Figure 4) and the baseline VAE (Figure S5) show good properties in the embedded space.

Then, considering only the learnt encoder as a nonlinear feature extractor, we inspected the latent space for the selected (unseen) compendia of real gene expression data. The embeddings are reported in Figures 6(a) and 6(b) for the VAE and GEESE, respectively.

Interestingly, the GEESE architecture shows a greater capability to generalise to unseen new data, and it is able to better spread the unseen data in the latent space. The baseline VAE, instead, collapses the majority of the new data in a very thin region of the latent space. We hypothesise that, in this context, the GSMM works as a prior, thus providing sounded built-in assumptions about the structure of the underlying data, and helps in making sense of noisy, high-dimensional measures.

4. Discussion and Conclusion

A fundamental question in biology is to understand what makes individuals, populations, and species different from each other. The notion of phenotype, i.e. observable attributes of an individual, is opposed to that of genotype, the inherited material encoded in genes. The ongoing quest of system biology is that of bridging the genotype–phenotype gap. Both gene expression microarrays and RNA-seq have been used to probe the transcriptional landscape of a biological sample. Notwithstanding, the prediction of a metabolic phenotype from gene expression levels is anything but a solved problem.

In this work, we tackled the problem of learning a meaningful latent space for gene expression data, using a deep generative model. In order to force the latent space to convey metabolic information, we

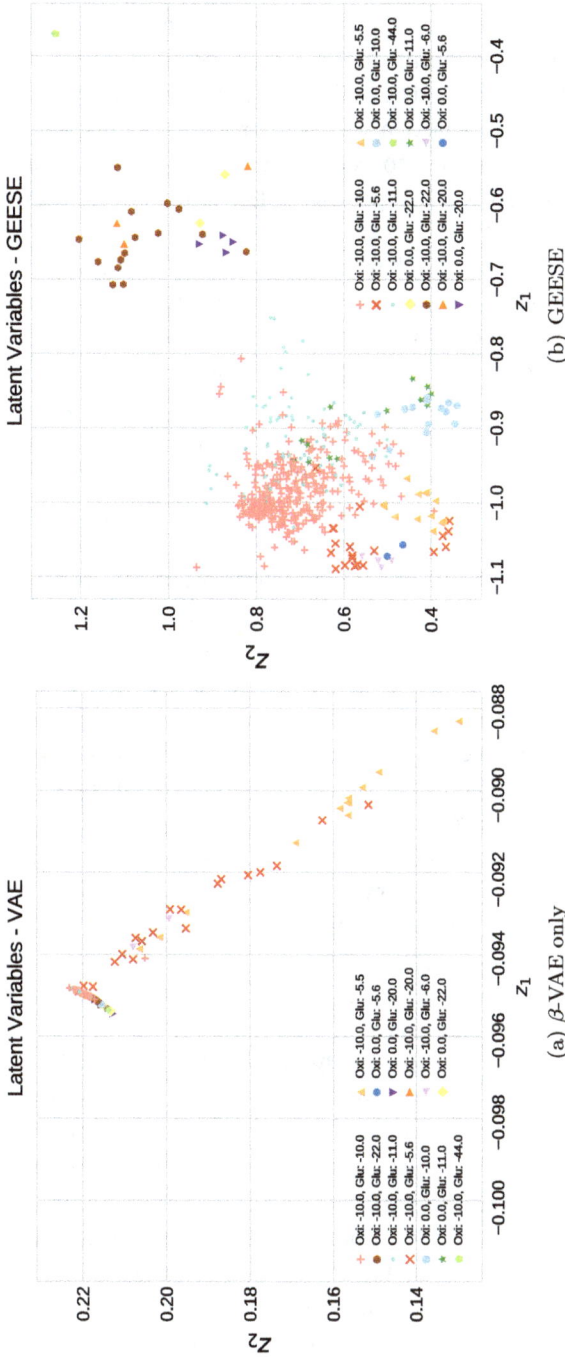

Fig. 6.   The latent spaces for (unseen) examples from the real dataset are shown for a baseline (VAE) (a) and our proposed architecture (GEESE) (b).

devised a specific framework, composed of a generative deep neural network and an approximation of a metabolic network-based flux balance analysis. We first trained the FBA approximator as a five-layered MLP; we then used a β-Variational Autoencoder (β-VAE), and we trained the model to reconstruct a gene expression vector that passing through a FBA produces the same flux distribution as the input one.

The learnt bidimensional manifold provides meaningful insights into the relationships between samples; first, the autoencoder is able to recognise gene expression vectors associated with different experimental conditions (e.g., aerobic/anaerobic and different values of glucose in the medium). Second, the autoencoder denoises the input data, while preserving the same metabolic phenotype. Third, the encoder maps a Pareto front of gene expression vectors into an oriented path in the bidimensional space (Figure 4). The oriented paths depict how the bacteria benefits from using different GE strategies to cope with varying environmental conditions; the overlap between strategies, notably when the environmental conditions are similar, buttresses the biological soundness of the inferred results. Indeed, the comparison with Figure S5 clearly shows how this information cannot be extracted by means as a standard AE. Fourth, GEEESE succeeds in identifying a set of specific genes that are characteristic of each of the experimental conditions, with minimal overlap among Pareto fronts and clear effect over optimisation. Finally, evaluating the learnt model on an unseen real dataset of gene expression microarray, we show that the proposed model achieves a better generalisation with respect to a baseline VAE, as pictured in Figure 6.

We state that constraining the reconstructed gene expression to approximate the original FBA output, we are driving the autoencoder to incorporate prior knowledge about the correlations between genes, thus helping in making sense of noisy, high-dimensional measures. The devised framework, dubbed GEEESE (Gene Expression latEnt Space Encoder), represents a step towards the understanding of the genotype–phenotype relationship. As GSMMs are becoming available for an increasing number of organisms, the applicability of the proposed model is broadening. Finally, we believe that our model provides a better understanding of different relevant conditions and a novel perspective of the problem of manifold learning in general.

Supplementary Figures

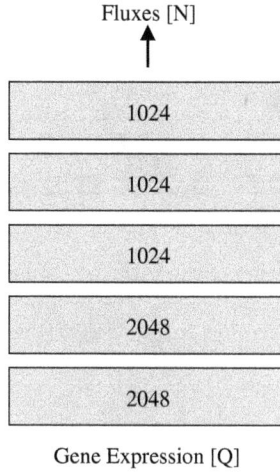

Fluxes [N]

1024
1024
1024
2048
2048

Gene Expression [Q]

Fig. S1. Architecture of the FBA approximator. Fully connected five-layered MLP with (2048,2048,1024,1024,1024) hidden dimensions respectively, and relu activation functions on all layers but the output, which has linear activation.

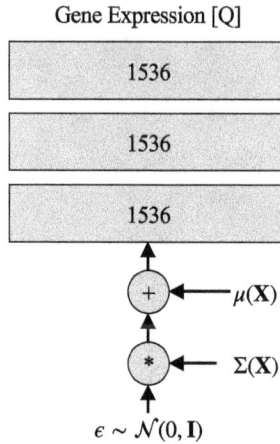

Gene Expression [Q]

1536
1536
1536

$+ \longleftarrow \mu(\mathbf{X})$

$* \longleftarrow \Sigma(\mathbf{X})$

$\epsilon \sim \mathcal{N}(0, \mathbf{I})$

Fig. S2. Decoder p architecture of the VAE model. Fully connected three-layered MLP with (1536,1536,1536) dimensions. The input is the sampled latent state $\mathbf{z}$ generated from the learned latent space, defined by the mean and standard deviation of the multivariate embedding gaussian (mu, Sigma).

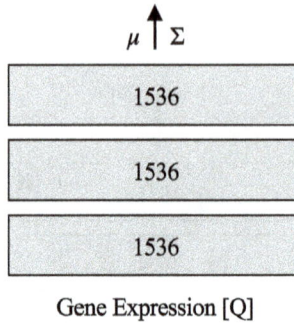

Fig. S3. Encoder q architecture of the VAE model. Fully connected three-layered MLP with (1536,1536,1536) dimensions. The output are the mean and standard deviation of the multivariate embedding gaussian (mu, Sigma) defining the latent space.

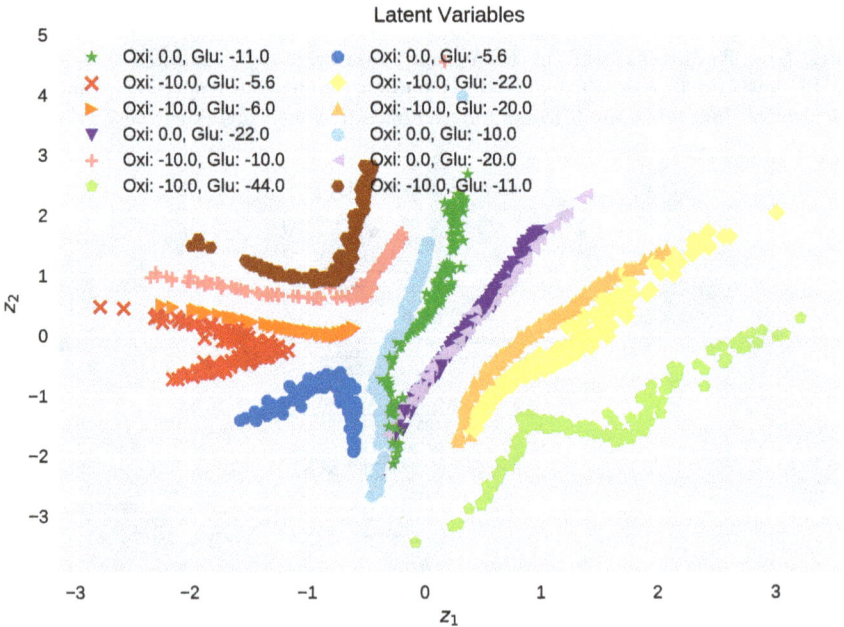

Fig. S4. Latent space learned by the VAE, capturing the different experimental conditions as partially overlapping curves or Pareto fronts.

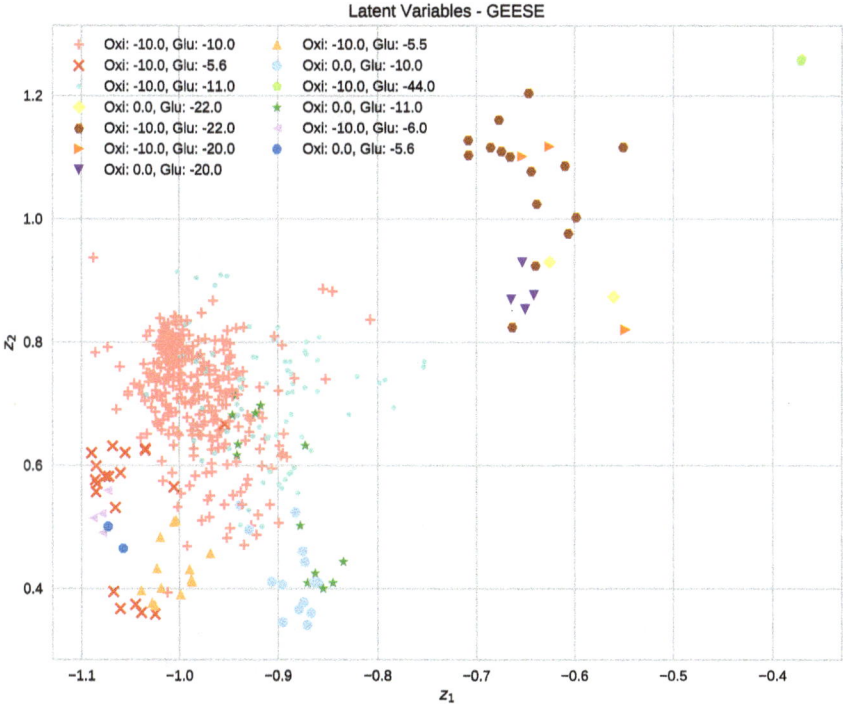

Fig. S5.   Latent space learned by the VAE without the FBA module. The experimental conditions are still separated by the embeddings, but the Pareto front structure is not preserved.

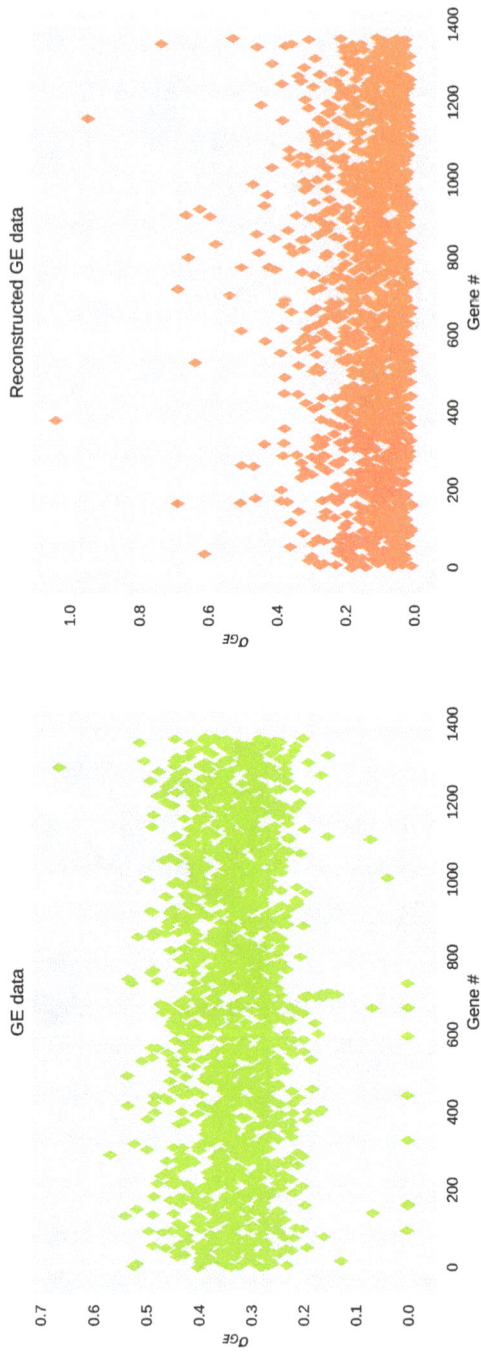

Fig. S6. Standard deviation of the original and reconstructed gene expression. The reconstructed gene expression show greater compactness when compared to the original version.

References

1. F. G. Vital-Lopez, A. Wallqvist, and J. Reifman, Bridging the gap between gene expression and metabolic phenotype via kinetic models, *BMC Syst. Biol.* **7**(1), 63 (2013). doi: 10.1186/1752-0509-7-63. https://doi.org/10.1186/1752-0509-7-63.
2. R. Lowe, N. Shirley, M. Bleackley, S. Dolan, and T. Shafee, Transcriptomics technologies, *PLOS Comput. Biol.* **13**(5), 1–23 (2017). doi: 10.1371/journal.pcbi.1005457. https://doi.org/10.1371/journal.pcbi.10 05457.
3. J. Shi and Z. Luo, Nonlinear dimensionality reduction of gene expression data for visualization and clustering analysis of cancer tissue samples, *Comput. Biol. Med.* **40**(8), 723–732 (2010). doi: https://doi.org/10.1016/j.compbiomed.2010.06.007. http://www.sciencedirect.com/science/article/pii/S0010482510000958.
4. C. Fefferman, S. Mitter, and H. Narayanan, Testing the manifold hypothesis, *J. Amer. Math. Soc.* **29**(4), 983–1049 (2016). doi: 10.1090/jams/852. https://doi.org/10.1090/jams/852.
5. D. P. Kingma and M. Welling, Auto-Encoding Variational Bayes, *ArXiv e-prints* (2013).
6. I. Goodfellow, J. Pouget-Abadie, M. Mirza, B. Xu, D. Warde-Farley, S. Ozair, A. Courville, and Y. Bengio. Generative adversarial nets. In *Advances in Neural Information Processing Systems,* (eds.) Z. Ghahramani, M. Welling, C. Cortes, N. D. Lawrence, and K. Q. Weinberger, 27, pp. 2672–2680. Curran Associates, Inc. (2014). http://papers.nips.cc/paper/5423-generative-adversarial-nets.pdf.
7. H. Shao, A. Kumar, and P. T. Fletcher, The Riemannian geometry of deep generative models, *ArXiv e-prints* (2017).
8. T. Y. Kim, S. B. Sohn, Y. B. Kim, W. J. Kim, and S. Y. Lee, Recent advances in reconstruction and applications of genome-scale metabolic models, *Curr. Opin. Biotech.* **23**(4), 617–623 (2012). doi: https://doi.org/10.1016/j.copbio.2011.10.007. http://www.sciencedirect.com/science/article/pii/S0958166911007038.
9. Y. Bengio, A. Courville, and P. Vincent, Representation learning: A review and new perspectives, *IEEE Trans. Pattern Anal. Mach. Intell.* **35**(8), 1798–1828 (2013). doi: 10.1109/TPAMI.2013.50.
10. I. Higgins, L. Matthey, A. Pal, C. Burgess, X. Glorot, M. Botvinick, S. Mohamed, and A. Lerchner, β-VAE: Learning Basic Visual Concepts with a Constrained Variational Framework, *ICLR2017* (2017).
11. G. P. Way and C. S. Greene. Extracting a biologically relevant latent space from cancer transcriptomes with variational autoencoders. In

Biocomputing 2018, pp. 80–91. World Scientific (2017). doi: 10.1142/ 9789813235533_0008. https://www.worldscientific.com/doi/abs/10.11 42/9789813235533_0008.

12. T. R. Maarleveld, R. A. Khandelwal, B. G. Olivier, B. Teusink, and F. J. Bruggeman, Basic concepts and principles of stoichiometric modeling of metabolic networks, *Biotechnol. J.* **8**(9), 997–1008 (2013). doi: 10.1002/biot.201200291. https://onlinelibrary.wiley.com/doi/abs/10.1 002/biot.201200291.

13. J. D. Orth, I. Thiele, and B. Ø. Palsson, What is flux balance analysis?, *Nature biotechnology.* **28**(3), 245–248 (2010). doi: 10.1038/nbt.1614. http://dx.doi.org/10.1038/nbt.1614.

14. A. Varma and B. O. Palsson, Stoichiometric flux balance models quantitatively predict growth and metabolic by-product secretion in wild-type escherichia coli w3110., *Appl. Environ. Microbiol.* **60**(10), 3724–3731 (1994). http://aem.asm.org/content/60/10/3724.abstract.

15. K. J. Kauffman, P. Prakash, and J. S. Edwards, Advances in flux balance analysis, *Curr. Opin. Biotechnol.* **14**(5), 491–496 (2003). doi: https://doi.org/10.1016/j.copbio.2003.08.001. http://www.sciencedire ct.com/science/article/pii/S0958166903001174.

16. E. J. O'Brien, J. M. Monk, and B. O. Palsson, Using genome-scale models to predict biological capabilities, *Cell* **161**(5), 971–987 (2015). doi: https://doi.org/10.1016/j.cell.2015.05.019. http://www.sciencedir ect.com/science/article/pii/S0092867415005681.

17. D. Molenaar, R. van Berlo, D. de Ridder, and B. Teusink, Shifts in growth strategies reflect tradeoffs in cellular economics, *Mol. Syst. Biol.* **5**(1) (2009). doi: 10.1038/msb.2009.82. http://msb.embopress.org/con tent/5/1/323.

18. A. E. M. Joo Sang Lee, Takashi Nishikawa, Why optimal states recruit fewer reactions in metabolic networks, *Discrete Contin. Dyn. Syst.-A.* **32**(1078-0947_2012_8_2937), 2937 (2012). doi: 10.3934/dcds.2012. 32.2937. http://aimsciences.org//article/id/56288123-03cd-44fa-96f2-c564d8db5fe2.

19. J. Costanza, G. Carapezza, C. Angione, P. Lió, and G. Nicosia, Robust design of microbial strains, *Bioinformatics.* **28**(23), 3097–3104 (2012). doi: 10.1093/bioinformatics/bts590. http://dx.doi.org/10.1093/bioinfo rmatics/bts590.

20. C. Angione and P. Lió, Predictive analytics of environmental adaptability in multi-omic network models, *Sci. Rep.* **5**, 15147 EP – (2015). http://dx.doi.org/10.1038/srep15147.

21. M. L. Mo, N. Jamshidi, and B. O. Palsson, A genome-scale, constraint-based approach to systems biology of human metabolism, *Mol. BioSyst.* **3**, 598–603 (2007). doi: 10.1039/B705597H. http://dx.doi.org/10.1039 /B705597H.

22. H.-J. Zimmermann, Fuzzy set theory, *Wiley Interdiscip. Rev.: Comput. Stat.* **2**(3), 317–332 (2010). doi: 10.1002/wics.82.

23. S. S. Kashaf, C. Angione, and P. Lió, Making life difficult for clostridium difficile: Augmenting the pathogen's metabolic model with transcriptomic and codon usage data for better therapeutic target characterization, *BMC Syst.Biol.* **11**(1), 25 (2017). doi: 10.1186/s12918-017-0395-3. https://doi.org/10.1186/s12918-017-0395-3.

24. H. Firczuk, S. Kannambath, J. Pahle, A. Claydon, R. Beynon, J. Duncan, H. Westerhoff, P. Mendes, and J. E. McCarthy, An in vivo control map for the eukaryotic mrna translation machinery, *Mol. Syst. Biol.* **9**(1) (2013). doi: 10.1038/msb.2012.73. http://msb.embopress.org/content/9/1/635.

25. J. J. Faith, B. Hayete, J. T. Thaden, I. Mogno, J. Wierzbowski, G. Cottarel, S. Kasif, J. J. Collins, and T. S. Gardner, Large-scale mapping and validation of escherichia coli transcriptional regulation from a compendium of expression profiles, *PLOS Biology.* **5**(1), 1–13 (2007). doi: 10.1371/journal.pbio.0050008. https://doi.org/10.1371/journal.pbio.0050008.

26. K. Deb, A. Pratap, S. Agarwal, and T. Meyarivan, A fast and elitist multiobjective genetic algorithm: Nsga-ii, *IEEE Trans. Evol. Comput.* **6**(2), 182–197 (2002). doi: 10.1109/4235.996017.

27. C. P. Burgess, I. Higgins, A. Pal, L. Matthey, N. Watters, G. Desjardins, and A. Lerchner, Understanding disentangling in β-VAE, *ArXiv e-prints* (2018).

28. I. Higgins, L. Matthey, X. Glorot, A. Pal, B. Uria, C. Blundell, S. Mohamed, and A. Lerchner, Early visual concept learning with unsupervised deep learning, *ArXiv e-prints* (2016).

Chapter 6

Deep Learning in Cheminformatics

Alessio Micheli* and Marco Podda[†]

*Department of Computer Science, University of Pisa,
Largo Bruno Pontecorvo 3, 56127 Pisa, Italy*
**alessio.micheli@unipi.it*
[†]*marco.podda@di.unipi.it*

Deep Learning (DL) is among the most promising modeling techniques to tackle hard Cheminformatics problems, whose solutions continue to have profound humanitarian and societal implications. This chapter covers two relevant applications of deep learning in the Cheminformatics landscape. The first is QSAR/QSPR analysis, which concerns the prediction of chemical properties or biological activity of molecular structures. Along with a review of the main results obtained through the use of deep learning in the field, we provide an overview of neural network models capable of processing structured data, such as sequences, trees, and graphs, which allow one to represent the rich structure of chemical data for predictive purposes. The second is *de novo* drug design, which concerns the generation of novel molecular structures with desired chemical properties to speed up the drug discovery pipeline. Here, we present the family of deep generative models for molecule generation, by which it is possible to learn the distribution of molecules from data and to generate novel chemical structures through sampling.

1. Introduction

The term *Cheminformatics* refers to the inter-disciplinary field that integrates studies in chemistry with the advancements of biological screening and computer-driven techniques to facilitate the development of novel chemical compounds. Cheminformatics is applied extensively in domains, such as environmental and biomedical sciences. Research in Cheminformatics encompasses technologies and problems from traditional chemistry and novel tools for data analysis, including library design and virtual screening, machine learning (ML) and data mining, molecular graphics, and simulation technology. In this chapter, we focus on its application to medicine, where Cheminformatics is applied to accelerate *drug discovery*, i.e., the process of designing and discovering candidate drug compounds with desired chemical properties (e.g., bioresponse). Drug discovery is part of the more complex process of *drug development*, whose aim is to bring new pharmaceuticals to the market. The possibility to expedite the discovery of new compounds has enormous scientific, humanitarian, and economic benefits. In fact, the development of pharmaceuticals that safely and effectively treat diseases or disorders is a costly process. In 2010, it was estimated that the development of a new prescription drug takes an average of 13 years at the cost of approximately 1.8 billion USD.[1] Moreover, there is a constant need to cope with new or evolving diseases, which require fast and effective responses from the medical community, increasing the urgency to accelerate the drug discovery cycle. Besides, research in the field is also motivated by the need to improve the percentage of compounds with real therapeutic value and to reduce undesirable side effects of drugs.

Drug discovery is a sequential process that goes from identifying a biological target for which treatment is needed to selecting a set of *lead* compounds that display activity against the target. This process requires to perform several biological *in vivo* or *in vitro* assays. However, these experiments have several drawbacks that make them unsuitable in many cases. For example, *in vivo* experimentation is considered controversial in some contexts (e.g., research and testing on animals). Moreover, in general, both *in vivo* and *in vitro* experiments are expensive, time-consuming, and infeasible on a large scale. Computational (or *in silico*) methodologies like ML and DL,[2] more recently, offer the opportunity to address all these issues simultaneously and are thus being increasingly studied by researchers in the field.[3-5] As two examples of drug discovery-related tasks where ML and DL have had a noticeable impact, we cite *Virtual Screening*,[6] i.e., the identification of active compounds against a target through computational methods, and *Absorption, Distribution, Metabolism,*

Excretion, Toxicity (ADMET) analysis,[7] which is required to filter out molecules with undesirable side effects.

To present applications of DL in Cheminformatics, and more specifically concerning the drug discovery landscape, we concentrate on two areas that directly impact the speed and reliability at which promising compounds are selected for further development. Specifically, we focus on *Quantitative Structure Activity/Property Relationship* (QSAR/QSPR) analysis, where a functional mapping from chemical structure to chemical properties is sought, and *de novo drug design*, where the functional mapping is reversed, i.e., the objective is to find an inverse relationship from desired chemical properties to suitable chemical structures. There are three reasons why we selected these two particular topics to talk about DL in drug discovery:

- Together, they cover the largest area in the field where DL methodologies have been applied extensively.
- While related, the two problems are fundamentally distinct: QSAR/QSPR analysis deals with *predictive* tasks, while *de novo* drug design is a *generative* problem. This represents an opportunity to give the reader a broad perspective on how different learning paradigms (supervised and unsupervised, respectively) can be tackled seamlessly with DL approaches.
- A specific motivation to choose QSAR/QSPR analysis is that, while QSAR/QSPR analysis has significantly been impacted by ML advancements, ML research has at the same time progressed thanks to QSAR/QSPR. An example is ML for structures, whose research was driven, among others, by the demanding challenges related to QSAR/QSPR analysis, such as handling chemical graphs. Neural networks for graphs[8] are an outstanding product of this symbiosis. These models have recently been rediscovered in the area of DL and are now actively applied in drug discovery research and Cheminformatics in general. Thus, specifically to QSAR/QSPR analysis, we choose this topic for its importance in the development of cutting-edge ML (and DL especially) research.

In the following section, we give a brief overview of the two topics of choice while we defer their extensive treatment to the subsequent sections.

1.1. QSAR/QSPR analysis

As we discussed previously, Cheminformatics can be used in drug discovery to help in making informed decisions about which compounds deserve a more in-depth analysis (i.e., a costly assay). Clearly, the availability of high-quality predictive models to test hypotheses prior to *in vivo* or *in vitro* experimentation is critical. For example, they could help select high-affinity ligands among a set of candidates, increasing the success rate of the following high-throughput screening experiments, or they could anticipate adverse health effects of pharmaceuticals, such as genotoxicity or carcinogenicity, without having to perform expensive ADMET assays.

QSAR/QSPR analysis is a relevant modeling methodology at the roots of such predictors. The underlying assumption of QSAR/QSPR is that chemical structure and chemical properties are related, and this relationship can be quantified. QSAR/QSPR analysis is especially useful when there is a collection of molecules with known properties or activity, but whose interactions (e.g., specifically to QSAR, between active molecules and their biological target) are not known in advance. Properties associated with these interactions are usually difficult to quantify precisely since they depend on a broad range of potential biological targets and mechanisms. To this end, QSAR/QSPR analysis methods allow learning a model of the structure–activity or structure–property relationship from a collection of known samples. The learned model can then be used to infer an estimation of the behavior of other similar compounds not yet measured. Since structure plays a primary role in QSAR/QSPR methods, the treatment of chemical structures (such as molecular graphs) is of fundamental importance, as detailed in Section 3. Various analytical tools from statistics and ML are used in QSPR/QSAR analysis, including predictive modeling (classification and regression), visualization, and exploratory data analysis (e.g., principal components and cluster analysis). Given their reasonably general nature of property/activity estimators, QSAR/QSPR models are used ubiquitously in many stages of drug discovery.

1.2. De novo drug design

While QSAR/QSPR methodologies address the problem of estimating chemical properties and/or potential activity of drug candidates, they cannot answer the question of how such drug candidates can be produced. During the early stages of drug discovery, once a specific biological target is identified, it is *screened* against a *library* of potentially active compounds, that is, each compound's activity against the target is checked with *in vitro* or *in silico* methods (e.g., with QSAR methods).

This practice is arguably limited by aspects such as the library size, the implicit bias in its assemblage, as well as non-strictly chemical factors like the technological and financial resources of the laboratories that perform the experiments. In contrast, screening against *chemical space*, i.e., the subset of all possible compounds with potential activity, is computationally infeasible, as its size is estimated to be of the order of 10^{60}.[9] Nonetheless, the selection of candidate drugs is critical to succeeding in subsequent stages of the drug development process (e.g., clinical trials): to avoid unexpected side effects such as toxicity, the candidate should be endowed with a specific set of chemical properties from the start. As such, strategies to find potentially active drug candidates outside of the ones found in screening libraries are researched continuously. The term *de novo* drug design[10] refers to a plethora of methodologies that seek to solve this problem by studying how to generate candidate drugs that meet a set of chemical desiderata.

The ultimate objective of *de novo* drug design is to "generate" (or more precisely, select) a drug-like compound out of chemical space by specification. Such specification contains the needed chemical properties that the candidate must meet in order to be, for example, active against the target and very unlikely to produce side effects such as adverse drug reactions. In this sense, QSAR/QSPR analysis is useful to identify the most important properties that make a molecule "druggable", while other ML or Computational Intelligence tools like generative models or genetic algorithms can be used to generate interesting compounds from chemical space.

1.3. *Overview of this chapter*

In Section 2, we recap some concepts of molecules that will be useful throughout. Moreover, we describe several ways to represent the information contained in molecules, such as molecular graphs, molecular fingerprints, SMILES strings, and other structured data. In Section 3, we dive into DL for QSAR/QSPR: in particular, we provide a historical perspective on how the field has evolved from using "flat" molecular representations to approaches that allow for the direct processing of the molecular structure. In Section 4, we discuss DL models for *de novo* molecular design by providing an overview of their architectural components and how they can be used effectively. Finally, in Section 5, we discuss where these approaches are headed in the near and not-so-near future.

2.   Molecules and Their Representation

In this section, we present some concepts about molecules that are functional to our discussion. In particular, we describe the various forms in which the information contained in molecules can be represented. It turns out that, while a graph can most expressively and concisely encode the molecular structure, other representations can be useful for the tasks presented in this chapter, such as molecular descriptors, molecular fingerprints, SMILES, and other structured representational forms.

2.1.   *Definitions*

A key concept in Cheminformatics is the notion of *compound*, a group of atoms held together by the electrostatic attraction among the electrons surrounding the nuclei of the atoms. Depending on how this attraction is originated, we distinguish *ionic* and *covalent* bonds. An ionic bond between two neutrally charged atoms is formed whenever one loses an electron and the other acquires it. The resulting charge imbalance creates attraction. Covalent bonds are instead formed whenever one or more pairs of electrons are shared between the two atoms. Compounds formed only by covalent bonds are called *molecules*. In our treatment of the subject, we focus on molecules rather than compounds; for colloquial reasons, we will sometimes slightly abuse their definitions and refer to molecules using both terms.

2.2.   *Chemical and structural formulae of molecules*

To convey information about the composition of a molecule, often its *chemical formula* is given. A chemical formula concisely reports the number of atoms constituting the molecule. For example, the chemical formula of aspirin is $C_9H_8O_4$, indicating that it contains nine Carbon (C) atoms, eight Hydrogen (H) atoms, and four Oxygen (O) atoms. However, molecules naturally contain several other information that chemical formulae cannot convey. A more comprehensive representation of the molecule is given by its *structural formula*, which represents the arrangement of atoms through a *molecular graph* (also called Lewis structure) in which atoms are nodes, and bonds are links between them. Usually, nodes in the molecular graph are labelled with the corresponding atom symbol or atomic number, while links are labelled with their bond type. The molecular graph can also represent a molecule's *stereochemistry*, i.e., its 3D structure, and several other useful information pieces.

2.3. *Molecular descriptors*

Molecules are associated with a large number of quantities, that can be assessed experimentally, called *molecular descriptors*. Descriptors can be broadly divided into three categories:

- *Experimental measurements*,[11] which quantify directly or by simulation the physical and chemical properties of atoms (or groups of atoms such as substituents), giving a partial description of the molecular structure; examples include polarization, molar refractivity, and hydrophobicity.
- *Theoretical descriptors*,[12–15] which are derived from the symbolic representation of a molecule. These descriptors encode morphological properties of the molecular graph (e.g., counting the number of paths of a given size or the number of rings); examples are topological and connectivity indices, number of rings, and many others.
- *Group contributions* such as *fragments*,[16] i.e., molecular substructures comprising individual atoms or simple atomic groups. Fragments usually coincide with portions of alkyl chains or with functional groups characterizing different classes of organic compounds.

For this chapter, we will limit our notions about descriptors to the concepts above. However, we refer the interested reader to the book by Todeschini *et al.*[17] for an extensive treatment of the subject.

2.4.　*Molecular fingerprints*

Molecular fingerprints[18, 19] are molecular representations that facilitate structural comparison among molecules and allow fast retrieval in large databases. Essentially, a fingerprint is a binary vector whose bits indicate the presence (1) or absence (0) of a particular structural feature. Depending on how these structural features are calculated, we distinguish *structural* and *hash* fingerprints. The bits of a structural fingerprint encode whether the molecule matches with a predefined set of substructures, that is, if these substructures are proper subgraphs of the molecular graph. Two examples are the Molecular ACCess System (MACCS) keys and the CACTVS substructure keys used in the PubChem database.

Hash fingerprints implement a different approach. To calculate one bit of a hash fingerprint, all linear substructures with N atoms rooted at a particular atom are enumerated (where N is usually chosen between 3 and 7). Each linear substructure is transformed into a string based on its structural properties and then turned into an integer i by passing it through a hash function. The corresponding ith position in the fingerprint bit vector is then set to 1. Prominent examples of this class of fingerprints are the Daylight Fingerprints and Extended Circular FingerPrints (ECFP).[20]

2.5.　*Other structural representations*

In Cheminformatics, many other representational forms of molecules have been developed, especially to represent some specific categories of molecules. For example, sugars are better represented using the Haworth projection, while the Fischer projection is useful to represent monosaccharides. One general-purpose representational form that is used in several Cheminformatics tasks is the Simplified Molecular Input Line Entry System (SMILES) encoding.[21] Essentially, this representation linearizes the molecular graph into a string of ASCII characters. A SMILES string is formed from a chemical graph by variations of the following general algorithm:

- First, all the hydrogen atoms are removed, and the molecular graph is transformed into a spanning tree by removing cycles (e.g., disconnecting rings). The disconnected bonds are marked with integers to allow their reconstruction.

- Then, the spanning tree is visited in depth-first order; each time a new atom is visited, the corresponding atomic symbol is added to the SMILES string. Tree branches are marked by parentheses.

Even though SMILES strings are essentially sequences of characters, they are generally considered structured representations of the molecular graph since they are constructed on its traversal. As a consequence of their construction method, SMILES strings are not unique, i.e., different SMILES strings can be associated with the same molecule by changing the root node of the spanning tree or the order in which cycles are broken. In fact, molecules with n atoms can be represented with at least n different SMILES strings. Indeed, most chemical packages include canonicalization algorithms that ensure that one molecule is associated with a unique SMILES string[22] (except few degenerate cases). Despite these issues, the SMILES encoding is widely adopted across the Cheminformatics landscape. For example, canonical SMILES are often used to index molecules in large databases.

Regarding other structured representations, labelled Directed Positional Acyclic Graphs (DPAGs) were employed in the pioneering studies that sought to predict QSAR/QSPR targets directly from the molecular structure (see Section 3.3). DPAG are also related to SMILES string: in fact, the tree traversed during the SMILES string construction is a sub-case of the DPAG type of data structure (DPAGs include the class of acyclic oriented graph where a total order is defined on the children of each node). As such, DPAGs can be considered an alternative way to represent molecules by sets of rules made in analogy to the SMILES approach. In Figure 1, we show several ways of representing molecules.

3. Deep Learning for QSAR/QSPR

This section presents QSAR and QSPR analysis, arguably the areas where ML has been applied more extensively. Our discussion follows a historical perspective, going from initial approaches that tackled these tasks without directly relying on molecular structure to first approaches for the direct treatment of structures for Cheminformatics, which progressively lead to methodologies for the treatment of

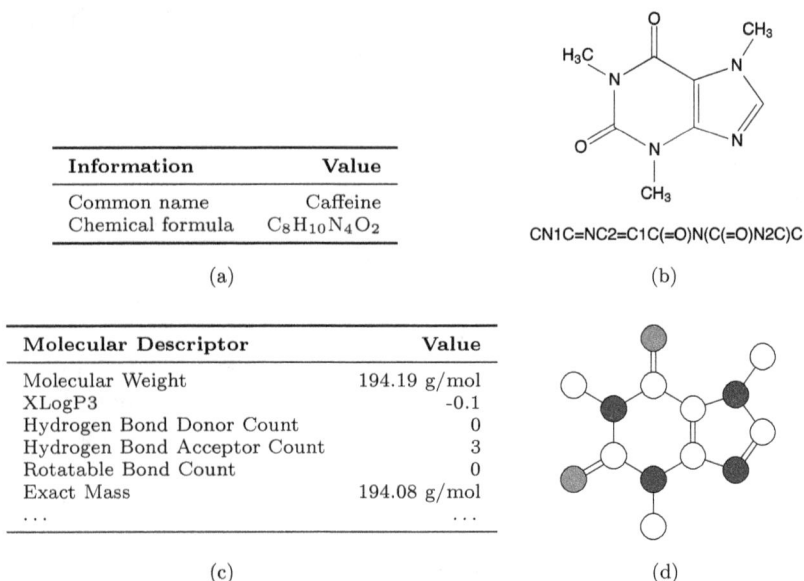

Information	Value
Common name	Caffeine
Chemical formula	$C_8H_{10}N_4O_2$

(a)

CN1C=NC2=C1C(=O)N(C(=O)N2C)C

(b)

Molecular Descriptor	Value
Molecular Weight	194.19 g/mol
XLogP3	-0.1
Hydrogen Bond Donor Count	0
Hydrogen Bond Acceptor Count	3
Rotatable Bond Count	0
Exact Mass	194.08 g/mol
...	...

(c)

(d)

Fig. 1. Different representational forms of the molecule of caffeine: (a) its chemical formula; (b) its 2D chemical representation subscripted by its SMILES encoding; (c) a subset of its possible molecular descriptors; (d) the corresponding molecular graph, where node shading indicates different atom types (N = dark grey, O = light grey, C = white), and double bonds are represented with two undirected edges connecting an atom pair. Note that hydrogen atoms are suppressed for a more concise representation, as their number can be inferred by valence rules.

general classes of graphs. For each step in our timeline, we describe traditional modeling approaches and their modern DL counterparts.

3.1. *Problem*

The basic assumption of QSPR/QSAR is that there exists a direct relationship between the chemical structure of a compound and its physical properties or its biological activity on a receptor, as shown schematically in Figure 2. Moreover, it is assumed that this relationship can be quantified. In other words, the objective of QSAR and QSPR approaches is to find a function $\mathcal{F}$ that satisfies the following relation:

$$\text{Property} = \mathcal{F}(\text{Structure}). \tag{6.1}$$

Structure $\mathcal{F}$ Property

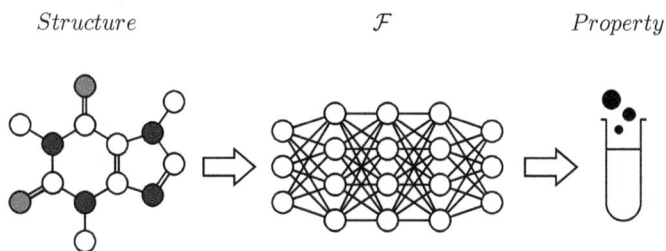

Fig. 2.   A schematic representation of the QSAR/QSPR analysis framework.

Here, Property represents an arbitrary chemical property of interest: for example, it might be activity against a biological target or other continuous quantities like solubility, polarizability, etc. Structure refers to any kind of representation that describes the molecular structure. To find an appropriate $\mathcal{F}$, two related sub-problems need to be solved sequentially:[23, 24]

- *feature representation*, i.e., finding an *encoding function* that maps the molecule into a set of features effective to solve the task;
- *mapping*, i.e., finding a (linear or nonlinear) *mapping function* that can predict a chemical or biological target of interest, given a proper encoding for a molecule.

3.2.   *Descriptor-based approaches*

The main problem in traditional approaches to QSPR/QSAR analysis is to find an effective numerical representation that retains the chemical and topological information present in chemical graphs and relates them to the target property or biological activity. This numerical representation is used by traditional mathematical models, e.g., multi-linear regression, to quantify the relationship of specific structural features of a compound with the target value.

Historically, a systematic approach to the treatment of structure–activity and structure–property relationships was mainly introduced by Hansch *et al.* in the 1960s,[25, 26] with the development of equations able to correlate the biological activity to numerical descriptors quantifying physical and chemical properties of biologically active compounds. Traditional approaches that follow this seminal approach are based on a case-dependent extraction of features, guided by domain knowledge, to obtain a set of suitable descriptors of the molecules (according to the taxonomy presented in Section 2.3), i.e., using a flat or vector/features-based representation of the problem domain (see Bianucci *et al.*[27] for a review). Then, these vectors are related to the target property, or biological activity by linear algebra or statistical techniques such as multiple linear regression, principal component analysis (PCA), partial least square (PLS),[28] or more powerful ML/Computational Intelligence techniques, such as genetic algorithms,[29, 30] feed-forward Neural Networks[31–33] (NNs) and support vector machines.[34, 35]

Even though NNs have been applied to descriptor-based representations since the 1990s, the first reported successful application of DL in QSAR/QSPR scenario dates back to 2012, where an ML research group without domain expertise in Cheminformatics won the Merck challenge on chemical compound activity using a multi-task Deep Neural Network (mt-DNN). A similar architecture to the winning solution was later described in 2015.[36] Since then, the mt-DNN paradigm has been extensively used to tackle QSAR/QSPR tasks.[37] It has been shown that massive mt-DNN architectures for QSAR perform in general better than single task ones[38] and also better than other ML algorithms such as random forests.[39] Among other architectures used for QSAR/QSPR tasks, Deep Belief Networks,[40, 41] Deep Autoencoders[42] (AEs), and Convolutional Neural Networks[43] have been used with success.

3.2.1. *Limitations*

Traditional, descriptor-based approaches to QSAR/QSPR problems break the feature representation problem described above in two sub-tasks: (1) finding the "right" information to capture structural aspects of the molecule that are relevant to the predictive task; (2) the encoding of such information in numerical form, which can be processed by a learning algorithm. Although this can be useful in many situations, the applicability of such approaches is limited whenever:

- Chemical descriptors are not available. For example, there are no known descriptors for inorganic metal complexes.
- The number and type of descriptors needed to solve a task are not known *a priori*. This might produce two opposite side effects: using

too few descriptors might result in poor predictive performance; conversely, using too many could result in unnecessarily noisy data, making learning difficult.

While these limitations affect the applicability of descriptor-based approaches on a specific task, a more general shortcoming that limits their use *across* tasks is that descriptors are not target-invariant. In other words, different tasks require their own specific sets of descriptors, which in turn means that whenever the target changes, a novel, complete and relevant set of descriptors must be chosen through trial and error, typically requiring some form of expert knowledge. Note that even resorting to feature selection approaches does not entirely solve the issue as the initial set of descriptors could not include the relevant information for the QSAR/QSPR analysis at hand. Besides these disadvantages, that call for adopting more flexible modeling strategies, traditional approaches leverage a somewhat underspecified representation of molecules. In fact, the structural richness of a molecule is more clearly and naturally conveyed by its molecular graph. These motivations ultimately lead to the development of a class of models to learn a direct mapping from the molecular graph to the target of interest.

3.3. *Recursive neural network-based approaches*

Pioneering approaches in the field of ML on graph data date back to 1997[44] (see the references therein for more details), where an architecture for the processing of structured data called *generalized recursive neurons* was first presented. A general framework for learning tree-structured data[45] (both from a connectionist and probabilistic perspective) was introduced in the following year, along with the first Cheminformatics application.[46] The two first-mentioned contributions describe what is now known as the Recursive Neural Network (RecNN) model. In essence, RecNNs "unfold" an NN over a structure of interest. A RecNN operates on each node of a tree (or DPAG) data structure according to this formulation:

$$h_n = f(x_n, h_{S(n)}), \tag{6.2}$$

$$y_n = g(x_n, h_n), \tag{6.3}$$

where f is an NN, g is a mapping (linear or nonlinear, generally another NN) to the output space, n is a generic tree node, x_n is its associated attribute (e.g., for molecules, its atom type), and h is used to denote encoding vectors, whose purpose is to keep track of the sub-structures visited so far. In practice, in Eq. (6.2), the encoding vector of a node is updated using f, according to its local information x_n and the encoding of the sub-tree $S(n)$, obtained by the set of encodings for the roots of the sub-trees of n. The node information and the updated encoding can be mapped by the function g to the output space, producing an output value y_n, as shown in Eq. (6.3). It is worthwhile to note that the functions f and g can be interpreted in the framework introduced in Section 3.1: the f function corresponds to the realization of the *encoding* function over a given structured representation of a molecule and g to the *mapping* function. To compute an encoding vector of the whole structure, the outputs at each node can be aggregated together (e.g., summed), or, more frequently, the encoding at the root node of the tree can be taken instead. The process is shown in Figure 3(b).

In Cheminformatics and QSAR/QSPR modeling particularly, the advent of RecNNs brought about a true shift in perspective. Different from traditional methods, the input of a RecNN is the varying-size

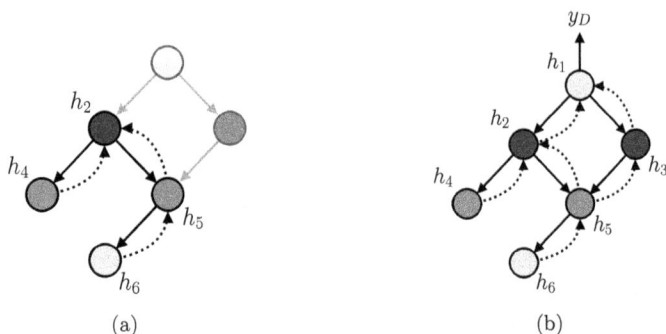

(a)   (b)

Fig. 3. The processing of a DPAG using a RecNN. Note that the attribute values (the x in Eq. (6.2)) are color-coded. Solid arrows denote DPAG dependencies, while dashed arrows denote encoding calculations. (a) An intermediate step of computation is shown, highlighting the *causality* principle. To compute the encoding of node 2, only the encoding vectors of nodes 4, 5, and 6 can be used since they are already computed. The encoding of the remaining nodes cannot be accessed by the model yet, and it is drawn shaded. (b) A situation at the end of structure traversal is shown, where the root node (1) encoding has been computed. At this point, the root node can be used to compute a whole DPAG-specific output y_D, i.e., a property or activity of interest for QSPR or QSAR, respectively.

structured representation of the molecules. Moreover, RecNNs do not require to solve the feature representation and mapping problems separately: instead, the encoding to numerical representations of chemical structures and the downstream regression or classification functions can be learned jointly (i.e., the functions f and g of Eqs. (6.2) and (6.3) are trained together as part of the same RecNN model). In other words, RecNNs can optimize a direct mapping from the structured domain input space to the activity/property output space. Finally, they learn *adaptively*, i.e., from data examples. This entails that a RecNN assigns numerical codes to chemical structures, which are optimized according to the predictive task. As such, similarities among molecules or the "topological index" computed by the internal layer are adapted by the model to the problem at hand.

Interestingly, RecNNs are also supported by distinguished theoretical results that support the generality of the encoding and characterize the kind of functions they can learn. Specifically, universal approximation theorems showing that RecNNs can approximate arbitrarily well any function from labeled trees to real values[47] and from labelled DPAGs to real values[48] have been proved.

The effectiveness of RecNNs has been assessed in a variety of radically different QSPR/QSAR problems, for instance, QSAR analysis for the prediction of the non-specific activity (affinity) towards the benzodiazepine/GABA receptor of a set of benzodiazepines[23, 27] and the prediction of A1 adenosine receptor ligands affinity towards the receptor,[49] QSPR analyses of alkanes,[27] thermodynamical properties of small molecules,[24] ionic liquids,[50] properties of polymers[51, 52] and copolymers,[53] and finally, for toxicity prediction.[54] In all these settings, RecNNs demonstrated competitive results in terms of accuracy with *ad hoc* traditional methods, paving the way for more advanced approaches that exploit the molecular structure in its general graph form. More recently, RecNNs have been applied to predict aqueous solubility in molecules[55] and in toxicity prediction and blood–brain barrier penetration.[56]

3.3.1. *Limitations*

The main limitation of RecNNs is the underlying assumption of causality, which implies that all the encodings of children nodes must be available to obtain the encoding of a node (see Figure 3(a)). This implies that encoding calculations must happen in order and constrains the applicability of RecNNs to restricted classes of graphs, where this order can be superimposed, such as trees or DPAGs (unless mutual dependencies are allowed considering dynamical systems, as discussed in the following section).

3.4. *Deep graph network-based approaches*

The study of efficient solutions to the treatment of general classes of graphs has been addressed by different authors. One recursive approach is to define a dynamical system based on contractive mappings that can be solved by relaxation techniques,[57] allowing one to treat cyclic graphs by a recursive model assuring the convergence by applying contractive constraints. A different approach, called NN4G,[58] is based on a constructive contextual processing for fairly general graph structures. In contrast to previous NNs for structures, this seminal approach relaxes the recursive assumption of causality, pioneering the current line of deep/convolutional NNs for graphs. Indeed, the methodology used in NN4G can be interpreted in terms of convolutional NNs. In particular, this can be seen if one constrains the local receptive field to the local topology of each node rather than to the local 2D kernel matrix used in image processing tasks. Approaches stemming from NN4G have been recently unified under the name of *Deep Graph Networks*[8] (DGNs). A simple formulation of how a DGN processes a graph G (slight variations are possible) at layer $\ell = 1, \ldots, L$ is as follows:

$$h_v^\ell = f^\ell(h_v^{\ell-1}, \sum_{u \in \mathcal{C}(v)} h_u^{\ell-1}), \qquad (6.4)$$

$$h_G^\ell = \sum_{v \in \mathcal{V}(G)} g(h_v^\ell), \qquad (6.5)$$

where g is any linear or nonlinear mapping, f is an NN, v and u are used to denote nodes belonging to the node set $\mathcal{V}(G)$, h indicates a context vector (again an encoding vector), and $\mathcal{C}(v)$ is the set of nodes connected to v in the graph. By convention, h_v^0 is a vector of node-specific features (e.g., atom type). In practice, in Eq. (6.4), the encoding of all the neighboring nodes $\mathcal{C}(v)$ is first aggregated together (in this case, with a sum); then, the encoding of the node is updated

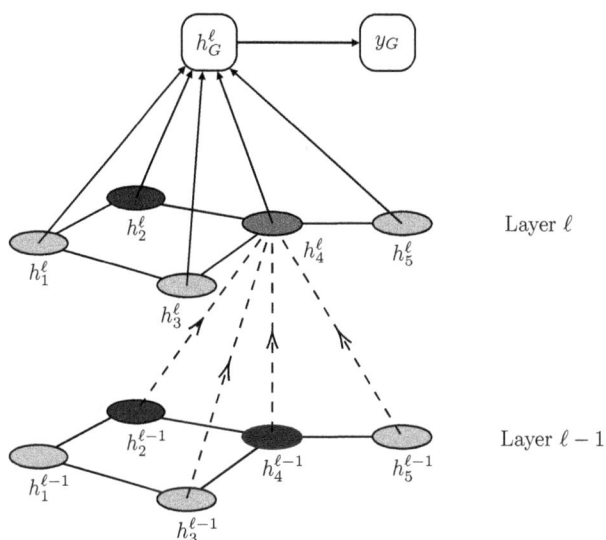

Fig. 4. The main mechanisms of DGNs on an example graph, where the node encodings are color-coded. Focusing on node 4, we see that it receives the encoded context from the previous layer (indicated by dashed lines), from itself and its neighboring nodes 2, 3, and 5. The same mechanism is applied to all nodes in the graph (not shown). Note how the encoding (the color) of h_4^ℓ is changed after the update. Finally, the contexts of nodes at layer ℓ are aggregated to form a layer-specific graph representation h_G^ℓ, which is used to compute an output y_G, e.g., biological activity or a chemical property associated with the graph.

by f using its current encoding and the aggregated encoding of its neighbors. The updated encoding vector becomes the input of the subsequent DGN layer, and the process is repeated for each of the L layers (realizing a context spreading over the graph[58]). Finally, as shown in Eq. (6.5), a layer-specific representation of the entire graph h_G^ℓ is computed by aggregating (e.g., with sum) the encodings obtained for each node. In Figure 4, this process is shown visually for two layers.

The line of research on DGNs has been rediscovered by the DL community in 2015. Since then, it has been used with success in many QSAR/QSPR tasks. One interesting application of DGNs has been to learn the so-called "neural fingerprints" which succeeded in predicting solubility and drug efficacy.[59] A DGN-based approach reportedly obtained competitive results with respect to multi-task deep networks, with way less thorough hyper-parameter tuning in several activity tasks.[60] More applications include log-partition coefficient prediction,[61] toxicity and adverse drug reaction prediction,[62, 63] and ADME analysis.[64] Finally, DGNs have also been combined with Neural Turing Machines,[65] outperforming non-DL competitors in nine activity prediction tasks.[66] Sun *et al.*[67] provide an extensive review of the application of DGNs to drug discovery.

4. Deep Learning for *De Novo* Drug Design

This section addresses *de novo* drug design, i.e., the production of suitable candidate molecules (*leads*) for drug discovery and development purposes. In Section 3, we discussed methodologies to predict chemical properties or biological activity from molecular structure. We focus on the design of molecules whose structure and chemical properties match an input specification. In Cheminformatics, this corresponds to the symmetrical problem, that QSAR/QSPR methodologies try to solve, known as the *inverse QSAR/QSPR* problem. Our goal in this discussion is not to review published methodologies (for which we have surveys such as Refs. 68 and 69); instead, we aim to provide the reader with the knowledge needed to read the current literature with a critical eye.

4.1. *Problem*

We define the inverse QSAR/QSPR problem as finding a function $\mathcal{F}^{-1}$ that satisfies the following:

$$\text{Structure} = \mathcal{F}^{-1}(\text{Property}), \qquad (6.6)$$

where we used the same names and the inverse function of Eq. (6.1) to emphasize the relationship with the forward QSAR/QSPR problems. A visual scheme of this concept can be seen in Figure 5.

The output space in *de novo* drug design is the whole chemical space: its sheer size implies that to solve an inverse QSAR/QSPR problem, finding a solution to the problem by enumerating all possible molecules is computationally infeasible. Hence, more sophisticated and "smart" search strategies are required.

Property $\mathcal{F}^{-1}$ Structure

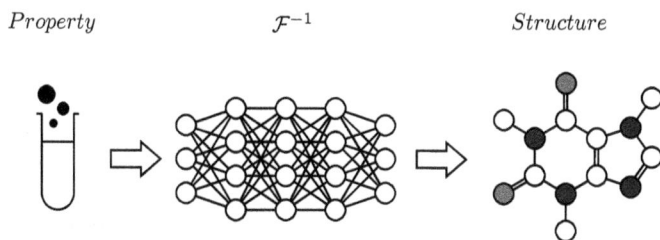

Fig. 5. A schematic representation of the *de novo* drug design. The inverse function $\mathcal{F}^{-1}$ emphasizes the relationship with QSAR/QSPR analysis.

From a probabilistic perspective, the problem is ascribable to learning a conditional distribution over the chemical space. This entails solving two non-trivial sub-problems:

- *Generation*, i.e., learning a meaningful and easy-to-sample distribution over the chemical space. The DL approach to this problem is to use Deep Generative Models (DGMs),[2] that is, models that parameterize a sampling process via deep neural networks.
- *Optimization*, i.e., biasing generation towards desired molecules. This requires applying techniques that allow the sampler to be more likely to choose useful molecules instead of useless ones.

DGMs have shown impressive results in generating images, sound, and text. In the case of molecules, however, there is an added layer of complexity due to the sample space's intrinsic nature. First, chemical space is a discrete object whose mathematical treatment is difficult. This implies that gradient-based optimization is not viable in most cases. Second, chemical space is sparse: a small move in chemical space (i.e., removing one atom from a molecule) might result in sampling a completely useless molecule. Third, conditioning over a set of desired molecules means that most points of chemical space will have zero probability, and only an infinitesimal part of it will actually contain interesting molecules. These reasons make generation and optimization two extremely challenging tasks.

4.2. *Architectures*

In inverse QSAR/QSPR, four DGM architectures are used: Recurrent Neural Networks[70] (RNNs), Variational Autoencoders[71]

(VAEs), Generative Adversarial Networks[72] (GANs), and Adversarial Autoencoders[73] (AAEs). For each of them, we give an intuitive view of their inner workings.

4.2.1. *Recurrent neural networks*

RNNs are a learning model explicitly designed to handle variable-length sequences. An RNN is an NN unfolded over the elements of a sequence (and in fact, they are a special case of RecNN applied to linear structures). To keep global information about the sequence, RNNs use an encoding vector updated after each element is processed. However, vanilla RNNs suffer from the vanishing and exploding gradient problems,[74] which limit their applicability to sequences with a short number of elements. For this reason, specific RNN variants designed to address these shortcomings, such as Long Short-Term Memory (LSTM) and Gated Recurrent Unit (GRU) networks, are often used instead. Here, we will use the term RNN to refer to any of these two variants for brevity. Although RNNs are a general framework that can be used to solve very different tasks on sequences, we focus our attention on *many-to-many* tasks, where the network returns an output for each sequence element. In this context, RNNs can be trained with "teacher forcing"[75] to maximize the probability of the training data, which corresponds to the following objective function:

$$\mathcal{L}_{\mathrm{RNN}} = -\sum_{t=1}^{n} \log g(f(x_t, h_{t-1})), \qquad (6.7)$$

where n is the length of the sequence, f is the unfolded NN, x_t is the generic sequence element at time step t, h_{t-1} is the encoding vector at time step $t-1$ (by convention, h_0 is usually a zero vector), and g is an output NN.

4.2.2. *Variational autoencoders*

A VAE is an encoder–decoder architecture where a set of latent variables models the latent space. The model jointly learns the posterior over the latent space through an encoder that transforms a data point into a latent vector and a generative model of the data through a decoder that performs the inverse mapping from latent space to data space. Precisely, VAEs optimize the following lower bound of the log-likelihood of the data:

$$\mathcal{L}_{\text{VAE}} = \mathbb{E}_{z \sim q(z|x)}[\log p(x \mid z)] - \text{KL}[q(z \mid x) \| p(z)], \qquad (6.8)$$

where x is a data point (a molecule) and z is its latent representation. For example, z can be the encoding vector of an RNN in the case of SMILES or the graph representation computed by a DGN. In Eq. (6.8), the leftmost term is the expectation of the decoder $p(x \mid z)$ under the posterior learned by the encoder $q(z \mid x)$, also known as the decoder's *reconstruction error*. The rightmost term is the Kullback–Leibler (KL) divergence of the posterior and some easy-to-sample prior distribution $p(z)$. It is a *regularization term* that forces the learned encoding distribution to be similar to the prior. If the prior is an isotropic Gaussian, this term is given in closed form.

4.2.3. *Generative adversarial networks*

GANs are implicit generative models, i.e., they learn to sample from a data distribution without explicitly optimizing a log-likelihood term in the objective function. In other words, they only learn a method to sample from the target distribution. A GAN is composed of two (usually deep) networks optimized jointly: a *generator*, which maps points sampled from a prior to data points, and a *discriminator* trained to distinguish between samples coming from the true data distribution and samples coming from the generator. The discriminator tries to maximize the ability to distinguish between real and generated samples, while the generator tries to "fool" the discriminator by producing realistic-looking samples. GANs optimize the following *min–max* objective function until a Nash equilibrium is found:

$$\mathcal{L}_{\text{GAN}} = \min_{G} \max_{D} \mathbb{E}_{x \sim p_{\text{data}}(x)}[\log D(x)] + \mathbb{E}_{z \sim p(z)}[\log(1 - D(G(z)))], \qquad (6.9)$$

where G is the generator, D is the discriminator, $p_{\text{data}}(x)$ is the true data distribution, and $p(z)$ is the prior distribution.

4.2.4. *Adversarial autoencoders*

AAEs are a hybrid model between standard AEs and GANs. Basically, they consist of an AE where regularization is achieved through *adversarial learning.* More specifically, AAEs optimize the following objective function:

$$\mathcal{L}_{\text{AAE}} = \mathbb{E}_{z \sim q(z|x)}[\log p(x \mid z)] - \text{AL}(q(z \mid x), p(z)), \qquad (6.10)$$

where the first term is the reconstruction error (as in a VAE) and the second term is a GAN that uses the encoder as a generator, whose discriminator is trained to distinguish between latent codes produced by the encoder and samples drawn from a prior $p(z)$. The model is trained alternating between standard AE training and GAN training.

4.3. *Generation*

Here, we focus on the sub-problem of generation. As described in Section 4.1, this problem entails learning a properly specified *generative process*, i.e., a parameterized function by which a molecule is generated. In the case of likelihood-based generative models such as VAEs and AAEs, this function is implemented by the decoder, while in the case of GANs, it is implemented by the generator. The output of the generative process depends on the representation that the models are tasked to output. In particular, we examine two possible approaches: generating the SMILES string of the molecule or generating the molecular graph. The latter can be further split into learning a set of matrices associated with the molecular graph or generating the molecular graph through a sequence of *graph transformations*.

4.3.1. *SMILES-based generation*

SMILES strings are essentially sequences of ASCII characters. As such, a dataset of molecules represented as SMILES strings can be used to learn the corresponding *language model*, i.e., a probability distribution over sequences of SMILES characters. To be used by the RNN, SMILES strings need to be encoded in numerical form: for this, they are first decomposed into *tokens*: in the case of SMILES, each token is a single ASCII character. Then, a vocabulary $\mathcal{V}$ of unique tokens is constructed from the dataset. The ith token in the vocabulary is encoded as a one-hot vector of size $|\mathcal{V}|$, where all positions are 0 except position i set to 1. Thus, SMILES strings from a training dataset become sequences of one-hot vectors, whose likelihood is maximized during training by the RNN.

Generative process: After the language model is learned, the RNN can be sampled to generate SMILES strings character by character, i.e., the character sampled at time step t becomes the input at time step $t+1$. This generative process is called *auto-regressive* since the output at step t depends on all the previous outputs at steps $< t$.

4.3.2. *Matrix-based generation of molecular graphs*

Matrix-based approaches generate the information of the molecule in matrix form.[76,77] To do so, the molecular graphs in a dataset need to be encoded as matrices. For illustrative purposes, we consider the case where a training molecule is represented with three different matrices:

- a squared matrix $\mathbf{A} \in \mathbb{R}^{N \times N}$, where position (i, j) is 1 iff there is a bond between the ith and jth atoms;
- a matrix $\mathbf{N} \in \mathbb{R}^{N \times A}$, where the ith row is a one-hot vector that specifies the ith atom type;
- a matrix $\mathbf{E} \in \mathbb{R}^{N^2 \times B}$, whose kth row is a one-hot vector that specifies the bond type of the kth pair of atoms (with the convention that it is a zero vector if the kth pair is not connected).

Above, N is the number of atoms of the largest graph in the dataset, A is the number of atom types, and B is the number of bond types (we assume this is the only information we have about atoms and bonds for simplicity). After the molecules are encoded in such form, the model can be trained to minimize a suitable objective function between the training matrices and the network's outputs. Standard objective functions for this task are maximum likelihood or various forms of matrix similarity.

Generative process: To generate a molecular graph, one first needs to sample the adjacency matrix entry by entry. Once the graph structure is determined, the two remaining matrices can be sampled according to different setups. For example, one could first sample bond types and then sample atom types conditioned on bond information.

4.3.3. *Incremental generation of molecular graphs*

Recently, a novel class of generative processes has been presented.[78] Briefly, graph generation is formulated as a sequence of actions that progressively transform an initially empty graph into the desired one. This assumes that molecules are first encoded as graphs and then into sequences of actions. The objective function is a composite loss that maximizes the likelihood of the sequence of actions in the dataset.

Generative process: Since each decision taken to transform the graph is implemented as an NN with probabilistic outputs, sampling a graph amounts to sampling hard decisions from all the architectural components. One crucial step to take into account is that each decision is conditioned on the graph's state up to that point. Binary decisions (e.g., add one more node) can be sampled from sigmoidal outputs, while multinomial decisions (e.g., which bond type to assign to an edge) can be sampled from the corresponding categorical distributions. Finally, note that this generative process is auto-regressive because the actions taken at one step depend on the actions taken at the previous steps. An example of one step of the generative process is shown in Figure 6.

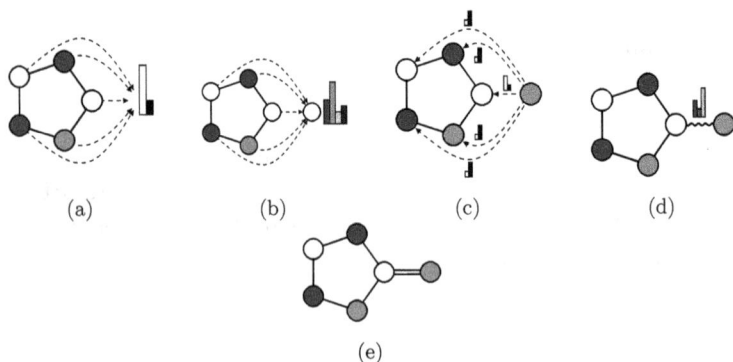

Fig. 6.   One step of incremental graph generation. (a) It is decided whether to add an atom based on the current graph state; (b) the new atom is initialized using the current state, and its type is sampled; (c) it is decided how and to which atoms the new atom will be connected; (d) a bond type for each new bond is sampled. In (e), the graph obtained after the incremental step is shown.

4.3.4. *Discussion*

Generating molecules as SMILES strings was the first successful application of DGMs to the task of molecular generation. With SMILES, generation is fast and uses language models, which are now very thoroughly studied and optimized by the DL community. However, SMILES generators often display problems as regards *chemical validity*,[79] i.e., they struggle with long-term dependencies (such as opened parentheses to close) and tend to produce invalid molecules. Indeed, much of the research regarding these methods is based on finding useful heuristics to keep high validity rates on generated molecules. Some attempts include making the model learn the grammar rules of SMILES instead of the language[80] or use techniques borrowed from the world of compilers like attribute grammars and syntax-directed translation.[81] Recently, methods based on SMILES sub-strings, rather than characters, have started to be developed.[82,83]

Graph-based methods are advantageous because they are based on the most natural form of molecular representation. It has also been shown that they are more likely to produce valid molecules than SMILES-based methods.[84,85] However, they also have shortcomings: one is that they are considerably slower to train and sample from than SMILES-based approaches. They also tend to focus on restricted subsets of chemical space, yielding molecules that lack diversity.[68] Matrix-based methods, in particular, cannot generalize to molecular graphs of arbitrary size (since the maximum size of the adjacency and node feature matrices is fixed in advance).[76] Incremental-based methods mitigate many issues of their matrix-based counterparts, even though they are still susceptible to higher duplicate rates compared to SMILES-based approaches.[68]

For all these three methodologies, the generative process is not permutation-invariant. SMILES strings are based on a fixed order induced by a particular DPAG. In matrix-based representations, shuffling the columns of the molecular graph's adjacency matrix or changing the sequence of graph transformations does not result in general in the same graph being generated. For these reasons, one of the most critical challenges in the field is how to design generative strategies that are invariant to permutations. Recently, the first attempt at solving the problem has been presented.[86]

4.3.5. *Sampling categorical distributions*

As we have seen, generating molecules requires sampling of multiple probability distributions. In the case of Bernoulli random variables (such as the outputs of sigmoid units), sampling corresponds to rounding to the nearest integer. In the case of categorical distributions, a straightforward approach is *greedy sampling*,[79] where the most probable token is chosen at each step. However, this might not be ideal in every situation, for example, RNNs are known to output very peaked probability distributions, resulting in low diversity among samples. *Simulated annealing* can be used to sample from the tails of the distribution more often. Other alternatives to greedy sampling have also been proposed in the literature.[83, 87, 88]

4.3.6. *Evaluation metrics*

There are several metrics under which the molecular generators can be evaluated. In principle, the ideal generator should possess the following qualities: it should output chemically valid molecules, i.e., molecules that make sense from a chemical point of view; it should output novel molecules, that is, molecules not present in the training dataset; it should output unique molecules, i.e., it should avoid repeating the same molecular patterns over and over. The last desired feature is directly related to the concept of diversity, which conveys a quite contrived notion. Ideally, generated molecules should be (i) structurally "different" enough from training molecules to span the largest possible chemical subspace and at the same time (ii) structurally "close" enough to possess similar interesting chemical properties. More precisely, the qualities mentioned above can be measured by the following metrics:

- *Validity*: This involves the ratio of chemically valid molecules out of the total number of generated molecules. In general, this metric can be assessed by validating the SMILES string associated with the molecule with third-party SMILES checkers.
- *Novelty*: This includes the percentage of "unseen" molecules generated out of the total number of molecules in the training set.
- *Uniqueness*: This includes the number of unique (not duplicated) molecules out of the total number of generated molecules.

- *Diversity*: As diversity is a complex concept, it cannot be measured by a single metric but rather by a set of them. *Internal* diversity can be measured by applying a distance function on all the possible pairs out of the set of generated molecules and averaging the result. Conversely, *external* diversity measures the diversity of each molecule in the generated set against its nearest neighbor in the training set. One distance function usually employed for this evaluation is the Tanimoto distance, a bitwise distance function defined over the molecular fingerprints associated with a molecule. Another recent metric is the Frechét ChemNet Distance,[89] which compares training and generates set by first feeding them to a pre-trained Deep Neural Network (ChemNet[90]) for property prediction and then comparing the statistics computed on the respective activation vectors at the penultimate layer.

Other useful evaluation metrics are based on the comparison of the distributions of chemical properties between the training set and the generated set, for example, quantifying their Kullback–Leibler or Wasserstein distances.

4.4. *Optimization*

We now shift our focus to the optimization problem described in Section 4.1. Specifically, we describe the methods to bias the generative process towards sampling molecules endowed with desired chemical properties, in other words, how to condition the generative process. Then, we review some standard techniques to accomplish this goal, highlighting their strengths and limitations as we discuss them. We conclude the discussion by presenting useful metrics that can be used to assess the results of the optimization.

4.4.1. *Conditional generation*

Conditional generation refers to the addition of vectors of desired chemical properties to the inputs of the generative process. In the case of discrete properties (e.g., the thresholded activity of the generated molecule against a biological receptor), these vectors are one-hot encoded. Conditional generation can be applied straightforwardly to any deep generative architecture. Regarding RNNs, the initial context vector can be (or can be concatenated to) the conditioning vector. For VAEs[91-93] and AAEs,[94] the same mechanism can be applied to the latent vector that initializes the decoder. In GANs,[95] the same principles can be applied to the vector sampled from the prior. Conditioning has been shown to be effective only in cases where the desired chemical property is discrete and one-hot encoded.[91] An undesirable drawback of this technique is that the data distribution and the distribution of the conditioning vectors are not independent. Another issue with this kind of approach is that the model can incur in low novelty scores because it tends to place more "emphasis" on the conditioning vector rather than the latent vector, as doing so solves an easier task.[68]

4.4.2. *Latent space optimization*

Latent space optimization methods optimize the desired chemical properties of molecules directly in latent space. As such, they require an encoder–decoder architecture. Basically, the model is jointly trained with a predictor that takes points in latent space and predicts their chemical properties.[84] This forces the latent space to be organized not only by structural similarity but also by chemical property. Multiple optimization is enabled by training multiple predictors for different chemical properties; however, multiple optimization usually causes unstable training, as each predictor tries to minimize its objective function. When learned properly, the latent space can be used to perform tasks such as linear interpolation between molecules[79] or latent optimization using gradient ascent.[84] One downside of this technique is that there is no known way to enforce chemical validity on latent space directly; thus, these models tend to produce invalid molecules unless proper countermeasures are taken at sampling time. For SMILES-based generation, this issue has been partially solved by enforcing validity with syntax-aware molecular representations[81] or by using constrained Bayesian optimization.[96] In graph-based iterative methods, masking is often used to prevent undesired graph transformations.[85,86]

4.4.3. *Reinforcement learning*

Reinforcement learning[97] approaches are based on training the DGM decoder as an *agent* that performs *actions* on the molecule. Each action moves the agent in a novel *state*. The state is evaluated by a *value function*, while the action is given a *reward* or *penalty*. The objective is to find an optimal *policy* (sequence of actions) that yields maximal reward: as the process is iterated, the sampler learns policies that maximize the expected reward. Actions are specific to the kind of generative process used: for SMILES strings, an action could mean appending one token to the string being generated.[98] Alternatively, in graph-based iterative generation, it could correspond to performing a certain transformation.[99] The reward function is usually related to the chemical properties that are being optimized or to favor chemically valid molecules rather than invalid ones.[98, 100] Multiple optimization can be achieved by combining several metrics into a weighted reward function. Reinforcement learning is usually applied to SMILES language models without latent space[101] and GANs.[77, 102] One problem with these approaches is that even though they tend to generate molecules with optimized properties, they often lack structural coherence compared to the training molecules.

4.4.4. *Transfer learning*

Transfer learning builds on the idea that a model can be *pre-trained* on a reasonably general task with a large dataset to learn task-agnostic features. Once the model is learned, it is *fine-tuned* (specialized) on a task of interest.[103] Thus, the fine-tuning task does not need large quantities of data, as most of the features were already learned during pre-training. In particular, auto-encoding tasks have been used for pre-training.[83] This technique fits *de novo* generative scenarios where many molecules are available for training, but only a handful of them have the desired characteristics. Transfer learning is almost always beneficial, and it is often used in combination with other optimization methods. However, pre-training requires extensive datasets (not always available) and a considerable amount of computational resources.

4.4.5. *Evaluation metrics*

To evaluate performances on the optimization task, one intuitive metric to compute is *success*, that is, the ratio of molecules in the generated set that displays the desired characteristics given as input. Regarding biological activity, knowing exactly whether the generated molecule is active or not requires lab experiments or clinical trials. In these cases, the ground truth activity is approximated by a pre-trained QSAR/QSPR predictor. For the optimization of continuous properties, an often employed performance metric is *improvement*, which measures the average increase or decrease of the property obtained in the generated set compared to the training set. Note that success and improvement should be evaluated after having cleaned the generated set from duplicates to avoid biased results.

5. Conclusions

This chapter has discussed two key applications of Cheminformatics for drug discovery: QSAR/QSPR analysis and *de novo* drug design. QSAR/QSPR analysis was presented from a historical perspective, which examined the progressive development of ML models for the treatment of structured data, up to describing the possibility of predicting the activity/property values directly from the chemical graphs. These techniques are now at the forefront of DL. Moreover, we presented *de novo* drug design under the lens of DGMs, which are considered by many as the key technology that will lead to the next innovative breakthrough in the field. As computational methods applied in this field, QSAR/QSPR analysis and *de novo* drug design substantially contribute to the process of drug discovery and development, providing a series of advantages with respect to *in vivo* and *in vitro* experimentation. As examples, we recall how using *in silico* methods such as Virtual Screening and computational ADMET analysis can provide accurate predictions, or useful insights, of many interesting chemical properties of molecules. This, in turn, allows researchers to understand the behavior of newly discovered compounds as they process through the drug development pipeline. These advantages are measured in terms of economic value and carry profound humanitarian implications, implying that constant progress is mandatory. Despite being strictly related, these two topics are sharply distinct as regards the challenges to be addressed to make drug discovery more efficient and effective.

QSAR/QSPR analysis is a mature field that has been employed since the 1960s as a tool to assess the chemical properties of molecules from known samples. The main challenges in this field relate to the development of even more powerful models and how to improve the predictive performance of already existing models to improve their reliability. One other related challenge is interpretability: we expect future modeling approaches to be interpretation-driven to improve the quality of decision-making driven by QSAR/QSPR analysis. The last 20 years of the history of QSAR/QSPR analysis have undoubtedly been tied with ML, as the inherent problem of handling molecular graphs was a significant promoter of the furtherance that lead to advanced ML models for structures. Similarly, the increased interaction between the DL on graphs and QSAR/QSPR analysis communities might drive an intensive innovation process, resulting in a mutual benefit.

De novo design is a relatively younger research area, in particular as regards the use of DL. In light of the recent successes obtained by DGMs on various tasks such as image generation, research in their application to inverse QSAR/QSPR problems has seen an unprecedented increase. Nonetheless, there is much room for improvement. Among the many aspects that need further study, the ones on which research should focus in the short term are the development of novel generative processes of molecular graphs and the improvement of optimization techniques to achieve a more focused generation towards desired molecular properties. In the medium-long term, innovation may also come from the development of novel DGMs. Recently, one promising candidate to be the next breakthrough methodology in this research field is the generative model based on normalizing flows.[104] We anticipate that their application to inverse QSAR/QSPR problems will see a rapid increase in the years to come.

The power of DL is opening new possibilities as regards novel fields of application not only in these two areas but also more generally in Cheminformatics. Among these, we cite biomaterial design and self-assembly molecules. At the crossroad between Cheminformatics and Medicine, one research area where the application of DL is gaining momentum concerns the integrated analysis of genomic, clinical, and chemical information for personalized medicine purposes. From a more general perspective, while ML methods are powerful, they also require a careful evaluation of the predictive accuracy to be deployed in out-of-sample scenarios. In this sense, a rigorous and principled approach to validation is now a must in these applications, more so in light of their crucial role in tasks that affect human health, among other aspects. In particular, we advocate in favor of a high-level education in ML, especially for researchers that seek to apply it in their field of competence, as is often the case in the QSAR/QSPR world. This discussion is closely related to the principles agreed by EC/OECD member states about the validation of QSAR models for regulatory purposes. On the ML side, and particularly within the specific world of DL on graphs, steps to move in the right direction have been taken,[105] but a widespread, collective effort is needed to reach higher standards.

Another pressing issue that needs to be addressed in the future concerns the standardization and public availability of chemical datasets. Online, open access to large and well-documented datasets has been a traditional issue in Cheminformatics. A large part of Cheminformatics research has been traditionally carried out in pharmaceutical companies or with industry support. Thus, it is not typically as visible or accessible as comparable research in related fields such as bioinformatics (see public data sources like GeneBank, PDB, Swissprot, etc.). In this sense, public agencies have already started to work towards this goal, e.g., in the USA, the National Institutes of Health (NIH), the National Cancer Institute (NCI), and the Environmental Protection Agency (EPA) for toxicity, as well as ECHA REACH for EU.

To conclude, the ultimate questions of QSAR/QSPR analysis and *de novo* drug design are yet to be answered in full. How to relate chemical structure to biological properties and vice versa remain to be hard and challenging tasks. In the following years, we foresee the increasing role of DL as a tool to look for answers.

References

1. A. Hopkins, Drug discovery: Predicting promiscuity, *Nature* **462** (7270), 167–168 (2009).
2. I. Goodfellow, Y. Bengio, and A. Courville, *Deep Learning*. MIT Press, Cambridge, MA (US) (2016).
3. J. Vamathevan, D. Clark, P. Czodrowski, I. Dunham, E. Ferran, G. Lee, B. Li, A. Madabhushi, P. Shah, M. Spitzer, and S. Zhao, Applications of machine learning in drug discovery and development, *Nat. Rev. Drug Discov.* **18**(6), 463–477 (2019).

4. S. Ekins, A. Puhl, K. Zorn, T. Lane, D. Russo, J. Klein, A. Hickey, and A. Clark, Exploiting machine learning for end-to-end drug discovery and development, *Nat. Mater.* **18**(5), 435–441 (2019).
5. H. Chen, O. Engkvist, Y. Wang, M. Olivecrona, and T. Blaschke, The rise of deep learning in drug discovery, *Drug Discov. Today* **23**(6), 1241–1250 (2018).
6. J. Melville, E. Burke, and J. Hirst, Machine learning in virtual screening, *Comb. Chem. High Throughput Screen.* **12**(4), 332–343 (2009).
7. J. Mitchell, Machine learning methods in chemoinformatics, *WIREs Comput. Mol. Sci.* **4**(5), 468–481 (2014).
8. D. Bacciu, F. Errica, A. Micheli, and M. Podda, A gentle introduction to deep learning for graphs, *Neu. Net.* **129**(September), 203–221 (2020).
9. P. Kirkpatrick and C. Ellis, Chemical space, *Nature* **432**(7019), 823–823 (2004).
10. P. Gantzer, B. Creton, and C. Nieto-Draghi, Inverse-qspr for de novo design: A review, *Mol. Inform.* **39**(4) (2020).
11. H. Kubinyi. In *Burger's Medicinal Chemistry and Drug Discovery*, Vol. 1, pp. 528–530. John Wiley & Sons, Inc., Hoboken, NJ (US) (1995), 5th edn.
12. L. Hall and L. Kier. The molecular connectivity Chi indexes and kappa shape indexes in structure-property modeling. In *Reviews in Computational Chemistry*, Chapter 9, pp. 367–422 (1991).
13. D. Rouvray. Should we have designs on topological indices? In *Chemical Applications of Topology and Graph Theory*, pp. 159–177, Elsevier, Amsterdam (NE) (1983).
14. V. Magnuson, D. Harris, and S. Basak. Topological indices based on neighborhood symmetry: Chemical and biological application. In *Chemical Applications of Topology and Graph Theory*, pp. 178–191, Elsevier, Amsterdam (NE) (1983).
15. M. Barysz, G. Jashari, R. Lall, V. Srivastava, and N. Trinajstic. On the Distance Matrix of Molecules Containing Heteroatoms. In *Chemical Applications of Topology and Graph Theory*, pp. 222–230, Elsevier, Amsterdam (NE) (1983).
16. A. Ben-Naim, *Solvation Thermodynamics*. Plenum Press, New York, NY (US) (1987).
17. R. Todeschini, V. Consonni, R. Mannhold, H. Kubinyi, and H. Timmerman, *Handbook of Molecular Descriptors*. Wiley, Weinheim (DE) (2008).
18. J. Auer and J. Bajorath, Molecular similarity concepts and search calculations, *Methods Mol. Biol.* **453**, 327–347 (2008).

19. G. Maggiora, M. Vogt, D. Stumpfe, and J. Bajorath, Molecular similarity in medicinal chemistry, *J. Med. Chem.* **57**(8), 3186–204 (2014).
20. D. Rogers and M. Hahn, Extended-connectivity fingerprints, *J. Chem. Inf. Comput. Sci.* **50**(5), 742–54 (2010).
21. D. Weininger, SMILES. A chemical language and information system. 1. Introduction to methodology and encoding rules, *J. Chem. Inf. Comput. Sci.* **28**, 31–36 (1988).
22. D. Weininger, A. Weininger, and J. L. Weininger, Smiles. 2. Algorithm for generation of unique smiles notation, *J. Chem. Inf. Comput. Sci.* **29**(2), 97–101 (1989).
23. A. Micheli, A. Sperduti, A. Starita, and A. Bianucci, Analysis of the internal representations developed by neural networks for structures applied to quantitative structure-activity relationship studies of benzodiazepines, *J. Chem. Inf. Comput. Sci.* **41** (2001).
24. L. Bernazzani, C. Duce, A. Micheli, V. Mollica, A. Sperduti, A. Starita, and M. R. Tiné, Predicting physical-chemical properties of compounds from molecular structures by recursive neural networks, *J. Chem. Inf. Comput. Sci.* **46**(5), 2030–2042 (2006).
25. C. Hansch and T. Fujita, RHO-SIGMA-PI analysis. A method for the correlation of biological activity and chemical structure, *J. Chem. Inf. Model.* **86**(8), 1616–1626 (1964).
26. C. Hansch, P. Maloney, T. Fujita, and R. Muir, Correlation of biological activity of phenoxyacetic acids with Hammett substituent constants and partition coefficients, *Nature* **194**, 178–180 (1962).
27. A. Bianucci, A. Micheli, A. Sperduti, and A. Starita, Application of cascade correlation networks for structures to chemistry, *Appl. Intell.* **12**, 115–145 (2000).
28. H. Kubinyi and U. Abraham. Practical problems in PLS analysis. In *3D-QSAR in Drug Design. Theory Methods and Application*, pp. 717–7256. ESCOM, Leiden (1993).
29. D. Rogers and A. Hopfinger, Application of genetic function approximation to quantitative structure-activity relationships and quantitative-property relationships, *J. Chem. Inf. Comput. Sci.* **34** (4), 854–866 (1993).
30. S. So and M. Karplus, Evolutionary optimization in quantitative structure-activity relationship: An application of genetic neural networks, *J. Med. Chem.* **39**(7), 1521–1530 (1996).
31. J. Burns and G. Whitesides, Feed-forward neural networks in chemistry: Mathematical system for classification and pattern recognition, *Chem. Rev.* **93**(8), 2583–2601 (1993).
32. B. Bakshi and U. Utojo, A common framework and overview for the unification of neural, chemometric and statistical modeling methods, *Anal. Chim. Acta.* **384**, 227–247 (1999).

33. V. Kvasnička and J. Pospichal, Application of neural networks in chemistry. Prediction of product distribution of nitration in a series of monosubstituted benzenes, *J. Mol. Struct.* **235**, 227–242 (1991).

34. A. Demiriz, K. Bennett, C. Breneman, and M. Embrechts. Support vector machine regression in chemometrics. In *Computing Science and Statistics: Proceedings of Interface* (2001).

35. O. Ivanciuc, Structure-odor relationships for pyrazines with support vector machines, *Internet Electron. J. Mol. Des.* **1**(5), 269–284 (2002).

36. G. Dahl, N. Jaitly, and R. Salakhutdinov, Multi-task neural networks for qsar predictions, *arXiv preprint* (2014).

37. S. Sosnin, M. Vashurina, M. Withnall, P. Karpov, M. Fedorov, and I. V. Tetko, A survey of multi-task learning methods in chemoinformatics, *Mol. Inf.* **38**(4), 1800108 (2019).

38. B. Ramsundar, B. Liu, Z. Wu, A. Verras, M. Tudor, R. Sheridan, and V. Pande, Is Multitask Deep Learning Practical for Pharma? *J. Chem. Inf. Comput. Sci.* **57**(8), 2068–2076 (2017).

39. J. Ma, R. Sheridan, A. Liaw, G. Dahl, and V. Svetnik, Deep neural nets as a method for quantitative structure-activity relationships, *J. Chem. Inf. Model.* **55**(2), 263–274 (2015).

40. F. Ghasemi, A. Dehnavi, A. Fassihi, and H. Pérez Sánchez, Deep neural network in QSAR studies using deep belief network, *Appl. Soft Comput.* **62**, 251–258 (2018).

41. F. Ghasemi, A. Fassihi, H. Pérez Sánchez, and A. Dehnavi, The role of different sampling methods in improving biological activity prediction using deep belief network, *J. Comput. Chem.* **38**(4), 195–203 (2017).

42. X. Li, Y. Xu, L. Lai, and J. Pei, Prediction of human cytochrome P450 inhibition using a multitask deep autoencoder neural network, *Mol. Pharm.* **15**(10), 4336–4345 (2018).

43. Q. Cui, S. Lu, B. Ni, X. Zeng, Y. Tan, Y. Chen, and H. Zhao, Improved prediction of aqueous solubility of novel compounds by going deeper with deep learning, *Front. Oncol.* **10**, 121 (2020).

44. A. Sperduti and A. Starita, Supervised neural networks for the classification of structures, *IEEE Trans. Neural Netw.* **8**(3), 714–735 (1997).

45. P. Frasconi, M. Gori, and A. Sperduti, A general framework for adaptive processing of data structures, *IEEE Trans. Neural Netw.* **9**(5), 768–86 (1998).

46. A. Bianucci, A. Micheli, A. Sperduti, and A. Starita, Quantitative structure-activity relationships of benzodiazepines by recursive cascade correlation. In *IJCNN Proc.*, pp. 117–122 (1998).

47. B. Hammer, Learning with recurrent neural networks. In *Lecture Notes in Control and Information Sciences*, Vol. 254, pp. 357–368 (1999).

48. B. Hammer, A. Micheli, and A. Sperduti, Universal approximation capability of cascade correlation for structures, *Neural Comput.* **17**(5), 1109–1159 (2005).

49. A. Micheli, A. Sperduti, A. Starita, and A. Bianucci, Design of new biologically active molecules by recursive neural networks. In *IJCNN Proc.*, Vol. 4, pp. 2732–2737 (2001).

50. R. Bini, C. Chiappe, C. Duce, A. Micheli, R. Solaro, A. Starita, and M. Tiné, Ionic liquids: Prediction of their melting points by a recursive neural network model, *Green Chem.* **10**, 306–309 (2008).

51. C. Duce, A. Micheli, A. Starita, M. Tiné, and R. Solaro, Prediction of polymer properties from their structure by recursive neural networks, *Macromol. Rapid Commun.* **27**(9), 711–715 (2006).

52. C. Bertinetto, C. Duce, A. Micheli, R. Solaro, A. Starita, and M. Tiné, Prediction of the glass transition temperature of (meth)acrylic polymers containing phenyl groups by recursive neural network, *Polymer* **48**, 7121–7129 (2007).

53. C. Bertinetto, C. Duce, A. Micheli, R. Solaro, and M. Tiné, QSPR analysis of copolymers by recursive neural networks: Prediction of the glass transition temperature of (meth)acrylic random copolymers, *Mol. Inform.* **29**(8–9), 635–643 (2010).

54. C. Bertinetto, C. Duce, R. Solaro, M. Tiné, A. Micheli, K. Héberger, A. Miličević, and S. Nikolić, Modeling of the acute toxicity of benzene derivatives by complementary QSAR methods, *MATCH — Commun. Math. Comput. Chem.* **70**(3), 1005–1021 (2013).

55. A. Lusci, G. Pollastri, and P. Baldi, Deep architectures and deep learning in chemoinformatics: The prediction of aqueous solubility for drug-like molecules, *J. Chem. Inf. Comput. Sci.* **53**(7), 1563–75 (2013).

56. G. Urban, N. Subrahmanya, and P. Baldi, Inner and outer recursive neural networks for chemoinformatics applications, *J. Chem. Inf. Comput. Sci.* **58** (2018).

57. F. Scarselli, M. Gori, A. Tsoi, M. Hagenbuchner, and G. Monfardini, The graph neural network model, *IEEE Trans. Neural Netw.* **20**(1), 61–80 (2009).

58. A. Micheli, Neural network for graphs: A contextual constructive approach, *IEEE Trans Neural Netw.* **20**(3), 498–511 (2009).

59. D. Duvenaud, D. Maclaurin, J. Aguilera-Iparraguirre, R. Gómez-Bombarelli, T. Hirzel, A. Aspuru-Guzik, and R. P. Adams. Convolutional Networks on Graphs for Learning Molecular Fingerprints. In *NIPS Proc.* (2015).

60. S. Kearnes, K. McCloskey, M. Berndl, V. Pande, and P. Riley, Molecular graph convolutions: Moving beyond fingerprints, *J. Comp. Aid. Mol. Des.* **30**(8), 595–608 (2016).

61. S. Ryu, Y. Kwon, and W. Kim, A Bayesian graph convolutional network for reliable prediction of molecular properties with uncertainty quantification, *Chem. Sci.* **10**, 8438–8446 (2019).
62. H. Altae-Tran, B. Ramsundar, A. Pappu, and V. Pande, Low data drug discovery with one-shot learning, *ACS Cent. Sci.* **3** (2016).
63. J. Li, D. Cai, and X. He, Learning graph-level representation for drug discovery, *arXiv preprint* (2017).
64. K. Liu, X. Sun, L. Jia, J. Ma, H. Xing, J. Wu, H. Gao, Y. Sun, F. Boulnois, and J. Fan, Chemi-net: A graph convolutional network for accurate drug property prediction, *arXiv preprint* (2018).
65. A. Graves, G. Wayne, and I. Danihelka, Neural turing machines, *arXiv preprint* (2014).
66. T. Pham, T. Tran, and S. Venkatesh. Graph memory networks for molecular activity prediction. In *ICPR Proc.*, pp. 639–644 (2018).
67. M. Sun, S. Zhao, C. Gilvary, O. Elemento, J. Zhou, and F. Wang, Graph convolutional networks for computational drug development and discovery, *Brief. Bioinform.* (2019).
68. D. Elton, Z. Boukouvalas, M. Fuge, and P. Chung, Deep learning for molecular design: A review of the state of the art, *Mol. Syst. Des. Eng.* **4**, 828–849 (2019).
69. D. Schwalbe-Koda and R. Gómez-Bombarelli, Generative models for automatic chemical design, *arXiv preprint* (2019).
70. J. Elman, Finding structure in time, *Cogn. Sci.* **14**, 179–212 (1990).
71. D. Kingma and M. Welling, Auto-encoding variational bayes, *ICLR* (2014).
72. I. Goodfellow, J. Pouget-Abadie, M. Mirza, B. Xu, D. Warde-Farley, S. Ozair, A. Courville, and Y. Bengio. Generative Adversarial Nets. In *NIPS Proc.*, pp. 2672–2680 (2014).
73. A. Makhzani, J. Shlens, N. Jaitly, and I. Goodfellow. Adversarial Autoencoders. In *ICLR* (2016).
74. Y. Bengio, P. Simard, and P. Frasconi, Learning long-term dependencies with gradient descent is difficult, *IEEE Trans. Neural. Netw.* **5**(2), 157–66 (1994).
75. R. Williams and D. Zipser, A learning algorithm for continually running fully recurrent neural networks, *Neural Comput.* **1**(2), 270–280 (1989).
76. M. Simonovsky and N. Komodakis. GraphVAE: Towards Generation of Small Graphs Using Variational Autoencoders. In *ICANN Proc.* (2018).
77. N. D. Cao and T. Kipf, MolGAN: An implicit generative model for small molecular graphs, *arXiv preprint* (2018).
78. D. Johnson. Learning Graphical State Transitions. In *ICLR* (2017).

79. R. Gómez-Bombarelli, J. Wei, D. Duvenaud, J. Hernández-Lobato, B. Sánchez-Lengeling, D. Sheberla, J. Aguilera-Iparraguirre, T. Hirzel, R. Adams, and A. Aspuru-Guzik, Automatic chemical design using a data-driven continuous representation of molecules, *ACS Cent. Sci.* **4**(2), 268–276 (2018).

80. M. Kusner, B. Paige, and J. Hernández-Lobato. Grammar variational autoencoder. In *ICML Proc.*, Vol. 70, pp. 1945–1954 (2017).

81. H. Dai, Y. Tian, B. Dai, S. Skiena, and L. Song. Syntax-directed variational autoencoder for structured data. In *ICLR* (2018).

82. M. Podda, D. Bacciu, and A. Micheli. A deep generative model for fragment-based molecule generation. In *AISTATS Proc.* (2020).

83. P. Maragakis, H. Nisonoff, B. Cole, and D. Shaw, A deep-learning view of chemical space designed to facilitate drug discovery, *arXiv preprint* (2020).

84. W. Jin, R. Barzilay, and T. S. Jakkola. Junction tree variational autoencoder for molecular graph generation. In *ICML Proc.*, pp. 2328–2337 (2018).

85. Q. Liu, M. Allamanis, M. Brockschmidt, and A. Gaunt. Constrained graph variational autoencoders for molecule design. In *NeurIPS Proc.*, pp. 7795–7804 (2018).

86. B. Samanta, A. D. De, G. Jana, P. Chattaraj, N. Ganguly, and M. Gomez-Rodriguez, NeVAE: A deep generative model for molecular graphs, *arXiv preprint* (2018).

87. W. Kool, H. Van Hoof, and M. Welling. Stochastic beams and where to find them: The Gumbel-top-k trick for sampling sequences without replacement. In *ICML Proc.*, Vol. 97, pp. 3499–3508 (2019).

88. A. Holtzman, J. Buys, L. Du, M. Forbes, and Y. Choi, The curious case of neural text degeneration, *arXiv preprint* (2019).

89. K. Preuer, P. Renz, T. Unterthiner, S. Hochreiter, and G. Klambauer, Fréchet chemnet distance: A metric for generative models for molecules in drug discovery, *J. Chem. Inf. Comput. Sci.* **58**(9), 1736–1741 (2018).

90. G. Goh, C. Siegel, A. Vishnu, and N. Hodas, ChemNet: A transferable and generalizable deep neural network for small-molecule property prediction, *arXiv preprint* (2017).

91. J. Lim, S. Ryu, J. Kim, , and W. Kim, Molecular generative model based on conditional variational autoencoder for de novo molecular design, *J. Chem.* **10**(1), 31 (2018).

92. Y. Li, L. Zhang, and Z. Liu, Multi-objective de novo drug design with conditional graph generative model, *J. Chem.* **10**(1), 33 (2018).

93. W. Jin, R. Barzilay, and T. Jaakkola, Hierarchical graph-to-graph translation for molecules, *arXiv preprint* (2019).

94. S. Hong, S. Ryu, J. Lim, and W. Kim, Molecular generative model based on an adversarially regularized autoencoder, *J. Chem. Inf. Comput. Sci.* **60**(1), 29–36 (2020).

95. O. Méndez-Lucio, B. Baillif, D. Clevert, D. Rouquié, and J. Wichard, De novo generation of hit-like molecules from gene expression signatures using artificial intelligence, *Nat. Commun.* **11**(1), 10 (2020).

96. R. Griffiths and J. Hernández-Lobato, Constrained Bayesian optimization for automatic chemical design using variational autoencoders, *Chem. Sci.* **11**, 577–586 (2020).

97. R. Sutton and A. Barto, *Reinforcement Learning: An Introduction*, second edn. MIT Press, Cambridge, MA (US) (2018).

98. M. Olivecrona, T. Blaschke, O. Engkvist, and H. Chen, Molecular de novo design through deep reinforcement learning, *arXiv preprint* (2017).

99. J. You, B. Liu, R. Ying, V. Pande, and J. Leskovec. Graph Convolutional Policy Network for Goal-Directed Molecular Graph Generation. In *Neur IPS Proc.*, pp. 6412–6422 (2018).

100. N. Ståhl, G. Falkman, A. Karlsson, G. Mathiason, and J. Boström, Deep reinforcement learning for multiparameter optimization in de novo drug design, *J. Chem. Inf. Comput. Sci.* **59**(7), 3166–3176 (2019).

101. M. Popova, M. Shvets, J. Oliva, and O. Isayev, Molecular RNN: Generating realistic molecular graphs with optimized properties, *arXiv preprint* (2019).

102. G. Guimaraes, B. Sanchez-Lengeling, C. Outeiral, P. C. Farias, and A. Aspuru-Guzik, Objective-reinforced generative adversarial networks (ORGAN) for sequence generation models, *arXiv preprint* (2017).

103. M. Segler, T. Kogej, C. Tyrchan, and M. Waller, Generating focused molecule libraries for drug discovery with recurrent neural networks, *ACS Cent. Sci.* **4**(1), 120–131 (2018).

104. I. Kobyzev, S. Prince, and M. Brubaker, Normalizing flows: An introduction and review of current methods, *arXiv preprint* (2019).

105. F. Errica, M. Podda, D. Bacciu, and A. Micheli, A fair comparison of graph neural networks for graph classification. In *ICLR* (2020).

Chapter 7

Deep Learning Methods for Network Biology

Lorenzo Madeddu[†,§] and Giovanni Stilo[*,‡,¶]

*†Sapienza University of Rome,
Piazzale Aldo Moro, 5, 00185 Roma RM, Italy
‡University of L'Aquila, 19 Piazza Santa Margherita,
2 Palazzo Camponeschi, 67100 L'Aquila AQ, Italy
§madeddu@di.uniroma1.it
¶giovanni.stilo@univaq.it*

Lives on earth are regulated by a complex system of interactions. Modelling these interactions through the network paradigms allows researchers to discover and understand the fundamental molecular mechanisms which drive the biological processes and lead to human diseases. The advancement made in the development of sequencing technologies has produced a growing amount of biological data. The aforementioned preconditions are at the base of a flourishing production of deep learning methods able to cope with the complexity and data abundance of this domain. For these reasons, this chapter provides a comprehensive overview of the recent advancements in the deep learning network-based approaches focusing on biology, medicine and pharmacological crucial research problems. At first, the needed biological and network science backgrounds are presented. Second, a comprehensive overview of the biological networks and resources is provided. Finally, we discuss the most recent methods in the field, organising them into three broad categories: the interactome, the network pharmacology, and the frontier biological problems.

---

*This author's work is partially supported by Territori Aperti, a project funded by Fondo Territori Lavoro e Conoscenza CGIL CISL UIL and by SoBigData-PlusPlus H2020-INFRAIA-2019-1 EU project, contract number 871042.

197

1. Introduction

The last decades are characterised by the advance of high-throughput technologies, such as yeast two-hybrid screening and next-generation sequencing. This advancement in technologies has boosted the creation of large omics datasets (i.e., molecular data) which helped one to reveal and understand the complex interconnections among all the subparts[a] of an organism.

In this context, researchers need new *"holistic"* tools to cope with the dimensionality and complexity of the biological data. The response to this demand, as we will see, is the modelisation offered by the Networks formalism. Biological networks, such as protein–protein interaction network, are new representations of *"omics"* data and combine network science and biology approaches to analyse the interconnection of biological processes. The study of the structures and functions of the biological networks is known as Network Biology or Systems Biology. The study of the pathogenic behaviour and drug processes in biological networks is referred to as Network Medicine. Systems biology and network medicine are keys to the following: (i) understanding the biological mechanisms and (ii) addressing challenges on both diagnostic and therapeutic aspects. The research literature has studied biological networks by using a plethora of graph-mining and classic machine learning approaches. However, diving into the complexity of the molecular interconnections across several levels of the organism's organisation is challenging. To overcome these limitations, researchers are adopting new powerful strategies in network biology and network medicine. Adoption of deep learning techniques in biology allows us to explore the latent mechanisms and untangle the intricate molecular interconnections that standard approaches are not able to. Lately, promising deep learning methods in graph mining, such as Graph Convolutional Networks (GCN),[1] have been successfully applied to biological networks to solve problems, such as drug repurposing[2] and identification of new disease genes.[3]

This chapter discusses the deep learning network-based approaches applied to both network biology and network medicine.

---

[a]In a modelisation of the organism as a system.

The chapter is organised as follows. Section 2 provides the fundamental knowledge about networks theory (Section 2.1), learning problems on networks (Section 2.2) and ground concepts of systems biology (Section 2.3). Section 3 describes in a formal way the most important biological networks (Section 3.1) and the publicly available resources (Section 3.2). In Sections 4–6, the most recent deep learning-based methods — organised by the tackled problem and the used data — are presented. Lastly, Section 7 discusses the future directions and concluding remarks.

2. Background Knowledge

In this section, a comprehensive summary of the key aspects related to network biology is presented. More precisely, in Section 2.1, the fundamental network concepts are briefly introduced. Section 2.2 describes the learning/prediction problems in network science. Finally, in Section 2.3, the most important biological concepts are summarised.

2.1. *Network background and formalisation*

In this section, we summarise the following network concepts and properties most useful in network biology:

Network: A simple network or graph is a mathematical formalism that allows describing in an abstract and concise way both the components of a system and their interactions. Formally, a graph $G = (V, E)$ is defined as a tuple containing the two sets V and E. V is the set of objects called nodes or vertices of the graph. The set of edges $E \subseteq \{(u, v)|u, v \in V\}$ contains the relationships among the objects of the system. Edges — also called links or ties — can be either *directed* or *undirected*.

Directed edges are necessary to describe asymmetrical relationships. Having a relationship among nodes i and j does not imply having the same relationship between nodes j and i. On the other hand, the *undirected* case implies that the relationships in the system are symmetrical. It is not necessary to distinguish the relationship among nodes i and j from the one from node j to i. Collection of

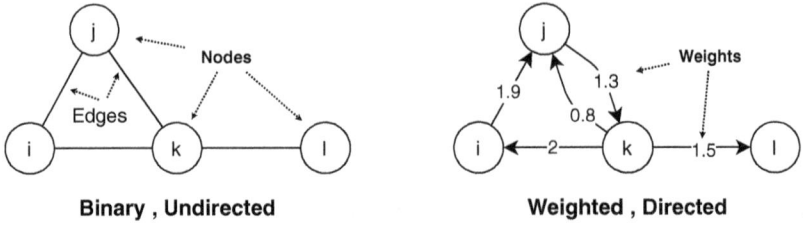

Fig. 1. Examples of several types of simple networks.

differences between the *importance* of each relationship is useful to define a weighting function $w(e) : E \to \mathbb{R}$, which returns values of the edges according to the semantics of the system. When a weighting function is defined, we call the graph a *weighted* one. Each simple graph (*binary*) is described by a square matrix A — called the adjacency matrix — of sizes $|V| \times |V|$, where its element A_{ij} contains 1 if there exists an edge from vertex i to vertex j or 0 otherwise. When the weighting function $w(e)$ is defined, the elements A_{ij} of the adjacency matrix are equivalent to the values of the weighting function $w(i, j)$ or zero otherwise. A graphical representation of a simple binary undirected graph and a weighted directed one is depicted in Figure 1.

The *complex systems* or the heterogeneous networks — where different information is associated with the system components and several kinds of relationships exist — can be modelled in many ways. They can be modelled as a decorated graph with categorical and/or numerical attributes on both edges and vertices. To encode this information with the graph, several (one for each attribute) mapping functions are defined. Later on, we will refer to this kind of graph as one with *attributes*.

The *bipartite* graph contains two distinct kinds of vertices, and no two vertices within the same set are adjacent. A bipartite graph $G = (V, U, E)$ is defined as a triple containing the three sets V, U and E. V and U are two disjoint sets of vertices: $V \cap U = \emptyset$. The set of edges $E \subseteq \{(u, v)| \quad (u \in V \cap v \in U) \cup (v \in V \cap u \in U)\}$ contains the relationships among the two different kinds of vertices. The bipartite graph is a special case of a k-partite graph, where $k = 2$.

Other Important Network Concepts and Properties:

Degree: The node's degree is the number of edges (incoming and/or outgoing in the directed case) of a node.

Path/diameter: A path, or walk, is a sequence of nodes in which every node is adjacent to the next one in the sequence. The diameter is the longest path between any pair of nodes.

Hub: A hub is a node which exposes a degree higher than the average degree of the network (normally, it is a property analysed in the directed graphs considering only the out-degree).

Connected graph: A graph is strongly connected if a path exists for any pair of its nodes.

Induced sub-graph: An induced sub-graph H is a graph containing a node subset of V and all the edges among them. Let G be the initial graph; $H = (V_H \subseteq V, E_H = \{(u,v)|u,v \in V_H \ and \ (u,v) \in E\})$.

Motif: A motif is a recurrent and statistically significant partial sub-graph. Note that the motifs differ from graphlets since they can be partial sub-graphs, whereas motifs are induced sub-graphs.

Community: The definition of *"community"* may change according to the application domain. From a network perspective, usually, a community is a locally dense sub-graph where the edge density among the inside community nodes is higher than the edge density among the inside community nodes and outside ones.

Random network: A random network is a network generated by a random distribution probability (e.g., Erdős–Rényi model[4]). A node $v \in V$ is connected to another node of the network following a certain probability p.

Scale-free network: A scale-free network is a network whose degree distribution follows the power-law distribution.[5]

Small-world network: A small-world network is a network in which any pair of nodes is connected to the other nodes of the network by a *small*, proportional to $log(|V|)$, path.[6]

2.2. *Learning problems on networks*

Networks are mathematical tools used to study and predict properties in the domain applications related, but not limited, to social behaviours, economic events, biology processes, traffic flow and internet connections. Despite the differences, every application on these domains is reducible to the same general network prediction tasks:

Node classification: Typically, a class is used to group a collection of nodes that expose similar characteristics. The classes are typically referred by unique textual descriptions, namely, labels or tags. Using nodes which are already classified, it is possible to train a classifier which captures some knowledge. A trained classifier can be used to assign a class to an unknown node. For instance, we would like to learn which proteins are related to a certain disease. The classification tasks can be either binary or multi-class (a given data instance may be assigned to one or many classes, respectively).

Link prediction: A fundamental problem with networks is that the link information in the graph may be of doubtful quality or not present at all. Thus, inferring the existences of edges between nodes has been referred to as link prediction.[7] Link prediction is a challenging problem that has been studied in various guises in different domains. The prediction of a link can be solely based on the structural information (graph associations) or also on the attribute information.

Community detection: Community detection refers to the procedure of identifying groups (sub-graphs) of tightly interacting vertices (i.e., nodes) in the network.

Representation learning: Representation learning is about deriving a succinct representation of the input data (graph in our settings[8]). This succinct representation allows one to achieve better performances (of the classification/prediction task) or to reduce the computational complexity. There exist many representation learning approaches: in deep learning, the representation is typically achieved by the composition of multiple nonlinear transformations (hidden layers) of the input data.

2.3. *Ground concepts of systems biology*

Hereafter, we present the fundamental biological concepts necessary to understand the papers collected in this chapter. Note that in network biology, the following biological/molecular concepts are normally organised in databases, which collect this information in one place. For a complete overview of these databases, see Section 3.2. The biological concepts are tightly interconnected. We decided to present at first the most important or general ones and then, going further, all the others. For this reason, we invite the reader to go through all the sections in order to gain a better understanding of all the ground concepts.

Cells: Cells are building blocks of the structure of an organism. A cell is a structure containing DNA, cytoplasm, cellular structures (e.g., ribosomes) and several molecules (e.g., proteins), all surrounded by a membrane. The specialisation of a cell (in terms of functionality) is determined by the gene expression. A collection of cells that work together to accomplish the same function is called a tissue.

Biological pathway: A biological pathway is an ordered sequence of actions among molecules (e.g., proteins or complexes) in a cell that leads to the creation of product or changes the cellular state. For example, a pathway could lead to the synthesis of a molecule, regulate genes, or spur a cell to move. The most common pathway types are metabolic pathways, gene regulation pathways, and signal transduction pathways. A metabolic pathway is a series of chemical reactions occurring within a cell. Gene regulation pathways turn genes on and off. The signal transduction pathway is a series of intracellular molecular events as a response to the activation of a cell's receptor by an extracellular signal. Enzymes, usually proteins, are involved in almost all metabolic pathways to accelerate chemical reactions.

Proteins: Proteins are large molecules composed by amino acids. They are responsible for biological processes in the cell. The sequence of amino acids and the environment determine both the protein's three-dimensional structure and its specific function. The instructions to build the sequence of amino acids of a protein are stored in the genes. As a convention, proteins are classified by family and domain. A *protein family* is a group of proteins sharing a common evolutionary origin reflecting a related set of functions or/and structural similarities. *Domains* are a compact way to describe the three-dimensional structure of a protein in structural units (responsible for a particular function or interaction). Another important aspect related to proteins is their ontological organisation. The *GO-terms* are proteins/genes ontological concepts organised into the three fundamental facets: molecular activities, cellular structures and biological processes.

Protein–protein interaction (PPI): PPI is a physical interaction which takes place in a cell among the structural region of two proteins. A PPI is responsible for the biological processes and can be permanent, as in the case of the *protein complexes*[b] or can be transient as in the case of the signals. PPIs are essential to understand how molecular biological processes are carried out.

Deoxyribonucleic acid (DNA): DNA *"is a complex and hereditary molecule that contains all of the information necessary to build and maintain an organism"*.[c] All organisms have a full copy of the DNA held within every cell. The DNA is composed of a chain of linked blocks called nucleotides. Each nucleotide is characterised by one of the four chemical bases: adenine (A), guanine (G), cytosine (C), and thymine (T).[d] The ordered sequence — constituted by about three billion of base pairs — encodes the information necessary to make the essential molecules such as proteins. The DNA is a string of roughly three billion characters, where the alphabet is {A, C, G, T}.

Gene: A gene is a section (contiguous subsequence) of the DNA that encodes information of a functional unit. The Human Genome Project[e] estimated that humans have between 20,000 and 25,000 genes. Mutations in the DNA cause diverse versions of the genes, namely, *alleles*. The information stored in genes — such as the rest of the DNA — contribute to regulating the mechanisms behind the protein synthesis.

Genotype and phenotype: The *genotype* is the collection of an organism's genes. The term *phenotype* refers to the observable traits of an organism. The phenotype is determined by the genotype, the gene expression and environmental factors.

Gene/protein nomenclature: Several committees are responsible for gene and protein nomenclature. Despite the standardization effort, the multitude of nomenclatures caused ambiguities.[f]

---

[b]Protein Complex (e.g., Haemoglobin) is an aggregation of proteins connected by PPIs.

[c]https://www.nature.com/scitable/topicpage/introduction-what-is-dna-65799 78/.

[d]https://ghr.nlm.nih.gov/primer/basics/dna.

[e]https://www.genome.gov/.

[f]https://www.uniprot.org/help/different_protein_gene_names.

The HUGO Human Gene Nomenclature Committee (HGNC)[g] is responsible for assigning names and symbols (shorter form of the names) to the human genes. Alternatively, the most popular nomenclatures in bioinformatics are the Entrez ID and the Ensembl ID.[h] UniProtKB complete the nomenclature overview, providing also the names for protein isoforms. In bioinformatics, Entrez and UniportKB are the most used nomenclatures for a programmatic access. The literature generally adopts the HGNC names or acronyms.

Gene expression: This is the cellular process of synthesising proteins or functional RNA. Gene expression is composed of two main steps: transcription and translation. The transcription is the process of transferring the information stored in a gene to the cytoplasm through the messenger-RNA (mRNA), which promotes the translation process. During the translation process, the read mRNA sequence in collaboration with the transfer-RNA (tRNA) allows us to assemble the protein.

Gene regulation: This is the process of controlling the gene expression profile in a cell. Gene regulation increases, decreases or suppresses the expression of genes. Since only a fraction of genes are expressed ("turned on"), the gene expression profile defines the type and the activities of a cell at a certain time. Mechanisms of gene expression control can occur at any step of the gene expression, but most commonly during the transcription process. *Transcription factors and microRNAs are key regulators of the gene expressions.* The *Transcription Factors* (TF) regulate the gene transcription (increase or decrease the amount of gene product of a gene). The *microRNAs* (miRNAs) regulate the gene expression at the post-transcription level by binding to target mRNAs preventing their expression. *Alternative splicing* is a regulation mechanism that enables the coding of multiple proteins (called protein isoforms) instead of one. Lastly, the long non-coding RNAs (lncRNAs), still under investigation, are involved in several molecular functions playing a key role in some cancer mechanisms.

Disease: A general definition states that the disease is any harmful deviation from the normal structural or functional state of an

---

[g]https://www.genenames.org/.

[h]https://m.ensembl.org/info/genome/genebuild/gene_names.html.

organism. The abnormal condition generates disorders in the whole organism or any of its parts. Generally, the disease is associated with certain signs and symptoms, and differs in nature from physical injury. The disease process is the result of complex dysfunctional mechanisms. As an example, a disease could alter the normal pathways causing patho-phenotypes.[i]

Virus: Virus is a submicroscopic infectious agent that can multiply only within the living cells of an organism. Consequently, a virus uses the chemical machinery of the living cells to continue to live and to reproduce itself. *Host-specific* viruses cause many common human infections and are also responsible for several diseases, for example, the common cold, caused by one of the rhinoviruses, and AIDS, caused by HIV. Viruses may have their genetic material (DNA or RNA).

Gene–disease association (or simply a disease gene): This happens when a gene or a gene product is involved in the disease process. A mutated gene which changes its expression may consequently change the produced proteins (and/or its quantity), thus drafting the basis of the dysfunctional process. For example, a mutation in *TP53* leads to several tumoral diseases, such as breast cancer, bladder cancer and lung cancer.[j]

Disease module: Some diseases are caused by more than one faulty gene product (disease gene or disease protein). Barabási *et al.*[9] have moved the focus from the disease genes to their complex set of interactions: *"a disease is rarely a consequence of an abnormality in a single gene product but reflects the perturbations of the complex intracellular network"*. The *disease module* is defined as the local neighbourhood of genes which linked to the same disease interact together and alter the normal structure and the biological functions.

Drug: In pharmacogenomics, a drug is a chemical compound which by interacting with specific molecules of the organism (e.g., enzymes or receptor proteins) produces therapeutic effects. A drug which

---

[i]https://www.genome.gov/about-genomics/fact-sheets/Biological-Pathways-Fact-Sheet.

[j]https://ghr.nlm.nih.gov/gene/TP53#conditions.

binds to a receptor (a protein family) changes its molecular structure and its functionalities. This change induces a signalling pathway within the cell or inhibits the functions of the receptor itself. The specific drug-induced alterations of the biological processes contrast the disease-induced ones, thus causing a therapeutic *"fixing"* effect.

We like to remark that in precision medicine,[k] it is fundamental to select those set of drugs which contrast the disease-altered biological processes and have a minimal or negligible impact on the other patient biological processes.

3. Biological Networks and Publicly Available Resources

In this section, we present the most common biological networks (Section 3.1) and an exhaustive collection of biological databases (Section 3.2).

3.1. *Biological networks*

Nodes of a molecular network usually represent genes, gene products or biological functions while edges define the molecular connections between these entities. In the following, we describe the most common types of biological networks, providing a complete explanation and a tabular description.

3.1.1. *Protein–protein interaction network*

Protein–protein interaction network (PIN), often referred to as interactome, is an undirected binary graph of PPIs where proteins are nodes and undirected edges are physical interactions. Contrary to the common convention, the PINs present an ambiguity to keep in mind. The absence of an edge may imply that the interaction between the two proteins does not exist or that the related lab test was not performed yet. Additionally, PIN nodes can be decorated with categorical attributes representing biological knowledge, such

---

[k]Precision medicine is an emergent approach to patient care that allows clinicians to select treatments that are most likely to help patients based on a genetic understanding of their disease.

as GO-terms, diseases relationships and other proteins features like domains. From the topological point of view, PINs have characteristics similar to those of scale-free[10] networks.[1] As reported by Jeong *et al.*[11] in PINs, the hubs are likely to be proteins which are essential for many fundamental life processes. Another typical property of the PIN is its modular organization.[10]

PINs are composed of modules, sub-graphs of proteins that tend to collaborate together in order to accomplish a biological function. Those modules play a key role in the life of an organism by enabling biological processes and by constituting protein complexes.

The PINs are mainly used to identify key proteins or modules essential for the development of biological processes like diseases.[9] Discovering such modules in the human PIN helps us to understand how diverse phenotypes might be linked at the molecular level. PINs and modules are key concepts which allow clinicians to investigate on co-morbidity and on drug repurposing.

We would like to remark that, notwithstanding the past decade witnessing systematic efforts to increase its coverage and accuracy, the human PIN remains highly incomplete and noisy.[12] For the aforementioned reasons, it is still an active and open research field.

Nodes:	Protein	Edges:	Physical interactions
Type:	Undirected	Weights:	Binary
Nodes Attributes:	Pathways, diseases, domains, families, tissues		
Edges Attributes:	Usually not present		

3.1.2. *Drug–target network*

A drug–target network (DTN) is a bipartite undirected network where one set of nodes is composed by drugs and the other set contains their target molecules. An edge/interaction is present when a drug has the tendency to bind to a target,[13] a protein (e.g., GPCR) peptide or nucleic acid. Furthermore, drugs can target several molecules at once, causing also adverse side effects to a patient.[14]

Since one of the main uses of DTN is in the field of drug repurposing, many networks also report categorical attributes. These

---

[1]Scale-free networks are also characterised by the presence of large hubs.

attributes constitute additional knowledge such as disease, protein domains, and drug pathway or categories. The DTN networks can also be expanded with protein–protein and drug–drug interactions. The drug repurposing approaches leverage enriched DTNs — with the functional and modular structures of the PINs — to achieve better performances.[2, 14, 15]

Another kind of network related to the DTN is the *drug–drug interaction (DDI) network*. In the DDI network, nodes are drugs, and the edges represent a change, often adverse, in the effect that one drug has on the target if combined with the other drug. For this reason, DDIs are usually employed to identify drugs' side effects and drive polypharmacy therapies. Similar to diseases, it has been observed that several drugs have an impact on the PIN neighbourhood of their targets. For example, a drug can be engineered to produce beneficial effects by interacting with proteins in the PIN neighbourhood of the disease proteins.[15]

Finally, the concept of drug–target module, hypothesised by Cheng *et al.* captures the tendency of proteins targeted by the same drug to form a localised neighbourhood as it happens in the case of the disease modules. An interesting property observed in polypharmacy is as follows: two drugs have a therapeutic effect only if the drug–target modules overlap with the disease module but not among them.

Nodes:	Drugs, Proteins	Edges:	Physical/Functional interactions
Type:	Undirected	Weights:	Binary
Nodes Attributes:	Diseases, protein features, drug features		
Edges Attributes:	Side effects		

3.1.3. *Gene expression network*

A Gene Co-Expression Network (GEN) is an undirected, often weighted, correlation network where nodes are genes and edges represent significant correlation in the expression between two genes. Gene nodes can be decorated with categorical attributes adding biological knowledge, such as diseases and GO-terms. GENs are typically constructed in two steps: in the first step, a correlation measure (Pearson or Spearman coefficients, mutual information, Euclidean distance) is computed between each pair of genes by using their expression data (Microarrays, RNA-Seq). In the second step, a significance threshold (a threshold cutoff or the Fishers Z-transformation) is applied over the previously computed correlation values in order to identify the co-expressed genes.

Studying GENs permits one to identify functionally related genes or co-expression module with key roles in biological pathways.[16]

We also want to highlight that, contrary to the PPI networks, the gene co-expression ones depend on the conditions (typically the temporal context) in which the samples have been collected.

Nodes:	Genes	**Edges:**	Correlations of gene expression
Type:	Undirected	**Weights:**	Real values
Nodes Attributes:	GO-Terms, diseases		
Edges Attributes:	Usually not present		

3.1.4. *Gene regulatory network*

A gene regulatory network (GRN) is a weighted, directed, bipartite network of gene regulatory dependencies. The interactions are between a *"regulator molecule"* (Transcription Factor, RNA, miRNA, etc.) and a *"regulated molecule"*, usually a gene. Nodes can either be characterised by other categorical attributes. The GRN captures the complex workflow of the gene regulation system. Studying the gene regulatory process allows the researchers to understand how molecular mechanisms work, thus identifying the key patterns and players which emerge in specific conditions like a disease state.[17]

Nodes:	TFs, RNAs, miRNAs, lncRNA, Genes	**Edges:**	Biological interactions
Type:	Directed	**Weights:**	Real values
Nodes Attributes:	GO-Terms, diseases		
Edges Attributes:	Usually not present		

3.1.5. *Brain network*

The connectome, also known as the brain network, is used to organise and represent information about functional or physical connectivity among different brain regions.[18] As often observed in several biological networks, as well as in the brain one, it is possible to recognise the scale-free topology.[19] Other studies have also found out that the connectome exposes some similarities with the small-world network model[20] and have identified some recurrent structural motifs.[21] Moreover, a brain network exposes modular structures related to cerebral functions[22] as[m] those that typically are present in the PIN networks.

To understand how the connectome was built, we must consider the different techniques employed to detect the brain zones and understand how they interact with one another. The two most popular ones are as follows: (i) the structural magnetic resonance imaging (sMRI or MRI) which detects anatomical structures and provides a map of physical neural connections and (ii) the functional magnetic resonance imaging (fMRI) which allows one to track the oxygen changes associated with blood flow helping to build the brain's activity map.

The analysis of brain networks led to great advancements in the research areas pertaining to degenerative brain-related diseases. For example, works[23] related to the study of Alzheimer's disease report evidence that the functional brain networks have structural properties that are less similar than those of the small-world model. This discovery allows a better understanding of the fact that Alzheimer's causes a disconnection among the distant brain zones.

Nodes:	Brain regions	Edges:	Physical connections
Type:	Undirected	Weights:	Binary
Nodes Attributes:	Usually not present		
Edges Attributes:	Usually not present		

3.2. *Publicly available resources*

Data collection (databases) constitutes a grounding block for deep learning methods. The network biology databases reflect the biological/molecular information of the organism, as presented in Section 2.3, by centralising them in one place. The databases can be classified into primary and secondary databases based on the experimental results submitted by researchers. They contain primary information (such as nucleotide or protein) and annotations, including bibliographies, functions, cross-references to other databases, and so forth. Secondary databases summarise the results from the analyses

---

[m]From the structural perspective.

(e.g., computational predictions) of primary databases. These analyses allow finding common features of biological classes, which can be used to classify unknown biological data. Databases that contain biological or medical information are usually classified as secondary ones. However, many databases have integrated both data from primary and secondary databases over the years, and thus, their classifications have become ambiguous.

It should be noted that the same biological information can be collected in several databases maintained by different national or transnational institutions: the National Institutes of Health (NIH) for the U.S. maintains the PubChem database and the European Bioinformatics Institute (EBI) for Europe maintains the corresponding one, ChEMBL.

In adjunction to the original article (containing the data description, structure and functionality of the database) exist dedicated journal issues (e.g., *Nucleic Acids Research*[n]), which annually reviews all the recently updated and available biological databases.

In Table 1, we present an exhaustive list of the publicly available databases. The table reports for each database its name, a description of the contained data and three binary columns which identify the primary databases and classify their content as features (attributes on nodes or edges) or/and associations (edges). The direct link to the original resource is provided; however, for purpose of readability, it is available only in the electronic format of the book. The table is organised by groups of databases[o]: gene/proteins, diseases, drugs, gene expression, gene regulation and pathways-related data. Following the authors' expertise and the recognised use of the databases, the most important databases have been underlined.[p]

---

[n]Freely accessible also on the Web.

[o]Note that a database can be present in more than one group.

[p]Due to several database versions released over the years, keeping track of citations in a precise way is a complicated task. Thus, the empty cells with dashes must be considered for advice.

Table 1. List of publicly available databases in network biology.

Database	Content description	Primary	Features	Associations	Website
Gene/Protein Data					
UniProt[24]	Proteins' additional information such as domains, families and sequences	—	Yes	—	http://www.uniprot.org
Gene Ontology (GO)[25]	Collection of ontological terms (GO-term) related to gene and gene products	—	Yes	—	http://www.geneontology.org
Human Protein Atlas[26]	Human protein distribution in cells, tissues, organs and cancer types	—	Yes	Yes	http://www.proteinatlas.org
BioGRID[27]	Large collection of PPIs	Yes	—	Yes	http://www.thebiogrid.org
IntAct[28]	Large collection of PPIs	Yes	—	Yes	http://www.ebi.ac.uk/intact/
DIP[29]	Collection of PPIs	—	—	Yes	http://dip.doe-mbi.ucla.edu
HPRD[30]	Collection of human only PPIs	Yes	—	Yes	http://www.hprd.org
HuRI[31]	Database of highly reliable PPIs	Yes	—	Yes	http://www.interactome-atlas.org
APID[32]	A database which contains PPIs collected from other several primary databases	—	—	Yes	http://apid.dep.usal.es
HIPPIE[33]	Collection of PPIs	—	—	Yes	http://cbdm-01.zdv.uni-mainz.de/~mschaefer/hippie/
CLAIRE-COVID	Protein-related data for COVID-19 tasks	—	Yes	Yes	http://github.com/CLAIRE-COVID-T4/covid-data
Disease Data					
ICD[34]	International classification of diseases	—	Yes	—	http://www.who.int/classifications/classification-of-diseases
SNOMED[35]	Modern disease taxonomy	—	Yes	—	http://browser.ihtsdotools.org/
MeSH[36]	Taxonomy of medical literature	—	Yes	—	http://www.nlm.nih.gov/mesh/meshhome.html

(*Continued*)

Table 1. (*Continued*)

Database	Content description	Primary Features	Associations	Website
UMLS[37]	Mapping among several medical terminologies	—	Yes	—	http://www.nlm.nih.gov/research/umls/index.html
DO[38]	Disease ontology and vocabularies with biomedical data	—	Yes	—	http://www.disease-ontology.org
HPO[39]	A phenotype ontology: contains symptom–disease associations	—	Yes	Yes	http://www.hpo.jax.org
MalaCards[40]	Data-mining-based human disease knowledge base	—	Yes	Yes	http://www.malacards.org
Orphanet[41]	European source for disease-related data (i.e., symptom–disease associations)	—	Yes	Yes	http://www.orpha.net/consor/cgi-bin/index.php
DisGeNET[42]	Large GDA collection: integrates multiple expert-curated and computational sources	—	—	Yes	http://www.disgenet.org
OMIM[43]	Disease vocabulary and expert-curated GDA collection	Yes	—	Yes	http://www.omim.org
ClinVar[26]	Collection of association between human variations and phenotypes	—	—	Yes	http://www.ncbi.nlm.nih.gov/clinvar/
PsyGeNET[44]	Collection of GDAs for psychiatric diseases	—	—	Yes	http://http://www.psygenet.org
HuGE Navigator[45]	Text-mining-based GDA	—	—	Yes	http://phgkb.cdc.gov/PHGKB/hNHome.action
COSMIC[46]	Collection of cancer-related GDAs	—	—	Yes	http://cancer.sanger.ac.uk/cosmic
CTD[47]	Literature-curated associations between drugs, genes and diseases	—	—	Yes	http://ctdbase.org/
GWAS Catalog[48]	Collection of GDA for gene variants from Genome-WAS	Yes	—	Yes	http://www.ebi.ac.uk/gwas/
GWASdb[49]	Collection of GDA for gene variants from Genome-WAS	Yes	—	Yes	http://jjwanglab.org/gwasdb
PheWAS[50]	Collection of GDA for gene variants from Phenome-WAS	Yes	—	Yes	http://phewascatalog.org
CLAIRE-COVID	Disease-related data for COVID-19 tasks	—	Yes	Yes	http://github.com/CLAIRE-COVID-T4/covid-data

Drug Data

Name	Description				URL
DrugBank[51]	Pharmaceutical knowledge base. Useful for DTIs/DIs/DDAs and drug side effects	—	Yes	Yes	http://www.drugbank.com
SIDER[52]	Drug-side effect association collection	—	Yes	Yes	http://sideeffects.embl.de/
ChEMBL[53]	European manually curated drug knowledge base. Useful for DTIs	Yes	Yes	Yes	http://www.ebi.ac.uk/chembl/
PubChem[54]	American manually curated drug knowledge base. Useful for DTIs	Yes	Yes	Yes	http://pubchem.ncbi.nlm.nih.gov
ChEBI[55]	Collection and ontology of small chemical compound (e.g., drugs)	—	Yes	—	http://www.ebi.ac.uk/chebi/
TTD[56]	Database of drug targets, targeted disease and pathway information	—	Yes	Yes	http://db.idrblab.net/ttd/
OFFSIDES[57]	Database of drug—side effect associations	—	Yes	Yes	http://tatonettilab.org/resources/tatonetti-stm.html
STITCH[58]	Collection of experimental-validated and computational-predicted DTIs	—	—	Yes	http://stitch.embl.de/
SuperPred[59]	Database of experimental-validated and computational predicted DTIs	—	—	Yes	http://prediction.charite.de
DGIdb[60]	Collection of DTIs collected from several sources	—	—	Yes	http://www.dgidb.org
TWOSIDES[57]	Collection of DTIs	—	—	Yes	http://tatonettilab.org/resources/tatonetti-stm.html
BindingDB[61]	Collection of DTIs with affinity measurements	Yes	—	Yes	http://www.bindingdb.org
PharmGKB[62]	Collection of DTIs with genetic variants	—	—	Yes	http://www.pharmgkb.org
CTD[47]	Database of literature-curated associations between drugs, genes and diseases (i.e., DDAs)	—	—	Yes	http://ctdbase.org/

(Continued)

Table 1. (*Continued*)

Database	Content description	Primary Features	Associations	Website
SuperTarget[63]	Database of DTIs with information about side effects, pathways and Gene Ontology terms	— Yes	Yes	http://insilico.charite.de/supertarget/index.php?site=about
Matador[63]	Collection of physical and functional, or indirect, DTIs	— —	Yes	http://matador.embl.de/
TDR targets[64]	Collection of drug–target resource for neglected human diseases	— —	Yes	http://tdrtargets.org/
DCDB[65]	Database of drug combinations (e.g., DIs)	— —	Yes	http://www.cls.zju.edu.cn/dcdb/
RepoDB[66]	Collection of repurposed drugs with indications (e.g., DDAs)	— —	Yes	http://portal.dbmi.hms.harvard.edu/projects/repoDB/
CLAIRE-COVID	Drug-related data for COVID-19 tasks	— Yes	Yes	http://github.com/CLAIRE-COVID-T4/covid-data
Gene Expression Data				
GEO[67]	American public collection of gene expressions data	Yes Yes	—	http://www.ncbi.nlm.nih.gov/geo/
ArrayExpress[68]	European public collection of gene expression data	Yes Yes	—	http://www.ebi.ac.uk/arrayexpress/
TCGA[69]	Repository of gene expression profiles associated with cancer	Yes Yes	—	http://www.cancer.gov/about-nci/organization/ccg/research/structural-genomics/tcga
Gene Regulation Data				
TransFAC[70]	Database of regulatory interactions	— Yes	Yes	https://genexplain.com/
GTRD[71]	Database of transcription factor binding sites	— Yes	—	http://gtrd.biouml.org/
TRRUST[72]	Manually curated collection of human and mouse regulatory networks	— —	Yes	http://www.grnpedia.org/trrust

Name	Description			URL
miRTarBase[73]	Collection of miRNA–gene associations	—	Yes	http://mirtarbase.cuhk.edu.cn/php/index.php
miRWalk[74]	Database of miRNA–gene associations	—	Yes	http://mirwalk.umm.uni-heidelberg.de/
miR2Disease[75]	Collection of miRNA–disease associations	—	Yes	http://www.mir2disease.org/
HMDD[76]	Collection of miRNA–disease associations	—	Yes	http://www.cuilab.cn/hmdd
miRCancer[77]	Database of miRNA–cancer associations	—	Yes	http://mircancer.ecu.edu/
PhenomiR[78]	miRNA knowledge base and collection of miRNA–disease associations	Yes	Yes	http://mips.helmholtz-muenchen.de/phenomir/
dbDEMC[79]	miRNA expression profiles in human cancers	Yes	—	http://www.picb.ac.cn/dbDEMC/
TCGA[69]	Collection of miRNA data in cancers	Yes	—	http://www.cancer.gov/about-nci/organization/ccg/research/structural-genomics/tcga
lncRNASNP2[80]	Database of miRNA–lncRNA associations	—	Yes	http://bioinfo.life.hust.edu.cn/lncRNASNP#!/
LncRNADisease[81]	Database of lncRNA–disease associations	—	Yes	http://www.cuilab.cn/lncrnadiseas e
LncRNA2Target[82]	Collection of lncRNA–protein associations	—	Yes	http://123.59.132.21/lncrna2target/
Pathway Data				
Reactome[83]	European-hosted pathway database	Yes	—	http://reactome.org/
KEGG[84]	Japanese-hosted pathway database	Yes	—	http://www.genome.jp/kegg/
WikiPathways[85]	Pathway database based on collaborative platform	Yes	—	http://www.wikipathways.org/
MSigDB[86]	Database-integrating pathways from other resources	Yes	—	http://www.gsea-msigdb.org/
Pathway Commons[87]	Database-integrating pathways from other resources	Yes	—	http://www.pathwaycommons.org/

4. Deep Learning for Interactome (I)

4.1. *PPI prediction (PPIP)*

Proteins play a key role in the biological processes. Having a complete collection of PPIs of an organism is crucial for the many molecular network studies (e.g., the disease gene identification or the drug–target association identification). Notwithstanding the time-consuming and labour-intensive dedication to the built of PPI detection systems, it is still necessary to put efforts to complete the PPI maps of several organisms. The protein–protein interaction identification task may help detect physical interactions which were not previously present among the proteins of an organism. The protein–protein interaction network (see Section 3.1.1), proteins, genes, gene expression and cells are the useful concepts presented in Section 2.3.

Three main experimental approaches are used to detect human protein–protein interactions: systematic experiments; literature curation; computational predictions. Systematic experiments, as Yeast two-Hybrid (Y2H) and Affinity-Purification with Mass-Spectrometry (AP-MS), are the most reliable approaches which provide diverse types of PPIs: Y2H detects binary interactions and AP-MS detects one-to-many (complexes) interactions.[12]

Notwithstanding their accuracy, systematic approaches are prone to identifying false positives and false negatives. As noted by Ref. 88, PPI collections built on a scientific literature review are richer but exposes a *lower quality* since the adopted methods are error-prone and can be affected by investigation biases. Computational approaches, on the other hand, are inexpensive — compared to the laboratory experiments — but due to their synthetic nature, the produced predictions must be validated with biological experiments. Several approaches were proposed in the recent years. The oldest and also one of the most used one as a comparison is node2vec: a skip-gram based approach — proposed in 2016 by Grover and Leskovec[89] — which learns the node network representation (embeddings), leveraging only structural information. Kishan et al.[90] (GNE) and Luo et al.[91] are based on a classic DNN approach. The most recent ones[92–94] are based on GNN. HO-VGAE, proposed by Xiao and Deng,[92] is also based on graph variational auto-encoder (GAE). Here, the aim of the authors is to predict PPIs by improving the GCN aggregation scheme in the GAE to explore higher-order neighbour-hoods of each node in the human PIN. Moreover, they integrate L3 principle, a recently discovered property of the human PIN.[95] In their comparative evaluation on the human PIN, HO-VGAE outperforms node2vec[89] by 3.4% AUPRC. Similar to the HO-VGAE, SkipGNN[93] improves the aggregation scheme to collect information from direct and second-order neighbours. It has been shown that similarity in second-order PPIs can be highly predictive of PPIs (i.e., L3 princi-ple).[95] In their comparative evaluation on the human PIN, SkipGNN outperforms node2vec[89] by 14.8% AUPRC and 15.1% AUROC. Simi-lar to HO-VGAE and SkipGNN, HOGCN[94] improves the aggregation scheme to collect information from direct k-order neighbours. In their comparative evaluation on the human PIN, HOGCN outperforms node2vec[89] by 15.7% AUPRC and 15.6% AUROC and SkipGNN by 0.9% AUPRC and 0.5% AUROC.

All the aforementioned approaches use solely the PPIs as input data with the exception of the method proposed by Kishan *et al.*[90] (GNE) which also uses gene expressions to build the gene representa-tion by integrating both the topological structure of the PIN and the gene expression. In their comparative evaluation on the yeast's PIN, GNE outperforms node2vec by 6% in AUROC and 12% in AUPRC. Unfortunately, these studies lack a common benchmark which per-mits a straight comparison. Each study, even if aligned from the point of view of the adopted evaluation measures, uses a PPI dataset often different from the other works. The most used evaluation measures are the AUROC and the AUPRC, an exception is made by Grover and Leskovec[89] who use solely the F-1 measure. For an additional overview of this subfield of studies, see the works of Lü and Zhou,[7] and Kovács *et al.*[95]

4.2. *Essential protein prediction (EPP)*

Essential genes or proteins are molecular components performing key biological processes for the growth and survival of an organ-ism. Furthermore, essential genes tend to be highly conserved in the evolutionary path of common species. For this reason, essen-tial proteins are employed in the gene–disease association discovery, drug development of antibiotics, and synthetic biology to assess the minimum set of the essential genes needed for the survival of an organism (i.e., essentialome).[96–98] The traditional biological discovery path used to find essential genes relies on time-consuming experiments, such as gene knockout, RNA interference, antisense RNA (asRNA) and transposon mutagenesis.[96,98] From a biological network perspective, the essential genes tend to be the hub nodes of the PIN network.[11] Since the PIN tends to be a scale-free network, the deletion of essential genes leads to the disruption of its connectivity and, consequently, produces instability in the organism.[99] However, if on the one hand essential proteins are strongly related to network topology, on the other hand, the noise and the incompleteness of the PINs limit the performance of classic network-based prediction methods.[96,97] Several computational approaches, based on deep neural network, were proposed in the recent years. The majority of them are based on node2vec in conjunction with other techniques, such as LSTM, CNN and GNN. Zeng *et al.*[100] propose an end-to-end model, based on node2vec and LSTM, to identify the essential proteins by jointly integrating *PIN, gene expression* and information on *subcellular localisation*. The produced classification of the essential proteins was tested on Yeast data using the F-measure, AUC, and AP measures. A similar approach was explored by Zeng *et al.*,[101] who use a CNN instead of LSTM, and by Zhang *et al.*,[102] who concatenate node2vec protein vectors and sequence data to feed a fully connected multi-layer neural network (DNN). We would like to note that Zhang *et al.* improve the overall performance of the EPP by exploiting protein sequence and topological features and by addressing the imbalanced learning problem by using a cost-sensitive training function. EPGAT, proposed by Schapke *et al.*,[97] is the most different one both in terms of method and used data. EPGAT constructs an attributed *PIN* network to apply a method based on a graph attention neural networks where they used a weighted binary cross-entropy (CE) function. The nodes of the PIN network are decorated with a feature vector based on *gene expression* profiles, *orthology information*, and *subcellular localisation*. Even if the aforementioned methods are exhaustively evaluated using several measures (e.g., accuracy, recall, precision, AUROC and AUPRC), they do not present a direct comparison with deep learning techniques. The main baseline methods used for comparison are the degree centrality and the support vector machine, but due to the use of different PIN data, it is not possible to highlight a common benchmark. For an additional overview of this subfield of studies, see the works of Li *et al.*[96] and Zhang *et al.*[98]

4.3. *Protein function prediction (PFP)*

As already stated, proteins carry out critical functions of an organism. However, the functions of almost all the proteins are largely unknown. According to Shehu *et al.*,[103] less than 1% of the proteins have reliable and detailed annotations in the Universal Protein (UniProt) database. Moreover, *"fundamental information is currently missing for 40% of the protein sequences deposited in the National Center for Biotechnology Information (NCBI) database"*. For the aforementioned reason and due to the growing gap between the number of proteins being discovered and their functional characterisation (in particular as a result of experimental limitations), completing the collection of the protein function has become a fundamental research problem to address. The first effort made by researchers to overcome this problem was to organise the protein functions in a structured and standardised way. The Gene Ontology (GO)[q] is a collection of three protein functions, hierarchical ontologies distinct by the biological aspect: cellular component, biological processes and molecular functions. Secondly, proposing a reliable prediction of protein function through computational methods has become crucial. In this direction, GraphSAGE, proposed by W. Hamilton *et al.*[104] presents an inductive framework that leverages node feature information to learn node embeddings. In this work, the authors use a PIN network only to prove the efficacy of their work. In 2018, M. Kulmanov *et al.* propose DeepGO,[105] a complex end-to-end deep learning method which exploits protein sequence features, topological cross-species PIN features and dependencies among GO classes to predict the protein function. The method is based on the concatenation of two deep neural networks, which combines the protein sequences and network representation, respectively. DeepNF, by Gligorijević *et al.*,[106] propose a network fusion method based on multimodal deep auto-encoder (MDA) to

---

[q]See Section 3.2 for additional details.

extract high-level features of genes from multiple heterogeneous inter-action networks (six different yeast protein–protein networks). The method uses the random walk with restart (RWR) to build a high-dimensional node embedding which, once it is reduced using an MDA, is used into an SVM classifier to predict the protein func-tions. Lastly, Fan *et al.* propose Graph2GO,[107] a model to predict protein functions (GO-terms) exploiting a *protein sequence similar-ity network* and a PIN with node attributes (amino acid sequence, subcellular location, and protein domains). The model uses two vari-ational graph auto-encoders (vGAEs) to learn latent representations for each protein and successively predict protein functions with a DNN. Graph2GO improves by 10.5% and 3.33% the micro-AUPRC and macro-AUPRC, respectively, when compared to deepNF. All works in the area use a combination of PPIs with attributes and normally prefer to use the precision, the recall and the F-measure as comparison metrics. To complete the overview of this subfield of stud-ies, readers are recommended to refer to the works of Shehu *et al.*,[103] Bonetta and Valentino.[108] The protein–protein interaction network (see Section 3.1.1) and the Proteins, PPI, Gene and Cells concepts (see Section 2.3) can be helpful concepts to better understand this section.

4.4. *Gene–disease association prediction (GDAP)*

The disease–gene identification consists of finding the gene or gene product involved in the origin of a genetic disease (i.e., disease gene). Traditional ways to assess the role of genes in diseases involve time-consuming and expensive[r] analyses, such as linkage analysis and genome-wide association studies (GWAS).[49]

Genome-wide association studies (GWAS) have led to large collec-tions of disease–gene associations available in public databases, such as OMIM[43] and DisGeNET.[42] The identification of disease genes pro-vides useful insights to understand disease mechanisms, design new therapies, improve disease prevention approaches and make an accu-rate risk factor evaluation. For this reason, computational methods in

---

[r]https://www.genome.gov/27541954/dna-sequencing-costs-data/.

this area of research have become increasingly prominent and widely proposed.

The computational approaches in this research area are mainly based on GNN and Skip-Gram using PPI and GDA data with enriched features. Agrawal et al.[109] use node2vec and a logistic regression to study how latent network structures of the human PIN are correlated with the disease module predictability. In HerGePred[110] (HDGN), a heterogeneous network is built by combining four types of relationships: *disease–gene*, *disease–symptom*, *gene–GO-terms*, gene–gene (*PPI*). Then it is applied in node2vec to learn the node embeddings. Finally, two distinct disease–gene rankings are produced leveraging the cosine similarity and an RWR-based approach. Similar to DeepWalk and node2vec, SmuDGE[111] performs random walks on heterogeneous networks (composed by PPI, disease–phenotypes and gene–phenotype associations) and then applies the Skip-Gram model to learn the disease and gene representations. SmuDGE uses two independent methods: (i) an unsupervised method based on the cosine similarity between embedding vectors and the query disease vector; (ii) a method based on a deep neural network which uses the gene and disease embeddings to perform the prediction. Another study based on node2vec is the work proposed by Ata et al.,[112] where they enrich the generated embeddings with around 500 *gene features* collected from UniProt. The enriched representation is used to train several binary classification models: SVM, generalized linear model (GLM), random forest (RF) and kNN. According to the authors, N2VKO outperforms plain node2vec by roughly 2.6% AUROC on six diseases. In HNEEM,[113]the authors construct a heterogeneous network based on *gene–disease* associations, *gene–chemical* associations and *disease–chemical* associations. Several models are then applied to learn different node embeddings: node2vec, DeepWalk, higher-order proximity preserved embedding (HOPE), semi-supervised depth model structural deep network embedding (SDNE),[114] graph factorization (GF)[115] and Laplacian eigenmaps (LE).[116] Finally, they predict the disease–gene association using a random forest-based approach. The method presented by Zhu et al.[117] uses a cascade of deep methods (DeepWalk with a graph convolution layer and a three-layer fully connected network) to predict the disease–gene associations. The presented approach uses a heterogeneous network that integrates a gene–gene network, disease–disease network and gene–disease network to outperform the prediction made by HerGePred by 11.7% AUPRC. HeteWalk[118] performs the Skip-Gram model on meta-path-controlled random walks which explore a weighted heterogeneous network of PPIs, miRNA–miRNA, disease–disease, gene–disease, gene–miRNA, miRNA–disease associations. Given a query disease, HeteWalk ranks genes according to the cosine similarity between their representations and the given disease vector. GCN-MF[119] extracts disease and gene features using the principal component analysis (PCA) and matrix factorisation methods on prior biological knowledge of diseases and genes. These features are then used to build a similarity network which in conjunction with the gene features are used to train a GCN model. A slightly different approach dgMDL is presented by Luo *et al.*[120] The method, based on a multi-modal deep belief net (DBN) first constructs a gene–gene similarity network and a disease similarity network based on PPIs and GO-terms data, respectively. Then, node2vec is applied to these networks to generate their latent representations. The generated embeddings are finally jointly used into a two-level DBNs. One of the most recent approaches is the Random Watcher Walker RW^2.[121] Madeddu *et al.* propose an unsupervised deep learning method that exploits both functional and connectivity patterns to predict the gene–disease associations. To do so, RW^2 collects the second-order random walk made over the gene attributes of the human PIN to learn Skip-Gram-based attribute representations. The final prediction is made using attribute representation which encompasses both structural and functional connectivity. The proposed framework allows one to integrate multiple sources of information without manipulating the original network topology, producing promising results. CIPHER-SC[122] uses an approach based on a graph convolution on a context-aware network with single-cell data. The heterogeneous network is composed by *ontological associations* and *biological relationships* from both public databases and single-cell data. The node2vec node representations are used into a deep neural network made with one GCN and one DistMult[123] layer. Authors compared CIPHER-SC to methods present in the literature (HerGePred, SmuDGE and GCN-MF), achieving an increment up to 8.02% in AUROC and 17.01% in AUPRC. Finally, HO-VGAE[94] and SkipGNN,[93] described in Section 4.1, improves the GNN's aggregation scheme to predict gene–disease associations. In their comparative evaluation on the GDAP problem, SkipGNN outperforms node2vec[89] by 8.7% AUPRC and 7.8% AUROC. HOGCN outperforms SkipGNN by 2.6% AUPRC and 2.4% AUROC.

It is also worth noting that this prediction problem is characterised by the absence of a sharp benchmark. All the methods can be distinguished mainly by the used data rather than the computational approach. Despite that, node2vec, AUROC and AUPRC represent the defacto baseline and measures for comparison. To complete the overview of this subfield of studies, readers are recommended to refer to the works of Luo *et al.*[124] and Kaushal *et al.*[125]

5. Deep Learning for Network Pharmacology (NP)

5.1. *Drug–target interaction prediction (DTIP)*

The drug–target association prediction is the task that consists in finding a molecule, usually a protein, which is bounded to a drug. There exist several wet-lab experiments to assess drug–target associations, but they are extremely expensive and time-consuming.[126] The identification of drug–target interactions is crucial for drug discovery and drug repurposing, and thus for the design of new therapies and development of Precision Medicine.

The most notable methods which rely on deep neural network techniques are the ones proposed by Zong *et al.*[127] and Wan *et al.*[128]

The first method[127] is a similarity-based drug–target one which first constructs a heterogeneous network of *drug–target, drug–disease* and *disease–target* associations. Then, the DeepWalk method is applied to the network to build node representation. Authors propose two rule-based inference methods to predict new drug–target associations: a drug-based similarity inference (DBSI) and a target-based similarity inference (TBSI) ones. The former, DBSI, predicts a new drug–target association (d_i, t_l) if the drug d_i is similar to the drug d_j and there exists an association among the drug d_j and the target t_l. On the other hand, TBSI predicts a new drug–target association (d_i, t_h) if there exists an association among the drug d_i and the target t_l and the target t_l is similar to the target t_h. The proposed method mainly takes advantage of the topological structure of biological networks to improve the predicted performances.

NeoDTI[128] is an end-to-end model to predict drug–target interactions from heterogeneous data. The method, first, constructs a network composed of other eight ones: drug–drug structure-based similarity, drug–side effect, drug–target, drug–drug, drug–disease, protein–protein sequence-based similarity, protein–disease and PIN. The proposed deep learning neural network framework takes in input the heterogeneous network to reconstruct the original eight networks adjacency matrices. Finally, NeoDTI predicts the drug–target interactions relying on the reconstructed network matrices.

Lastly, SkipGNN[93] and HO-VGAE,[94] described in Section 4.1, improves the GNN's aggregation scheme to predict drug–drug interactions. In their comparative evaluation on the DTIP problem, SkipGNN outperforms node2vec[89] by 15.7% on AUPRC and 20.2% on AUROC. HOGCN outperforms SkipGNN by 0.9% on AUPRC and 1.2% on AUROC.

The main advantages of the proposed methods are the integration of several sources of information to extract nonlinear patterns from the data. AUROC and AUPRC are the most used metrics in this research field. For an additional overview of this subfield of studies, refer to the works of Ezzat *et al.*,[126] Bagherian *et al.*[129] and Abbasi *et al.*[130]

5.2. *Drug–disease association prediction (DDAP)*

A drug–disease association (also named *drug repurposing*) is a synthetic representation of the therapeutic effect which a drug has on a certain disease. It is important to note that a disease is a complex process which has an impact on an organism by modifying its biological processes and thus must be distinguished from the drug–target interaction. Note that the drug discovery process, where a new drug is developed from scratch, is different from the drug repurposing one. Drug discovery is a time-consuming and expensive process while the repurposing process of an existing drug may drastically reduce costs and time of drug validation, especially if it is addressed by computational approaches.

The first solution to DDAP was proposed by Zeng *et al.* with DeepDR.[131] DeepDR is a network-based deep learning approach for drug repurposing which uses several biological networks: *drug–disease, drug–side effect, drug–target* and seven *drug–drug* networks. At first, DeepDR generates the low-dimensional representations capturing highly nonlinear patterns (drug embeddings) by using the DeepNF model (presented in Section 4.3) on nine drug-related networks. Then, the learned drug embeddings and drug–disease associations are used into a *collective variational auto-encoder*[132] to predict novel drug–disease associations. Similarly, the approach of Gysi *et al.*[2] learns disease and gene representations, applying the Decagon model (presented in Section 5.3) on four association networks (*protein–protein, drug–target, disease–protein, and drug–disease associations*) to predict the drug–COVID-19 associations. Lastly, Karimi *et al.* present a reinforcement learning-based approach, HVGAE.[133] The method learns disease and drug embeddings using a *hierarchical variational graph auto-encoder* with attentional pooling on PPI, gene–disease and disease–disease networks. The learned representations are used into a reinforcement learning model to identify the drug combinations which maximise the therapeutic efficacy. This work addresses the challenging problem of finding clinical indications for a set of drugs instead of repurposing a single drug as in the aforementioned works.

The most used metrics in this domain are AUROC and AUPRC. Unfortunately, it is not possible to recognise a common benchmark. An additional overview of this domain is presented in the works of Xue *et al.*[134] and Jarada *et al.*[135]

5.3. *Drug–drug interaction prediction (DDIP)*

The combined interactions of two or more drugs with individual biological processes may cause unexpected and critical health complications.[136] These complications, called adverse drug reactions (ADRs), are dangerous for the patient and expensive for the health system. A significative number of hospital admissions and medical errors are due by DDI.[137]

Notwithstanding the high demand for improving our understanding of DDIs, the current known side effects of these interactions are less than 1% of the total[138] and their prediction by clinical and wet-lab experiments are extremely expensive and hard to carry out.[139]

For the aforementioned reason, drug–drug interaction detection is a relevant task necessary for the success of patients' treatments.

Several computational classic machine learning approaches have been developed,[139, 140] the only three methods that can be highlighted as deep-based ones are Decagon,[136] SkipGNN[93] and HO-VGAE.[94]

The authors of Decagon present an *end-to-end multimodal graph auto-encoder* approach for predicting drug–drug associations and their side effects. The input of the model is a multimodal (heterogeneous) graph composed by *protein–protein interactions, drug–protein target interactions and polypharmacy side effects.* The drugs are the nodes and each side effect is an edge of a different type. The method is based on a novel convolutional neural network for multi-relational link prediction. Decagon addresses the problem of polypharmacy to find side effects of drug combinations, a task different from the one of finding a combined clinical treatment as in the work of Karimi *et al.*[133] (presented in detail in Section 5.2).

HO-VGAE[94] and SkipGNN,[93] presented in Section 4.1, improve the GNN's aggregation scheme to predict drug–drug interactions. In their comparative evaluation on the DDIP problem, SkipGNN outperforms node2vec[89] by 6.5% on AUPRC and 7.7% on AUROC. HOGCN outperforms SkipGNN by 3.1% on AUPRC and 2.5% on AUROC.

6. Deep Learning for Other Biological Problems (BIO)

6.1. *miRNA–disease association prediction (MDAP)*

The miRNA–disease association prediction (MDAP) is the task of identifying the interactions between microRNA (miRNA) and a disease. miRNAs play a key role in gene regulation with an important impact on biological processes and disease mechanisms. Several studies have shown the usefulness of miRNA–disease associations for personalised diagnosis and drug development.[141] Biological methods to assess miRNA–disease associations are reverse transcription–polymerase chain reaction, northern blotting and micro-array profiling.[142] However, these experiments, as often happen in the biological domain, are expensive and time-consuming. For this reason, applying computational methods, mainly based on CNN and GNN, will benefit the identification of new associations.

Xuan *et al.* present two works, namely, CNNMDA[143] and CNNDMP,[144] both based on a CNN. To overcome the limitation of classic computational methods of the area, the authors embed a higher number of miRNA–disease associations. The two methods mainly differ from the input data processing step needed by CNN. To extract network representations, CNNMDA uses the nonnegative matrix factorisation (NMF) and CNNDMP uses RWR. MDA-CNN[145] extracts network-based features by applying an autoencoder to a three-layer complex network which includes disease similarity network, miRNA similarity network and protein–protein interaction network. MDA-CNN predicts the miRNA–disease associations with a CNN which uses the learned low-dimensional representations as input. The authors of HGCNMDA[141] propose a method based on a heterogeneous network of *human PPIs, miRNA–disease, miRNA–gene, disease–gene* associations. The method first generates the gene embeddings by applying node2vec to the human PINs. Then, it uses a *graph convolutional layer* for every network in conjunction with the learned node embeddings. Finally, HGCN-MDA averages the resulting GCN representations to predict miRNA–disease associations in a link prediction setting. The first step of NIMCGCN[146] is based on the construction of miRNA–disease similarity networks. A GCN method is used to learn miRNA and disease latent representations. Lastly, the representations are used by a neural inductive matrix completion (NIMC) model to generate an association matrix which allows the prediction of miRNA–disease associations. Another GCN-based method (FCGCNMDA) is presented by Li *et al.*[147] It first constructs a complete network in which nodes represent miRNA–disease pairs. Then the miRNA–disease network along with a feature matrix (i.e., miRNA–disease association scores as node weights) are used by a two-layer GCN to predict new miRNA–disease associations. Lastly, GAMEDA[142] is a graph auto-encoder-based model which first collects the associations between miRNAs using a bipartite graph. The projected (in the same vector space) miRNA and disease nodes are then processed by a graph auto-encoder (GAE) to learn dense representations. Finally, GAEMDA uses the miRNA and disease embeddings with a *bilinear decoder* to reconstruct and predict new miRNA–disease associations.

The reference metrics used by these works are the AUROC and AUPRC. Generally, the works are not going to self-compare with the other methods in the same field of research. MDAP, as a new area of research, suffers by the absence of common benchmarks and the availability of comprehensive literature reviews.

6.2. *Disease analysis (DA)*

The discovery of the mechanisms of a complex disease, such as cancer or tumours, is dependent on the underlying interconnected molecular heterogeneous processes. In this context of analysis, GDAP methods, based solely on the analysis of the organism PIN, generally fail to identify the condition-specific disease drivers. In order to identify the drivers specific of a disease subtype or a patient, several works successfully integrate gene expression profiles with network biology. This integration helps clinicians to make a better diagnosis and select a patient personalised treatment. In this section, we discuss the recent works for the analysis of specific disease-related conditions using gene expression data and networks.

Rhee *et al.*[148] solve the patient classification problem proposing a method based on *relation network (RN)* and *graph convolution neural network (graph CNN)*. The method captures localised patterns of associating genes with graph CNN and then learns the relationship between these patterns with the RN. The proposed framework is applied to the human PIN and gene expression profiles of patients with breast cancer level 3 to classify the subtype of breast cancer according to the PAM50 scheme. The work proposed by Schulte *et al.*[149] tackles the problem of combining multiple omics data types into a single learning model. Their model uses gene expression data for cancer gene prediction by applying a GCN. The used attributed PIN is composed of nodes which have features vector extracted from the gene expression profiles in specific cancer condition. DeepDriver[150] uses a Deep CNN applied to a gene–gene similarity network and a gene features vector derived from *gene expression* data. Authors focused their approach on cancer specific genes. iSOM-GSN[151] uses the self-organizing maps (SOMs) algorithm to generate a gene–gene similarity network from gene expression data. Then, it enriches the adjacency matrix by integrating each gene with feature values of gene expression, DNA methylation and copy number alteration (CNA). Finally, they use the enriched obtained data into CNN to predict the disease states.

Due to the recent introduction of this research field and the limited amount of works present in the area, it is difficult to clearly identify a common set of evaluation measures and a common benchmark.

6.3. *Brain analysis (BA)*

The brain network (i.e., connectome, see Section 3.1.5) analysis is a new emergent field of study. Typically, it is used to understand the mechanisms of diseases, such as schizophrenia, depression, Alzheimer's and multiple sclerosis.[152] The connectome is characterised by complex interdependencies between brain regions. The relation between brain network structures and their functional roles is partially known. For this reason, applying computational approaches becomes necessary to improve their current understanding.

Two deep neural network-based methods can be identified in this field. The first one, proposed by Rosenthal *et al.*[152] uses node2vec to learn the low-dimensional network representations of brain regions to study their latent relationships. The latter, proposed by Lee *et al.*,[153] addresses the problem of analysing the natural organisation of the brain networks. The method uses a Graph Auto-Encoder (GAE), with non-negative weight constraints, to a *"structural"* brain network to learn low-dimensional representations of the nodes (brain zones). The non-negative weight constraint in the GAE is the most innovative contribution proposed by this method, which adds interpretability capabilities to the model.

We would like to note that this field of research is characterised by custom qualitative examinations rather than a clear benchmark and a precise set of evaluation measures.

7. Conclusion and Future Work

This chapter summarises the concepts, datasets, and techniques used by deep learning applications in network biology. A complete overview of the presented works with respect to the used base methods, data and evaluation measures are summarised in Table 2. The reviewed works have shown that it is now possible to delve deep into the biological network complexity in a more detailed way. Despite the impressive results achieved by deep learning techniques, future works will need to cope with data and method issues.

On the one hand, even if recent advancements in high-throughput technologies have produced a huge and growing quantity of biological data, these data are affected by the following quality and reliability problems:

Incompleteness: The biological networks are characterised by high incompleteness. As shown in Table 2, the most used network, with its attributes, is the human PIN known for its 20% only.[12] This data incompleteness strongly limits deep learning method performances.

Bias: Biological knowledge suffers from the study bias. Several PPI collections are strongly biased towards the most studied genes leading to network structures that are not representative of the topology of the complete human PIN.[9] Bias in biological networks is a critical issue because it influences the quality of the patterns extracted by network-based methods and hence their performance. Recently, Luck *et al.*[31] presented a human PIN obtained by a systematically, unbiased proteome-wide study.

Noise: Both literature-based data and high-throughput technologies are prone to generate false positives and false negatives.[92, 154] For this reason, biological interaction datasets must be completed by evidence/reliability scores.[28, 42]

Lack of negative knowledge: This is common practice in the biomedical literature (due to practical and economical reasons) to avoid discussion of the biological entities which are not interacting. The absence of these *"negative"* results create uncertainty about the absence of the interaction or the lack of knowledge about it.[121, 154] Machine learning methods achieve better performances if they can learn both from positive and negative samples. To solve this issue, negative knowledge is randomly sampled or generated with biological heuristics. However, these generation strategies may force one to consider an unknown positive interaction as a negative one, leading to lower quality of the model through overestimation of the performances.

On the other hand, future development of the computational methods in network biology must face the following open challenges:

Heterogeneous data: Heterogeneous data in network biology can be both node and edge features or whole additional networks. In the literature, given the complex and interconnected nature of biomedical entities and the aforementioned lack of knowledge in the biological datasets, there is no agreement on how heterogeneous data must be appropriately handled. As we have seen, several methods can differ solely on the techniques used to tackle this aspect. Modelling and integrating heterogeneous information, even if it is a difficult task, will be the key strategy to achieve better results.

Imbalanced learning: Problems in network biology are usually extremely imbalanced by their nature (e.g., PPIP). If not properly handled, this imbalance will affect the performances by producing overestimated evaluations.

Biological heuristics: Several graph deep learning methods in network biology are inspired by techniques developed for social networks. However, biological networks rely on different topological patterns. Recent studies[93] are facing this challenge by integrating the L3 principle[95] rather than the social homophily.[89]

To conclude, graph deep learning approach in network biology represents a powerful tool to unchain the hidden biology, medicine and pharmacology knowledge.

Table 2. Summary of surveyed works with respect to methods, data and evaluation measures.

Methods

Problems		DNN	Classic		Auto-encoder (AE)				DeepWalk	Skip-gram based Node2vec	Others	GNN
			CNN	LSTM	AE	VAE	MDA	GAE				
I	PPIP	90, 91						92				92–94
I	EPP	102	100									97
I	PFP	105	105				106					104
I	GDAP	111, 117, 120							113, 117	109, 110, 112, 113, 120, 122	110, 111, 113, 118, 121	93, 94, 117, 119, 122
NP	DTIP	128			101				127			93, 94
NP	DDAP					131	131	2, 133				2
NP	DDIP							136				93, 94, 136
BIO	MDAP		143–145		145			142		141		141, 146, 147
BIO	DA	150										148, 149
BIO	BA							153		152		

Data types

Problems		Gene/Protein		Drug				GDA	Disease	Features	Gene expression	Gene regulation	Pathways	Brain
		PPI	Features	DTI	DDI	DI	Features							
I	PPIP	89–94												
I	EPP	97, 100–102	97, 100, 102								90			
I	PFP	104–106	104–106								97, 100, 101			
I	GDAP	109–112, 117–122	110–112, 117, 120, 122	113	113		110, 111, 117, 119–122	93, 109–113, 117–120, 122	110, 111, 117–120, 122			118		
NP	DTIP	128	128	127, 128	93, 94, 127, 128	128		127, 128						
NP	DDAP	2, 133	133	2, 131	2, 131, 133	131		2, 133					133	
NP	DDIP	136		136		93, 94, 136								
BIO	MDAP	141					141–147	141		141–147		141–147		
BIO	DA	148, 149						148, 150			148–151			
BIO	BA													152, 153

Evaluation measures

Problems		Classic measures					Ranking/Thresholding measures						
		ACC.	RC.	PR.	F-1	MCC	F-1@K	PR@k	RC@k	AP	NDCG	ROC	PRC
I	PPIP				89			92				90, 91, 93, 94	90–94
I	EPP	100–102	100–102	100–102	100, 101					101, 102		97, 100–102	100–102
I	PFP	106			104, 106	105	105, 107	105, 107	105, 107	105		105, 107	106
I	GDAP	113	113	113	113	113	110, 117, 119	110, 117, 119	109, 110, 117, 119, 121	110, 117, 119	119	93, 94, 111–113, 118–120, 122	93, 94, 113, 122
NP	DTIP								127			93, 94, 127, 128	93, 94, 127, 128
NP	DDAP						133		131	2, 133		2, 131, 133	2, 131
NP	DDIP								136	136		93, 94, 136	93, 94, 136
BIO	MDAP	141, 142, 146	142, 145	142, 145	142, 145				143, 144			141–147	141, 143–145, 147
BIO	DA	148, 151	151	151	148, 151							149–151	149

References

1. T. N. Kipf and M. Welling, Semi-supervised classification with graph convolutional networks, *arXiv:1609.02907* (2016).
2. D. M. Gysi, Í. D. Valle, M. Zitnik, A. Ameli, X. Gan, O. Varol, H. Sanchez, R. M. Baron, D. Ghiassian, J. Loscalzo, *et al.*, Network medicine framework for identifying drug repurposing opportunities for COVID-19, *arXiv:2004.07229* (2020).
3. L. Madeddu, G. Stilo, and P. Velardi. Predicting disease genes for complex diseases using random watcher-walker. In *Proceedings of the 35th Annual ACM Symposium on Applied Computing* (2020).
4. P. Erdős and A. Rényi, On the evolution of random graphs, *Publ. Math. Inst. Hung. Acad. Sci.* **5**(1) (1960).
5. A.-L. Barabási and R. Albert, Emergence of scaling in random networks, *Science* **286**(5439) (1999).
6. D. J. Watts and S. H. Strogatz, Collective dynamics of small-world networks, *Nature* **393**(6684) (1998).
7. L. Lü and T. Zhou, Link prediction in complex networks: A survey, *Physica A: Stat. Mech. Appl.* **390**(6) (2011).
8. P. Goyal and E. Ferrara, Graph embedding techniques, applications, and performance: A survey, *Knowl.-Based Syst.* **151** (2018).
9. A.-L. Barabási, N. Gulbahce, and J. Loscalzo, Network medicine: A network-based approach to human disease, *Nat. Rev. Genet.* **12**(1) (2011).
10. A.-L. Barabasi and Z. N. Oltvai, Network biology: Understanding the cell's functional organization, *Nature Rev. Genet.* **5**(2) (2004).
11. H. Jeong, S. P. Mason, A.-L. Barabási, and Z. N. Oltvai, Lethality and centrality in protein networks, *Nature* **411**(6833) (2001).
12. K. Venkatesan, J.-F. Rual, A. Vazquez, U. Stelzl, I. Lemmens, T. Hirozane-Kishikawa, T. Hao, M. Zenkner, X. Xin, K.-I. Goh, *et al.*, An empirical framework for binary interactome mapping, *Nat. Methods* **6**(1) (2009).
13. M. AY, K.-I. Goh, M. E. Cusick, A.-L. Barabasi, M. Vidal, *et al.*, Drug–target network, *Nat. Biotechnol* **25**(10) (2007).
14. F. Cheng, I. A. Kovács, and A.-L. Barabási, Network-based prediction of drug combinations, *Nat. Commun.* **10**(1) (2019).
15. F. Cheng, R. J. Desai, D. E. Handy, R. Wang, S. Schneeweiss, A.-L. Barabási, and J. Loscalzo, Network-based approach to prediction and population-based validation of in silico drug repurposing, *Nat. Commun.* **9**(1) (2018).
16. P. Langfelder and S. Horvath, Eigengene networks for studying the relationships between co-expression modules, *BMC Syst. Biol.* **1**(1) (2007).

17. K. Glass, J. Quackenbush, D. Spentzos, B. Haibe-Kains, and G.-C. Yuan, A network model for angiogenesis in ovarian cancer, *BMC Bioinform.* **16**(1) (2015).

18. O. Sporns, *Networks of the Brain.* MIT press (2010).

19. V. M. Eguiluz, D. R. Chialvo, G. A. Cecchi, M. Baliki, and A. V. Apkarian, Scale-free brain functional networks, *Phys. Rev. Lett.* **94**(1) (2005).

20. D. S. Bassett and E. Bullmore, Small-world brain networks, *Neuroscientist* **12**(6) (2006).

21. O. Sporns and R. Kötter, Motifs in brain networks, *PLoS Biol.* **2**(11) (2004).

22. M. A. Bertolero, B. T. Yeo, and M. D'Esposito, The modular and integrative functional architecture of the human brain, *Proc. Natl. Acad. Sci.* **112**(49) (2015).

23. E. J. Sanz-Arigita, M. M. Schoonheim, J. S. Damoiseaux, S. A. Rombouts, E. Maris, F. Barkhof, P. Scheltens, and C. J. Stam, Loss of "small-world" networks in Alzheimer's disease: Graph analysis of fmri resting-state functional connectivity, *PLoS one.* **5**(11) (2010).

24. U. Consortium, UniProt: A worldwide hub of protein knowledge, *Nucleic Acids Res.* **47**(D1) (2019).

25. G. O. Consortium, The gene ontology resource: 20 years and still going strong, *Nucleic Acids Res.* **47**(D1) (2019).

26. M. Uhlén, L. Fagerberg, B. M. Hallström, C. Lindskog, P. Oksvold, A. Mardinoglu, Å. Sivertsson, C. Kampf, E. Sjöstedt, A. Asplund, *et al.*, Tissue-based map of the human proteome, *Science* **347**(6220) (2015).

27. R. Oughtred, J. Rust, C. Chang, B.-J. Breitkreutz, C. Stark, A. Willems, L. Boucher, G. Leung, N. Kolas, F. Zhang, *et al.*, The biogrid database: A comprehensive biomedical resource of curated protein, genetic, and chemical interactions, *Protein Sci.* (2020).

28. S. Orchard, M. Ammari, B. Aranda, L. Breuza, L. Briganti, F. Broackes-Carter, N. H. Campbell, G. Chavali, C. Chen, N. Del-Toro, *et al.*, The mintact project — intact as a common curation platform for 11 molecular interaction databases, *Nucleic Acids Res.* **42**(D1) (2014).

29. I. Xenarios, D. W. Rice, L. Salwinski, M. K. Baron, E. M. Marcotte, and D. Eisenberg, Dip: The database of interacting proteins, *Nucleic Acids Res.* **28**(1) (2000).

30. T. Keshava Prasad, R. Goel, K. Kandasamy, S. Keerthikumar, S. Kumar, S. Mathivanan, D. Telikicherla, R. Raju, B. Shafreen, A. Venugopal, *et al.*, Human protein reference database — 2009 update, *Nucleic Acids Res.* **37**(suppl_1) (2009).

31. K. Luck, D.-K. Kim, L. Lambourne, K. Spirohn, B. E. Begg, W. Bian, R. Brignall, T. Cafarelli, F. J. Campos-Laborie, B. Charloteaux, *et al.*, A reference map of the human binary protein interactome, *Nature* **580**(7803) (2020).

32. D. Alonso-López, F. J. Campos-Laborie, M. A. Gutiérrez, L. Lambourne, M. A. Calderwood, M. Vidal, and J. De Las Rivas, Apid database: Redefining protein–protein interaction experimental evidences and binary interactomes, *Database* **2019** (2019).

33. G. Alanis-Lobato, M. A. Andrade-Navarro, and M. H. Schaefer, Hippie v2. 0: enhancing meaningfulness and reliability of protein–protein interaction networks, *Nucleic Acids Res.* (2016).

34. P. Trott, Int. classification of diseases for oncology, *J. Clin. Pathol.* **30**(8) (1977).

35. K. A. Spackman, K. E. Campbell, and R. A. Côté. SNOMED RT: A reference terminology for health care. In *Proceedings of the AMIA Annual Fall Symposium* (1997).

36. C. E. Lipscomb, Medical subject headings (mesh), *Bull. Med. Libr. Assoc.* **88**(3) (2000).

37. O. Bodenreider, The unified medical language system (umls): integrating biomedical terminology, *Nucleic Acids Res.* **32**(suppl_1) (2004).

38. L. M. Schriml, C. Arze, S. Nadendla, Y.-W. W. Chang, M. Mazaitis, V. Felix, G. Feng, and W. A. Kibbe, Disease ontology: A backbone for disease semantic integration, *Nucleic Acids Res.* **40**(D1) (2012).

39. S. Köhler, N. A. Vasilevsky, M. Engelstad, E. Foster, J. McMurry, S. Aymé, G. Baynam, S. M. Bello, C. F. Boerkoel, K. M. Boycott, *et al.*, The human phenotype ontology in 2017, *Nucleic Acids Res.* **45** (D1) (2017).

40. N. Rappaport, N. Nativ, G. Stelzer, M. Twik, Y. Guan-Golan, T. Iny Stein, I. Bahir, F. Belinky, C. P. Morrey, M. Safran, *et al.*, Malacards: An integrated compendium for diseases and their annotation, *Database* **2013** (2013).

41. S. S. Weinreich, R. Mangon, J. Sikkens, M. Teeuw, and M. Cornel, Orphanet: a european database for rare diseases, *Nederlands tijdschrift voor geneeskunde* **152**(9) (2008).

42. J. Piñero, À. Bravo, N. Queralt-Rosinach, A. Gutiérrez-Sacristán, J. Deu-Pons, E. Centeno, J. García-García, F. Sanz, and L. I. Furlong, DisGeNET: a comprehensive platform integrating information on human disease-associated genes and variants, *Nucleic Acids Res.* (2016).

43. A. Hamosh, A. F. Scott, J. S. Amberger, C. A. Bocchini, and V. A. McKusick, Online Mendelian Inheritance in Man (OMIM), a knowledgebase of human genes and genetic disorders, *Nucleic Acids Res.* **33** (suppl_1) (2005).

44. A. Gutiérrez-Sacristán, S. Grosdidier, O. Valverde, M. Torrens, À. Bravo, J. Piñero, F. Sanz, and L. I. Furlong, Psygenet: A knowledge platform on psychiatric disorders and their genes, *Bioinformatics* **31**(18) (2015).

45. W. Yu, M. Gwinn, M. Clyne, A. Yesupriya, and M. J. Khoury, A navigator for human genome epidemiology, *Nat. Genet.* **40**(2) (2008).

46. J. G. Tate, S. Bamford, H. C. Jubb, Z. Sondka, D. M. Beare, N. Bindal, H. Boutselakis, C. G. Cole, C. Creatore, E. Dawson, *et al.*, Cosmic: The catalogue of somatic mutations in cancer, *Nucleic Acids Res.* **47**(D1) (2019).

47. A. P. Davis, C. J. Grondin, R. J. Johnson, D. Sciaky, R. McMorran, J. Wiegers, T. C. Wiegers, and C. J. Mattingly, The comparative toxicogenomics database: Update 2019, *Nucleic Acids Res.* **47**(D1) (2019).

48. D. Welter, J. MacArthur, J. Morales, T. Burdett, P. Hall, H. Junkins, A. Klemm, P. Flicek, T. Manolio, L. Hindorff, *et al.*, The NHGRI GWAS catalog, a curated resource of snp-trait associations, *Nucleic Acids Res.* **42**(D1) (2014).

49. M. J. Li, Z. Liu, P. Wang, M. P. Wong, M. R. Nelson, J.-P. A. Kocher, M. Yeager, P. C. Sham, S. J. Chanock, Z. Xia, *et al.*, GWASdb v2: An update database for human genetic variants identified by genome-wide association studies, *Nucleic Acids Res.* **44**(D1) (2016).

50. J. C. Denny, M. D. Ritchie, M. A. Basford, J. M. Pulley, L. Bastarache, K. Brown-Gentry, D. Wang, D. R. Masys, D. M. Roden, and D. C. Crawford, PheWAS: Demonstrating the feasibility of a phenome-wide scan to discover gene–disease associations, *Bioinformatics* **26**(9) (2010).

51. D. S. Wishart, Y. D. Feunang, A. C. Guo, E. J. Lo, A. Marcu, J. R. Grant, T. Sajed, D. Johnson, C. Li, Z. Sayeeda, *et al.*, Drugbank 5.0: A major update to the drugbank database for 2018, *Nucleic Acids Res.* **46**(D1) (2018).

52. M. Kuhn, I. Letunic, L. J. Jensen, and P. Bork, The sider database of drugs and side effects, *Nucleic Acids Res.* **44**(D1) (2016).

53. A. Gaulton, A. Hersey, M. Nowotka, A. P. Bento, J. Chambers, D. Mendez, P. Mutowo, F. Atkinson, L. J. Bellis, E. Cibrián-Uhalte, *et al.*, The ChEMBL database in 2017, *Nucleic Acids Res.* **45**(D1) (2017).

54. S. Kim, P. A. Thiessen, E. E. Bolton, J. Chen, G. Fu, A. Gindulyte, L. Han, J. He, S. He, B. A. Shoemaker, *et al.*, PubChem substance and compound databases, *Nucleic Acids Res.* **44**(D1) (2016).

55. K. Degtyarenko, P. De Matos, M. Ennis, J. Hastings, M. Zbinden, A. McNaught, R. Alcántara, M. Darsow, M. Guedj, and

M. Ashburner, ChEBI: A database and ontology for chemical entities of biological interest, *Nucleic Acids Res.* **36**(suppl_1) (2007).

56. Y. H. Li, C. Y. Yu, X. X. Li, P. Zhang, J. Tang, Q. Yang, T. Fu, X. Zhang, X. Cui, G. Tu, *et al.*, Therapeutic target database update 2018: Enriched resource for facilitating bench-to-clinic research of targeted therapeutics, *Nucleic Acids Res.* **46**(D1) (2018).

57. N. P. Tatonetti, P. Y. Patrick, R. Daneshjou, and R. B. Altman, Data-driven prediction of drug effects and interactions, *Science Transl. Med.* **4**(125) (2012).

58. M. Kuhn, C. von Mering, M. Campillos, L. J. Jensen, and P. Bork, Stitch: Interaction networks of chemicals and proteins, *Nucleic Acids Res.* **36**(suppl_1) (2007).

59. M. Dunkel, S. Günther, J. Ahmed, B. Wittig, and R. Preissner, Superpred: Drug classification and target prediction, *Nucleic Acids Res.* **36** (suppl_2) (2008).

60. K. C. Cotto, A. H. Wagner, Y.-Y. Feng, S. Kiwala, A. C. Coffman, G. Spies, A. Wollam, N. C. Spies, O. L. Griffith, and M. Griffith, DGidb 3.0: A redesign and expansion of the drug–gene interaction database, *Nucleic Acids Res.* **46**(D1) (2018).

61. M. K. Gilson, T. Liu, M. Baitaluk, G. Nicola, L. Hwang, and J. Chong, BindingDB in 2015: A public database for medicinal chemistry, computational chemistry and systems pharmacology, *Nucleic Acids Res.* **44**(D1) (2016).

62. M. Hewett, D. E. Oliver, D. L. Rubin, K. L. Easton, J. M. Stuart, R. B. Altman, and T. E. Klein, PharmGKB: The pharmacogenetics knowledge base, *Nucleic Acids Res.* **30**(1) (2002).

63. S. Günther, M. Kuhn, M. Dunkel, M. Campillos, C. Senger, E. Petsalaki, J. Ahmed, E. G. Urdiales, A. Gewiess, L. J. Jensen, *et al.*, SuperTarget and Matador: Resources for exploring drug-target relationships, *Nucleic Acids Res.* **36**(suppl_1) (2007).

64. F. Agüero, B. Al-Lazikani, M. Aslett, M. Berriman, F. S. Buckner, R. K. Campbell, S. Carmona, I. M. Carruthers, A. E. Chan, F. Chen, *et al.*, Genomic-scale prioritization of drug targets: The TDR targets database, *Nat. Rev. Drug Discov.* **7**(11) (2008).

65. Y. Liu, Q. Wei, G. Yu, W. Gai, Y. Li, and X. Chen, DCDB 2.0: A major update of the drug combination database, *Database* **2014** (2014).

66. A. S. Brown and C. J. Patel, A standard database for drug repositioning, *Sci. Data.* **4**(1) (2017).

67. T. Barrett, S. E. Wilhite, P. Ledoux, C. Evangelista, I. F. Kim, M. Tomashevsky, K. A. Marshall, K. H. Phillippy, P. M. Sherman, M. Holko, *et al.*, Ncbi geo: archive for functional genomics data sets — update, *Nucleic Acids Res.* **41**(D1) (2012).

68. N. Kolesnikov, E. Hastings, M. Keays, O. Melnichuk, Y. A. Tang, E. Williams, M. Dylag, N. Kurbatova, M. Brandizi, T. Burdett, *et al.*, Arrayexpress update — simplifying data submissions, *Nucleic Acids Res.* **43**(D1) (2015).

69. K. Tomczak, P. Czerwińska, and M. Wiznerowicz, The cancer genome atlas (tcga): An immeasurable source of knowledge, *Contemp. Oncol.* **19**(1A) (2015).

70. V. Matys, E. Fricke, R. Geffers, E. Gößling, M. Haubrock, R. Hehl, K. Hornischer, D. Karas, A. E. Kel, O. V. Kel-Margoulis, *et al.*, TRANSFAC®: Transcriptional regulation, from patterns to profiles, *Nucleic Acids Res.* **31**(1) (2003).

71. I. Yevshin, R. Sharipov, S. Kolmykov, Y. Kondrakhin, and F. Kolpakov, Gtrd: a database on gene transcription regulation — 2019 update, *Nucleic Acids Res.* **47**(D1) (2019).

72. H. Han, J.-W. Cho, S. Lee, A. Yun, H. Kim, D. Bae, S. Yang, C. Y. Kim, M. Lee, E. Kim, *et al.*, TRRUST v2: An expanded reference database of human and mouse transcriptional regulatory interactions, *Nucleic Acids Res.* **46**(D1) (2018).

73. H.-Y. Huang, Y.-C.-D. Lin, J. Li, K.-Y. Huang, S. Shrestha, H.-C. Hong, Y. Tang, Y.-G. Chen, C.-N. Jin, Y. Yu, *et al.*, miRTarBase 2020: Updates to the experimentally validated microrna–target interaction database, *Nucleic Acids Res.* **48**(D1) (2020).

74. C. Sticht, C. De La Torre, A. Parveen, and N. Gretz, miRWalk: An online resource for prediction of microrna binding sites, *PLoS One* **13** (10) (2018).

75. Q. Jiang, Y. Wang, Y. Hao, L. Juan, M. Teng, X. Zhang, M. Li, G. Wang, and Y. Liu, miR2Disease: A manually curated database for microrna deregulation in human disease, *Nucleic Acids Res.* **37** (suppl_1) (2009).

76. Z. Huang, J. Shi, Y. Gao, C. Cui, S. Zhang, J. Li, Y. Zhou, and Q. Cui, HMDD v3. 0: A database for experimentally supported human microrna–disease associations, *Nucleic Acids Res.* **47**(D1) (2019).

77. B. Xie, Q. Ding, H. Han, and D. Wu, miRCancer: A microrna–cancer association database constructed by text mining on literature, *Bioinformatics* **29**(5) (2013).

78. A. Ruepp, A. Kowarsch, and F. Theis. PhenomiR: Micrornas in human diseases and biological processes. In *Next-Generation MicroRNA Expression Profiling Technology*. Springer (2012).

79. Z. Yang, L. Wu, A. Wang, W. Tang, Y. Zhao, H. Zhao, and A. E. Teschendorff, dbDEMC 2.0: Updated database of differentially expressed miRNAs in human cancers, *Nucleic Acids Res.* **45**(D1) (2017).

80. Y.-R. Miao, W. Liu, Q. Zhang, and A.-Y. Guo, lncRNASNP2: An updated database of functional snps and mutations in human and mouse lncRNAs, *Nucleic Acids Res.* **46**(D1) (2018).

81. G. Chen, Z. Wang, D. Wang, C. Qiu, M. Liu, X. Chen, Q. Zhang, G. Yan, and Q. Cui, LncRNADisease: A database for long-non-coding rna-associated diseases, *Nucleic Acids Res.* **41**(D1) (2012).

82. L. Cheng, P. Wang, R. Tian, S. Wang, Q. Guo, M. Luo, W. Zhou, G. Liu, H. Jiang, and Q. Jiang, LncRNA2Target v2. 0: A comprehensive database for target genes of lncrnas in human and mouse, *Nucleic Acids Res.* **47**(D1) (2019).

83. A. Fabregat, S. Jupe, L. Matthews, K. Sidiropoulos, M. Gillespie, P. Garapati, R. Haw, B. Jassal, F. Korninger, B. May, *et al.*, The reactome pathway knowledgebase, *Nucleic Acids Res.* **46**(D1) (2018).

84. M. Kanehisa and S. Goto, Kegg: Kyoto encyclopedia of genes and genomes, *Nucleic Acids Res.* **28**(1) (2000).

85. D. N. Slenter, M. Kutmon, K. Hanspers, A. Riutta, J. Windsor, N. Nunes, J. Mélius, E. Cirillo, S. L. Coort, D. Digles, *et al.*, Wikipathways: A multifaceted pathway database bridging metabolomics to other omics research, *Nucleic Acids Res.* **46**(D1) (2018).

86. A. Liberzon, A. Subramanian, R. Pinchback, H. Thorvaldsdóttir, P. Tamayo, and J. P. Mesirov, Molecular signatures database (mSigDB) 3.0, *Bioinformatics* **27**(12) (2011).

87. I. Rodchenkov, O. Babur, A. Luna, B. A. Aksoy, J. V. Wong, D. Fong, M. Franz, M. C. Siper, M. Cheung, M. Wrana, *et al.*, Pathway commons 2019 update: Integration, analysis and exploration of pathway data, *Nucleic Acids Res.* **48**(D1) (2020).

88. M. E. Cusick, H. Yu, A. Smolyar, K. Venkatesan, A.-R. Carvunis, N. Simonis, J.-F. Rual, H. Borick, P. Braun, M. Dreze, *et al.*, Literature-curated protein interaction datasets, *Nat. Methods.* **6**(1) (2009).

89. A. Grover and J. Leskovec. node2vec: Scalable feature learning for networks. In *Proceedings of the 22nd ACM SIGKDD Int. Conference on Knowledge Discovery and Data Mining* (2016).

90. K. Kishan, R. Li, F. Cui, Q. Yu, and A. R. Haake, GNE: A deep learning framework for gene network inference by aggregating biological information, *BMC Syst. Biol.* **13**(2) (2019).

91. H. Luo, D. Wang, J. Liu, Y. Ju, and Z. Jin, A framework integrating heterogeneous databases for the completion of gene networks, *IEEE Access* **7** (2019).

92. Z. Xiao and Y. Deng, Graph embedding-based novel protein interaction prediction via higher-order graph convolutional network, *PLoS One* **15**(9) (2020).

93. K. Huang, C. Xiao, L. Glass, M. Zitnik, and J. Sun, SkipGNN: Predicting molecular interactions with skip-graph networks, *Sci. Rep.* **10** (2020).

94. K. KC, R. Li, F. Cui, and A. Haake, Predicting biomedical interactions with higher-order graph convolutional networks, *arXiv:2010.08516* (2020).

95. I. A. Kovács, K. Luck, K. Spirohn, Y. Wang, C. Pollis, S. Schlabach, W. Bian, D.-K. Kim, N. Kishore, T. Hao, *et al.*, Network-based prediction of protein interactions, *Nat. Commun.* **10**(1) (2019).

96. X. Li, W. Li, M. Zeng, R. Zheng, and M. Li, Network-based methods for predicting essential genes or proteins: A survey, *Brief. Bioinform.* **21**(2) (2020).

97. J. Schapke, A. Tavares, and M. Recamonde-Mendoza, Epgat: Gene essentiality prediction with graph attention networks, *arXiv:2007.09671* (2020).

98. X. Zhang, M. L. Acencio, and N. Lemke, Predicting essential genes and proteins based on machine learning and network topological features: A comprehensive review, *Front. Physiol.* **7** (2016).

99. R. Albert, H. Jeong, and A.-L. Barabási, Error and attack tolerance of complex networks, *Nature* **406**(6794) (2000).

100. M. Zeng, M. Li, Z. Fei, F. Wu, Y. Li, Y. Pan, and J. Wang, A deep learning framework for identifying essential proteins by integrating multiple types of biological information, *IEEE/ACM Transactions on Computational Biology and Bioinformatics* (2019).

101. M. Zeng, M. Li, F.-X. Wu, Y. Li, and Y. Pan, DeepEP: A deep learning framework for identifying essential proteins, *BMC Bioinform.* **20**(16) (2019).

102. X. Zhang, W. Xiao, and W. Xiao, DeepHE: Accurately predicting human essential genes based on deep learning, *PLOS Comput. Biol.* **16**(9) (09, 2020).

103. A. Shehu, D. Barbará, and K. Molloy. A survey of computational methods for protein function prediction. In *Big Data Analytics in Genomics*. Springer (2016).

104. W. Hamilton, Z. Ying, and J. Leskovec. Inductive representation learning on large graphs. In *Advances in neural information processing systems* (2017).

105. M. Kulmanov, M. A. Khan, and R. Hoehndorf, DeepGO: Predicting protein functions from sequence and interactions using a deep ontology-aware classifier, *Bioinformatics* **34**(4) (2018).

106. V. Gligorijević, M. Barot, and R. Bonneau, deepNF: Deep network fusion for protein function prediction, *Bioinformatics* **34**(22) (2018).

107. K. Fan, Y. Guan, and Y. Zhang, Graph2GO: A multi-modal attributed network embedding method for inferring protein functions, *GigaScience* **9**(8) (2020).

108. R. Bonetta and G. Valentino, Machine learning techniques for protein function prediction, *Proteins* **88**(3) (2020).

109. M. Agrawal, M. Zitnik, J. Leskovec, *et al.* Large-scale analysis of disease pathways in the human interactome. In *PSB* (2018).

110. K. Yang, R. Wang, G. Liu, Z. Shu, N. Wang, R. Zhang, J. Yu, J. Chen, X. Li, and X. Zhou, HerGePred: Heterogeneous network embedding representation for disease gene prediction, *IEEE J Biomed. Health Inform.* **23**(4) (2018).

111. M. Alshahrani and R. Hoehndorf, Semantic disease gene embeddings (smudge): phenotype-based disease gene prioritization without phenotypes, *Bioinformatics* **34**(17) (2018).

112. S. K. Ata, L. Ou-Yang, Y. Fang, C.-K. Kwoh, M. Wu, and X.-L. Li, Integrating node embeddings and biological annotations for genes to predict disease–gene associations, *BMC Syst. Biol.* **12**(9) (2018).

113. X. Wang, Y. Gong, J. Yi, and W. Zhang. Predicting gene–disease associations from the heterogeneous network using graph embedding. In *2019 IEEE Int. Conference on Bioinformatics and Biomedicine (BIBM)* (2019).

114. D. Wang, P. Cui, and W. Zhu. Structural deep network embedding. In *Proceedings of the 22nd ACM SIGKDD Int. conference on Knowledge discovery and data mining* (2016).

115. A. Ahmed, N. Shervashidze, S. Narayanamurthy, V. Josifovski, and A. J. Smola. Distributed large-scale natural graph factorization. In *Proceedings of the 22nd Int. conference on World Wide Web* (2013).

116. M. Belkin and P. Niyogi, Laplacian eigenmaps and spectral techniques for embedding and clustering, *Adv. Neural Inf. Process Syst.* **14** (2001).

117. L. Zhu, Z. Hong, and H. Zheng. Predicting gene–disease associations via graph embedding and graph convolutional networks. In *2019 IEEE Int. Conference on Bioinformatics and Biomedicine (BIBM)* (2019).

118. Y. Xiong, M. Guo, L. Ruan, X. Kong, C. Tang, Y. Zhu, and W. Wang, Heterogeneous network embedding enabling accurate disease association predictions, *BMC Med. Genom.* **12**(10) (2019).

119. P. Han, P. Yang, P. Zhao, S. Shang, Y. Liu, J. Zhou, X. Gao, and P. Kalnis. Gcn-mf: Disease–gene association identification by graph convolutional networks and matrix factorization. In *Proceedings of the 25th ACM SIGKDD Int. Conference on Knowledge Discovery & Data Mining* (2019).

120. P. Luo, Y. Li, L.-P. Tian, and F.-X. Wu, Enhancing the prediction of disease–gene associations with multimodal deep learning, *Bioinformatics* **35**(19) (2019).

121. L. Madeddu, G. Stilo, and P. Velardi, A feature-learning-based method for the disease-gene prediction problem, *Int. J. Data Min. Bioinform.* **24**(1) (2020).

122. Y. Zhang, L. Chen, and S. Li, CIPHER-SC: Disease–gene association inference using graph convolution on a context-aware network with single-cell data, *IEEE/ACM Trans. Comput. Biol. Bioinform* (2020).

123. B. Yang, S. W.-t. Yih, X. He, J. Gao, and L. Deng. Embedding entities and relations for learning and inference in knowledge bases. In *Proceedings of the Int. Conference on Learning Representations (ICLR) 2015* (May, 2015).

124. P. Luo, B. Chen, B. Liao, and F.-X. Wu, Predicting disease-associated genes: Computational methods, databases, and evaluations, *Wiley Interdisciplinary Reviews: Data Mining and Knowledge Discovery* (2020).

125. P. Kaushal and S. Singh, Network-based disease gene prioritization based on protein–protein interaction networks, *Netw. Model. Anal. Health Inform. Bioinform.* **9**(1) (2020).

126. A. Ezzat, M. Wu, X.-L. Li, and C.-K. Kwoh, Computational prediction of drug–target interactions using chemogenomic approaches: An empirical survey, *Brief. Bioinform.* **20**(4) (2019).

127. N. Zong, H. Kim, V. Ngo, and O. Harismendy, Deep mining heterogeneous networks of biomedical linked data to predict novel drug–target associations, *Bioinformatics* **33**(15) (2017).

128. F. Wan, L. Hong, A. Xiao, T. Jiang, and J. Zeng, NeoDTI: Neural integration of neighbor information from a heterogeneous network for discovering new drug–target interactions, *Bioinformatics* **35**(1) (2019).

129. M. Bagherian, E. Sabeti, K. Wang, M. A. Sartor, Z. Nikolovska-Coleska, and K. Najarian, Machine learning approaches and databases for prediction of drug–target interaction: A survey paper, *Brief. Bioinform.* (2020).

130. K. Abbasi, P. Razzaghi, A. Poso, S. Ghanbari-Ara, and A. Masoudi-Nejad, Deep learning in drug target interaction prediction: Current and future perspective, *Curr. Med. Chem.* **27** (2020).

131. X. Zeng, S. Zhu, X. Liu, Y. Zhou, R. Nussinov, and F. Cheng, deepDR: A network-based deep learning approach to in silico drug repositioning, *Bioinformatics* **35**(24) (2019).

132. Y. Chen and M. de Rijke. A collective variational autoencoder for top-n recommendation with side information. In *Proceedings of the 3rd Workshop on Deep Learning for Recommender Systems* (2018).

133. M. Karimi, A. Hasanzadeh, and Y. Shen, Network-principled deep generative models for designing drug combinations as graph sets, *Bioinformatics* **36**(Supplement_1) (2020).

134. H. Xue, J. Li, H. Xie, and Y. Wang, Review of drug repositioning approaches and resources, *Int. J. Biol. Sci.* **14**(10) (2018).

135. T. N. Jarada, J. G. Rokne, and R. Alhajj, A review of computational drug repositioning: strategies, approaches, opportunities, challenges, and directions, *J. Cheminformatics.* **12**(1) (2020).

136. M. Zitnik, M. Agrawal, and J. Leskovec, Modeling polypharmacy side effects with graph convolutional networks, *Bioinformatics.* **34** (13) (2018).

137. D. W. Bates, N. Spell, D. J. Cullen, E. Burdick, N. Laird, L. A. Petersen, S. D. Small, B. J. Sweitzer, and L. L. Leape, The costs of adverse drug events in hospitalized patients, *Jama* **277**(4) (1997).

138. N. Rohani and C. Eslahchi, Drug-drug interaction predicting by neural network using integrated similarity, *Sci. Rep.* **9**(1) (2019).

139. F. Cheng and Z. Zhao, Machine learning-based prediction of drug–drug interactions by integrating drug phenotypic, therapeutic, chemical, and genomic properties, *J. Am. Med. Inform. Assoc.* **21**(e2) (2014).

140. W. Zhang, H. Zou, L. Luo, Q. Liu, W. Wu, and W. Xiao, Predicting potential side effects of drugs by recommender methods and ensemble learning, *Neurocomputing* **173** (2016).

141. C. Li, H. Liu, Q. Hu, J. Que, and J. Yao, A novel computational model for predicting microrna–disease associations based on heterogeneous graph convolutional networks, *Cells* **8**(9) (2019).

142. Z. Li, J. Li, R. Nie, Z.-H. You, and W. Bao, A graph auto-encoder model for miRNA-disease associations prediction, *Brief. Bioinform.* (2020).

143. P. Xuan, H. Sun, X. Wang, T. Zhang, and S. Pan, Inferring the disease-associated miRNAs based on network representation learning and convolutional neural networks, *Int. J. Mol. Sci.* **20**(15) (2019).

144. P. Xuan, Y. Dong, Y. Guo, T. Zhang, and Y. Liu, Dual convolutional neural network based method for predicting disease-related miRNAs, *Int. J. Mol. Sci.* **19**(12) (2018).

145. J. Peng, W. Hui, Q. Li, B. Chen, J. Hao, Q. Jiang, X. Shang, and Z. Wei, A learning-based framework for miRNA-disease association identification using neural networks, *Bioinformatics* **35**(21) (2019).

146. J. Li, S. Zhang, T. Liu, C. Ning, Z. Zhang, and W. Zhou, Neural inductive matrix completion with graph convolutional networks for miRNA–disease association prediction, *Bioinformatics* **36**(8) (2020).

147. J. Li, Z. Li, R. Nie, Z. You, and W. Bao, FCGCNMDA: Predicting miRNA–disease associations by applying fully connected graph convolutional networks, *Mol. Genet. Genom.: MGG* (2020).

148. S. Rhee, S. Seo, and S. Kim. Hybrid approach of relation network and localized graph convolutional filtering for breast cancer subtype classification. In *Proceedings of the Twenty-Seventh Int. Joint Conference on Artificial Intelligence, IJCAI-18* (2018).

149. R. Schulte-Sasse, S. Budach, D. Hnisz, and A. Marsico. Graph convolutional networks improve the prediction of cancer driver genes. In *Int. Conference on Artificial Neural Networks* (2019).

150. P. Luo, Y. Ding, X. Lei, and F.-X. Wu, deepDriver: Predicting cancer driver genes based on somatic mutations using deep convolutional neural networks, *Front. Genet.* **10** (2019).

151. N. Fatima and L. Rueda, iSOM-GSN: An integrative approach for transforming multi-omic data into gene similarity networks via self-organizing maps, *Bioinformatics* **36**(15) (2020).

152. G. Rosenthal, F. Váša, A. Griffa, P. Hagmann, E. Amico, J. Goñi, G. Avidan, and O. Sporns, Mapping higher-order relations between brain structure and function with embedded vector representations of connectomes, *Nat. Commun.* **9**(1) (2018).

153. P. Lee, M. Choi, D. Kim, S. Lee, H.-G. Jeong, and C. E. Han. Deep learning based decomposition of brain networks. In *2019 Int. Conference on Artificial Intelligence in Information and Communication (ICAIIC)* (2019).

154. J. Loscalzo, *Network medicine.* Harvard University Press (2017).

Chapter 8

The Need for Interpretable and Explainable Deep Learning in Medicine and Healthcare

Alfredo Vellido[*,§], Paulo J. G. Lisboa[†,¶], and José D. Martín[‡,‖]

*Computer Science Department, IDEAI-UPC Research Center,
Universitat Politècnica de Catalunya — UPC BarcelonaTech
C. Jordi Girona, 1-3, Barcelona 08034, Spain
†School of Computer Science and Mathematics,
Liverpool John Moores University,
Byrom St., Liverpool L3 3AF, UK
‡Electronic Engineering Department, ETSE-UV,
University of Valencia,
Avgda. Universitat s/n, 46100 Burjassot, Valencia, Spain
§avellido@cs.upc.edu
¶p.j.lisboa@ljmu.ac.uk
‖jose.d.martin@uv.es

From the widespread implementation and use of electronic health records to basic research in omics science, from the popularization of health wearables to the digitalization of procedures at the point of care, the domains of medicine and healthcare are bringing data to the fore of their practice. The abundance of data in turn calls for methods that allow transforming such raw information into novel knowledge that is usable in the domain. These methods for data analytics can be provided by statistics and also from machine learning and its currently most popular incarnation: deep learning. Effective as the latter may prove itself to be, its practical application is curtailed by a limitation that is particularly sensitive in the medical domain: its lack of interpretability, leading to limited explainability. In this chapter, we aim to map the many aspects of this problem and review research aimed at overcoming it, paying special attention to three questions, namely, reliability of data-driven methods in the medical field, relevance of deep learning as one of the most appealing approaches within machine learning, and need of interpretability and explainability for an accepted application of deep learning to clinical problems.

1. Three Questions: From Data to Deep Learning

The availability of data is central to healthcare delivery and critical for medical and pharmaceutical research. Already, the ubiquity of data is extending the notion of healthcare beyond retrospective treatment of disease and towards proactive interventions through predictive models of disease progression that have the potential to reduce avoidable hospital admissions, for instance, with telehealth programmes for chronic diseases and with apps for lifestyle interventions and for self-management, which can ultimately reduce the prevalence and severity of illness. There is little doubt that rich datasets provide the most specific evidence base for healthcare delivery and monitoring.

Better use of data is arguably the cornerstone of sustainable healthcare for two main reasons: it is key to therapy optimization, from precision medicine to personalization of follow-up, essential elements to maximize the utility of clinical resources, and also essential for efficient out-of-hospital care, with an increasing role for ambulatory sensors including wearables and biofeedback, with applications to holistic care, from obesity to mental health and independent living in old age.

The growing role of data in medicine and healthcare raises three questions that are the focus of this chapter: Should we be concerned about data-driven delivery of healthcare? Is deep learning (DL) of particular value in this context? If so, how important is it to place a focus on explanation and interpretation?

(1) *To what extent should we be concerned with the idea of putting data at the core of medical and healthcare research?*

The application of data varies enormously across clinical domains, between in-hospital and out-of-hospital care, from lifestyle management to public health surveillance. This raises a broad range of issues, some of which are specific to particular uses of the data, for instance, around ethics and public acceptance. In this section, we focus on methodological questions that relate to the technical use of machine learning.

Let us begin answering this first question with a specific example: the critical care domain. The current critical care patient is intensively monitored through an array of sophisticated technologies. The intensive care unit (ICU) high-acuity patient is technologically dependent on life-sustaining devices, such as infusion pumps, mechanical ventilators, or catheters. Data captured by the bedside are conditioned by potentially swift changes in patient status and may go to enrich the electronic health record (EHR) and include monitoring device data (fluid intake and patient output, laboratory blood draw analyses, medical images, demographics, and so on). Most of these measurements are electronically stored, generating what we could call a "digital signature" of patient's stay at the ICU.

The critical care example is quite specific and involves the point of care in a clinical environment, with a very well-delimited data management scenario.[1] Data in medicine and healthcare occupy a much broader spectrum, though, which goes from the population at large to this clinical point of care. In the population extreme of the spectrum, we find the area of epidemiology, brought to the public attention by the COVID-19 pandemic, in which geo-localized traceability data become so relevant. The exploitation of geo-localized data using machine learning (ML) made early headlines with Google's (later heavily questioned by the medical establishment[2]) implementation of its Google Flu application. Note that the use of this type of data is also related to the increasingly popular use of health wearables, which has given rise to the area of mobile health (m-Health), a cornucopia of data production, amenable to analysis.[3]

Somewhere in between the general population and the point of care that we have exemplified in the critical care domain, we can place the public health administration, as well as professional organizations, as a sort of intermediating "data brokers". Healthcare authorities and medical associations, from the international down to the local level, must play a role in the implementation of health data policies and setting of standards. A relevant example of this is the design, standardization and increasing widespread use of EHR. Through the EHR, medical practitioners are allowed networked access to patients' data, which is often multi-modal and includes image, signal and text about patients' history, hospital admissions, treatment prescriptions, visitation notes, etc. Beyond individual use, EHRs are ideally suited for the creation of large and heterogeneous databases, which make them natural targets, for instance, for natural language processing ML analysis.[4]

A common thread in the use of ML in medicine is the reliance on observational data, distinct from the gold standard for the design of clinical interventions, namely, randomized control trials. The consequence of this is three-fold:

- First is the quality of data. Routinely acquired data often focus on auditing information to justify the choice of therapy rather than providing a comprehensive record that is consistent for all patients – to do this, which usually requires engagement in a prospective study. As a consequence, missing data are prevalent in some key variables and missingness can be informative, sometimes correlating with poor prognosis. Patients that are not very unwell have a full record showing that all of the variables are in or close to an acceptable range, but records for patients who are very unwell contain mainly the key indicators of severity of illness, which are sufficient to determine the choice of therapy. This requires careful handling of missing data that are not missing completely at random. DL models can use large data vectors, with less use of variable selection and less concern for sparse modelling. As a result, there can be a greater prevalence of missing values.
- The second natural consequence of observational data is lack of balance. Clinicians often need help with less prevalent events, such as sepsis or sudden deterioration in ICU, as in the earlier example. Unbalanced data can pose difficulties for DL classifiers if discriminant thresholds are fixed at 0.5. This is in contrast with probabilistic models, an example for medical statistics being logistic regression, which are generally well calibrated and, since they predict probability of class membership, can be thresholded at the prevalence of class in the whole populations. So, if sepsis is predicted with a given probability, the cut point for intervention can be set at the overall prevalence of sepsis, avoiding the need to rebalance the data.
- Third, there is potential for bias arising from confounders, that is to say variables that affect the data distribution and so impact

on the correlation between the measured inputs and outcome variables. This is the reason why data-based models using cohorts and cross-sectional data reflect associations and not causality, which requires data from active interventions followed up over time. Nevertheless, there is a concern among the medical community for the limitations inherent in evidence-based practice, founded on randomized controlled trials, as the patients recruited in such studies need to meet a range of criteria with many exclusions. Real patients often have comorbidities and other conditions that are excluded from typical randomized trials. Therefore, there is a real need for practice-based evidence, in other words, modelling of observational data, which brings up the issues discussed above.

All three threads, handling of missing values, data imbalance and inherent bias, apply to large datasets typical of data-based applications in medicine and healthcare. This has specific implications for the implementation of DL models and particularly in relation to interpretability. We consider these two points in Sections 2 and 3.

(2) *In this data-centered medical context, why should we pay particular attention to DL as it is just one approach in the overpopulated field of ML?*

Let us reflect for a moment about how a medical practitioner makes decisions (on diagnosis, prognosis, or course of treatment, for instance) on the basis of the available evidence. Specific information about a case is processed according to the individual's experience, provided by both training and practice at college, trained as a resident or during the professional career. This knowledge is bounded by human limitations in knowledge, augmented by the medical protocols and guidelines that result from the accumulated experience of the profession for a given problem and are meant to assist and guide medical decision-making. But let us consider again the critical care scenario or the analysis of EHRs considered in previous paragraphs. The large databases gathered over time from, perhaps, thousands of patients are well beyond the reach of the data processing capabilities of any individual expert. This is, instead, the domain of ML and similar (semi-)automated approaches, which can be employed to extract usable medical knowledge and assist medical decision-making.[5]

In previous paragraphs, EHRs have been mentioned as one of the most obvious medical data targets for ML. The intense attention currently given to this area of research has to do, precisely, with the fact that these data comply with most of the requirements for successful DL application: large datasets, heterogeneous unstructured data and complex multi-modal data combinations.[6] Methods from the fastly growing DL family are grabbing the headlines for their success in traditionally difficult medical problems,[7] but not without generating controversy on their wake.[8,9] The fact is that, even if ML has, for decades, shown its promise in medicine and healthcare, DL has moved center stage of ML due to its adequacy for medical image analysis (radiology)[10] and for data from the *omics* sciences.[11] Unfortunately, this reported success is clouded by problems such as the one that ultimately motivates this chapter.

In summary, DL has strong potential for modeling structured data, such as radiological images including multi-parametric data, physiological time-series, such as ECGs and Natural Language Processing (NLP). Applications to MRI, in particular, are progressing at an advanced pace.[12]

Looking beyond deep convolutional neural networks (CNN) and LSTM,[13] there is significant potential in coupling predictive models with reinforcement learning (RL) for treatment optimization, which has already demonstrated concrete improvements in care and quality of life in real-world clinical settings.[14] However, there is also evidence arising about overuse of DL with tabular data, that is to say flat data with a combination of continuous and discrete clinical indicators, typically used in patient stratification by diagnostic and prognostic outcomes. The review[15] indicates that DL is no better for tabular data than logistic regression in comparative evaluations that are demonstrably unbiased. Therefore, DL has real potential for outstanding performance for specialist applications involving data formats with inherent structure.

(3) *How important is it to consider the problems of model interpretability and explainability in the application of DL approaches to medical and healthcare problems?*

Many data scientists wonder why, if ML in general and DL in particular have been shown to excel in performance over the last decade, at least on paper, as tools for medical discovery and as decision-support systems, these techniques are only scantly seen to be applied in practice at the point of care. Beyond the domain's natural reluctance to embrace potentially disruptive technologies, this can at least partially be motivated by the existence of less obvious barriers to adoption,[16] including the risk of deskilling medical staff due to the introduction of semi-automated analytical processes, the analytical bias introduced by the data format requirements of ML methods, the inadequate handling of the uncertainty that is intrinsic to many medical observations and processes, and, finally, the object of this chapter, the difficulty of acceptance of models of the analyzed data that cannot be interpreted in a humanly understandable way and that, therefore, cannot be explained appropriately to the interested parties.

The drive for interpretable models is predicated on the need for responsible governance for the application of AI in high stakes decision-making.[17] Important components of this are, first, fairness and bias in decision support, in particular, where models can reflect bias that is inherent in data, e.g., the demonstration in Ref. [18] of a clear data artefact where the model indicates the reverse of clinical understanding about asthma as a risk factor for pneumonia. Second, legal requirements in the so-called "right to explanation" enshrined in the European General Data Protection Regulation (GDPR) whereby the subject of an action based on automated decision support has the legal right to request information about the logic used to make that decision.[19]

Complementary to the ethico-legal side, there are technical imperatives about arriving at the right predictions for the right reasons.[20] In particular, given that observational data may have artefactual effects and sometimes bias, it is important to have a mechanism to find and fix problems in the data. The simplest way to do this is with an interpretable model that makes clear what influence each input has to arrive at an individual prediction.

This last question is expanded in Section 2. This is followed by a taxonomy of the different approaches proposed to confer interpretability to DL methods, illustrated with examples from the recent literature.

2. Interpretability and Explainability in the Medical Context

A recent review of AI in radiology makes it clear that interpretable models are needed in order to gain the trust of experts.[12] This is a *sine qua non* for end-user acceptance in the medical domain.

Another medical area where ML is making strong strides, as mentioned in the introduction, is epidemiology.[21] Let us bring up the current COVID-19 pandemic situation, in which data scientists are striving to complement the strictly medical research advances. As an example, and just considering the specific area of prognosis, a recent systematic review[22] identified 50 published prognostic models for predicting mortality risk or progression to severe disease. But, from a data-centric viewpoint, this pandemic involves other challenges, such as, for instance, vaccination management. Even if safe and effective COVID-19 vaccines are tested and quickly approved for use, they are unlikely to be available immediately in amounts sufficient to vaccinate the whole population. Therefore, vaccines will almost certainly be available only in limited supplies and different cohorts of the population will have to be prioritized for vaccine access.

Data-driven models could be employed by public health authorities as a guide to the allocation process of a vaccine with an initial limited availability. A model of this type, called COVER, has recently been proposed[23] and it was built using a sizeable patient database. The perfect setting for a DL approach, perhaps. Instead, authors resort to an LASSO-regularized logistic regression. This choice is no surprise for at least two reasons though: (i) because the medical data analysis domain is quite familiarized with logistic regression methods and (ii) because a logistic regression model is straightforwardly interpretable in terms of the covariates used for prediction.

This example is just an illustration of a more general conundrum: if this data-rich environment is ripe for ML/DM to thrive, why is it that these approaches have only superficially penetrated medical practice, despite their maturity, after decades of research and development?

It is argued here that the main reasons behind this have less to do with data science maturity and technological readiness than with with adoption and implementation challenges that, unless resolved, will not allow ML and specially not DL to be adopted in routine medical practice beyond a reduced number of niche applications. One and perhaps the main of these challenges is the intrinsic lack of interpretability and, therefore, explainability of many ML techniques.[24] The ML "black-box syndrome" challenge has been discussed for decades in the medical domain,[25] but has not entered the mainstream discussion until recently.[26] DL methods are seen as an exacerbated case of *black box*, and, paradoxically, it is the interest they have raised in the medical domain that has led to the intensification of the related discussion.

Many medical practitioners should be familiar with this problem: an ML/DL-based system may yield results that, despite their quality, cannot be used in full because they are not likely to be amenable to comprehensible description. In many medical decision-making contexts, this might pose an insurmountable barrier for adoption, as the medical expert could not trust to implement a decision related to diagnosis, prognosis or, for instance, as in our initial example, vaccine delivery prioritization, which cannot be explained to either the patient, the other medical experts, or the health authorities.

This barrier could be seen as colliding with practical healthcare delivery or medical ethics, but also, more pragmatically, as colliding with the law. In Europe, this directly relates to the recent implementation of the European Union directive for GDPR which mandates a "right to explanation" of all decisions made by "automated or artificially intelligent algorithmic systems".[19] Article 13 of this directive states that a designated "data controller" is legally bound to provide requesting citizens with "meaningful information about the logic involved, as well as the significance and the envisaged consequences of such processing [automated decision making, as described in its Article 22] for the data subject". The ripples of this directive have reverberated through the medical community. Actors in data-dependent fields such as health-related academia and biobanks have engaged in a legal debate concerning data reuse in research, and, as described in Ref. [27], these actors have built an "argumentative repertoire" defending their side on issues of data sharing and biobank-related data governance. As stated in Ref. [28], at least part of the concerns have to do with data pseudonymization and anonymization, as with the broader issue of data ownership. Beyond that, though, a big question mark is placed over the aforementioned "right to explanation": if medical decision-making *must* be explained upon legal request, who would dare using *black-box* methods as the foundations of such decision-making?

Much research has been devoted to imbue ML/DL methods with the interpretability qualities they lack from inception, so that even complex predictive models can ultimately be explained in human understandable terms, and most of this research proposes methods to somehow replicate human interpretation procedures, as we illustrate in some detail in the following section. This brings another element to the discussion, which has been broached in Ref. [29], the need to integrate the available human medical knowledge into the ML/DL models, creating frameworks for machine–human interaction that put the medical expert (and not the models) at the center of the interpretability process.[30] As argued in Ref. [31], the understanding of the requirements about model interpretability depend upon who will receive the explanation. If the medical expert is the conduit of medical decision, this person should be the one evaluating the interpretation and conveying the explanation. Again, as stated in Ref. [31], "the purpose of the explanation is to overcome an ethical problem; namely, to establish meaningful human control over that decision by allowing one to confirm that the reasons for a decision are in line with domain-specific norms and best practices".

One of the reasons why ML-based systems need to be interpretable in the medical and healthcare domains has to do with the idea that interpretability is required when there is some form of incompleteness (or gap of knowledge) in the formulation of a problem,[26] for instance, resulting from a mismatch between the data modelling objectives and the medical goals. Note that the latter are often mediated by clinical guidelines, which are an *open guide for the practitioner when dealing with specific problems*; therefore, guidelines are the distillation of interpretable rules guiding specific processes: nothing but prior knowledge-based procedural decision-making pipelines. An upwards trend in ML-based medical data analytics is that of the "analytical pipeline" and, related to it, automated ML or AutoML,[5] which even addresses the possibility of automated pipeline optimization. Not too different, in fact, to the time-honored concept of medical decision-support systems (MDSS), which have made inroads in at least a few specific domains[32,33] and whose barriers to adoption have for long been the subject of research.[34] What is worth highlighting here is the many commonalities between ML-based data analytics and medical guidelines conveyed in the concept of pipeline, which could be key to dress DL with the interpretability clothes required to enter the reality of the point of care.

Ultimately, not only is interpretability important in medicine and healthcare, it also needs to be carefully tailored to the specific application and, moreover, algorithm transparency to the user can be measured. The survey of method and metrics in Ref. [35]sets out specific, measurable criteria, to assess the extent to which explanations and interpretations of machine learning methods are appropriate and effective for the end user.

3. Making Deep Learning Interpretable in the Medical Domain: Approaches

Machine explanation, that is to say the explanation of individual predictions by ML models including DL models, is a current area of very active research. Some of the most commonly used approaches involve attribution of influence to particular inputs to produce a saliency map, e.g., Local Interpretable Model-agnostic Explanations (LIME[36]). The main limitation of this method is that the explanations are local not global. However, this limitation does not detract from the significant utility of the approach.

There are comprehensive reviews of methods for explanation and interpretation. The difference between the two is that explanation normally works backwards from the prediction to quantify the influence that each input variable or combination of variables had in the prediction, similar to a sensitivity map,[37] whereas interpretation is about understanding the cause of a model output, in some way weighting each input according to its importance to the prediction.[38]

Taxonomies of Explainable Artificial Intelligence (XAI) methods with reasons for interpretability have been recently reviewed,[39] being especially interesting how they can be formulated in the case of DL applied to the medical field.[40,41] Not only does interpretability play a crucial role on an accepted application of DL-based approaches in Medicine, but they also need to be reliable. These two concepts, interpretability and reliability are indeed closely linked to each other, since it is necessary to understand how models work in order to claim a proper justification of how trustworthy they are.[42] In this framework, the mathematical and technical training of medical staff seems essential to facilitate the acceptance and understanding of relatively complex mathematical models, such as those based on DL.

Reliability is a particularly key aspect when developing DL models and interpreting them, especially for sensitive tasks, such as those affecting human well-being in which it is crucial to avoid unsafe decisions and actions.[43] Before implementing an ML system, it is necessary to validate its behavior and ensure that it will perform as expected in a real-world environment. The verification of this reliability can make use of XAI, focused on exposing complex models to humans in a systematic and interpretable manner.

XAI visualization techniques, like the integrated gradient attribution method and the SmoothGrad noise reduction algorithm, can be used to gain an insight into the features learned by very deep models, as the acclaimed convolutional neural networks are,[44] thus putting light into the DL black box and allowing its interpretability. In this sense, some remarkable clinical studies in the fields of ophthalmology and oncology have been carried out.[45, 46]

Explainability will likely be a legal requirement of automated or semi-automated MDSS in the near future, particularly when the impact of DL on human life might be relevant, e.g., in medical diagnoses and treatments. This is one of the cornerstones of a real practical application of DL to the medical field and will involve not only ML and medical practitioners but also lawyers and experts in regulations so that all of them can come up with a solution that is accurate, understandable by clinicians, and legally compliant. However, experts coming from such different fields may have very different views and biases and it may well be difficult to achieve a consensus easily. The reason for that is partially due to the fact that most of the XAI approaches are based on too technical solutions, only within the grasp of DL experts able to manipulate the corresponding mathematical functions. A complementary approach that can be helpful in order to make XAI to be easier to handle is represented by symbolic Artificial Intelligence, where symbols act as translators between humans and deep learning;[47] in particular, Knowledge Graphs (KGs) and their underlying semantic technologies.

4. Conclusions

Endowing ML models with interpretability and explainability is a *sine qua non* for advancing their integration into medical practice. Arguably, this need is heightened for DL methods that, regardless of their performance, can be seen as extreme cases of *black-box* data modelling. Note, though, that arguments against the adequacy of explicability in AI, or highlighting the contradictions and underspecifications that sometimes predominate in interpretability discourses have been put forward,[31,48] for instance, arguing about "the fact that AI is used for many low-risk purposes for which it would be unnecessary to require that it be explicable". Although this objection may be justified up to a point, it applies only to low-risk decision-making, which is often not the case in medical decision-making. For decision makers in life or death situations where confidence is critical, the benefits of artificial intelligence can be out of reach without interpretability.[49]

It is also argued that[31] "[a] principle requiring explicability would prevent us from reaping the benefits of AI used in these situations [...] the explanations given by explicable AI are only fruitful if we already know which considerations are acceptable for the decision at hand. If we already have these considerations, then there is no need to use contemporary AI algorithms because standard automation would be available. In other words, a principle of explicability for AI makes the use of AI redundant". We reckon that this objection is incorrect. The purpose of ML, as an instantiation of AI, is to make the quantification of risk more accurate than is currently possible. An interpretable model can be as accurate but will likely be sparse in comparison with a DL model with all of the available variables. In reality, it comes down to the signal in the noise. By selecting variables with the best signal-to-noise ratio, the model is not only smaller but also less disrupted by chance effects. As a result, a sparse mode can, and in general, will outperform a model with "junk" variables added in. Therefore, interpretability need not get in the way of performance and can even enhance it.[17]

We want to conclude stressing the importance of understanding interpretability and explainability for DL models applied to medical problems as an issue that is only partially technical,[30] thus arguing that more attention should be paid to the articulation of problem-specific requirements from the medical expert viewpoint, elucidating how these requirements can make DL modelling compatible with guidelines-based medical decision-making reasoning and compliant with current data protection regulations.

We think that after a golden decade of DL, when models were increasingly accurate and able to solve problems that were deemed as unapproachable so far, the next decade will be especially devoted to extracting understandable information from DL approaches, particularly in fields, such as medicine, where explainability, interpretability and reliability are crucial to allow real implementations and daily-practice applications on a routine basis.

References

1. C. V. Cosgriff, L. A. Celi, and D. J. Stone, Critical care, critical data, *Biomed. Eng. Comput. Biol.* **10**, 1–7 (2019).
2. D. Lazer, R. Kennedy, G. King, and A. Vespignani, Big data - the parable of Google Flu: Traps in big data analysis, *Science* **343**, 1203–1205 (2014).
3. S. Erdeniz, I. Maglogiannis, A. Menychtas, A. Felfernig, and T. Tran, Recommender systems for IoT enabled m-health applications, In (eds.) L. Iliadis, I. Maglogiannis, and V. Plagianakos, *Artificial Intelligence Applications and Innovations. AIAI 2018*, vol. 520, *IFIP Advances in Information and Communication Technology*, pp. 227–237. Springer, Cham (2018).
4. P. B. Jensen, L. J. Jensen, and S. Brunak, Mining electronic health records: Towards better research applications and clinical care, *Nat. Rev. Genet.* **13**(6), 395–405 (2012).
5. J. Waring, C. Lindvall, and R. Umeton, Automated machine learning: Review of the state-of-the-art and opportunities for healthcare, *Artif. Intell. Med.* **104**, 101822 (2020).
6. J. R. Ayala Solares, F. E. Raimondi, Y. Zhu, F. Rahimian, D. Canoy, J. Tran, A. C. Gomes, A. H. Payberah, M. Zottoli, M. Nazarzadeh, N. Conrad, R. Kazem, and G. Salimi-Khorshidi, Deep learning for electronic health records: A comparative review of multiple deep neural architectures, *J. Biomed. Inform.* **101**, 103337 (2020).
7. N. Tomašev, X. Glorot, J. W. Rae, M. Zielinski, H. Askham, A. Saraiva, A. Mottram, C. Meyer, S. Ravuri, Protsyuk, A. Connell, C. O. Hughes, A. Karthikesalingam, J. Cornebise, H. Montgomery, G. Rees, C. Laing, C. R. Baker, K. Peterson, R. Reeves, D. Hassabis, D. King, M. Suleyman, T. Back, C. Nielson, J. R. Ledsam, and S. Mohamed, A clinically applicable approach to continuous prediction of future acute kidney injury, *Nature* **572**, 116–119 (2019).
8. H. Shah, The DeepMind debacle demands dialogue on data, *Nat. News* **547**(7663), 259 (2017).
9. J. A. Kellum and A. Bihorac, Artificial intelligence to predict AKI: Is it a breakthrough? *Nat, Rev. Nephrol.* **15**, 663–664 (2019).
10. M. De Bruijne, Machine learning approaches in medical image analysis: From detection to diagnosis, *Med. Image Anal.* **33**, 94–97 (2016).

11. D. Bacciu, P. J. Lisboa, J. D. Martín, R. Stoean, and A. Vellido. Bioinformatics and medicine in the era of deep learning. In *Procs. of the 26ᵗʰ European Symposium on Artificial Neural Networks, Computational Intelligence and Machine Learning (ESANN)*, pp. 345–354, Bruges, Belgium (2018).

12. M. Reyes, R. Meier, S. Pereira, C. Silva, F. Dahlweid, H. Tengg-Kobligk, R. Summers, and R. Wiest, On the interpretability of artificial intelligence in radiology: Challenges and opportunities, *Radiol.: Artif. Intell.* **2**, e190043 (2020).

13. O. Pellicer-Valero, I. Cattinelli, L. Neri, F. Mari, J. Martín-Guerrero, and C. Barbieri, Enhanced prediction of hemoglobin concentration in a very large cohort of hemodialysis patients by means of deep recurrent neural networks, *Artif. Intell. Med.* **107**, 101898 (2020).

14. P. Escandell-Montero, M. Chermisi, J. M. Martínez-Martínez, J. Gómez-Sanchis, C. Barbieri, E. Soria-Olivas, F. Mari, J. Vila-Francés, A. Stopper, E. Gatti, and J. D. Martín-Guerrero, Optimization of anemia treatment in hemodialysis patients via reinforcement learning, *Artif. Intell. Med.* **62**(1), 47–60 (2014).

15. E. Christodoulou, J. Ma, G. Collins, E. Steyerberg, J. Verbakel, and B. Van Calster, A systematic review shows no performance benefit of machine learning over logistic regression for clinical prediction models, *J. Clin. Epidemiol.* **110**, 12–22 (2019).

16. F. Cabitza, R. Rasoini, and G. F. Genisi, Unintended consequences of machine learning in medicine, *JAMA* **318**(6), 517–518 (2017).

17. C. Rudin, Stop explaining black box machine learning models for high stakes decisions and use interpretable models instead, *Nat. Mach. Intell.* **1**, 206–215 (2019).

18. R. Caruana, Y. Lou, J. Gehrke, P. Koch, M. Sturm, and N. Elhadad. Intelligible models for healthcare: Predicting pneumonia risk and hospital 30-day readmission. In *Procs. of the 21ˢᵗ ACM SIGKDD International Conference on Knowledge Discovery and Data Mining*, pp. 1721–1730 (2015).

19. B. Goodman and S. Flaxman, European Union regulations on algorithmic decision making and a "right to explanation", *AI Mag.* **38** (2017).

20. A. Ross, M. Hughes, and F. Doshi-Velez. Right for the right reasons: Training differentiable models by constraining their explanations. In *Procs. of the Twenty-Sixth International Joint Conference on Artificial Intelligence (IJCAI 17)*, pp. 2662–2670 (2017).

21. J. Wiens and E. Shenoy, Machine learning for healthcare: On the verge of a major shift in healthcare epidemiology, *Clin. Infect. Dis.* **66**, 149–153 (2018).

22. L. Wynants, B. Van Calster, G. Collins, *et al.*, Prediction models for diagnosis and prognosis of Covid-19: Systematic review and critical appraisal, *BMJ* **369**, m1328 (2020).

23. R. Williams, A. Markus, C. Yang, and *et al.* Seek COVER: Development and validation of a personalized risk calculator for COVID-19 outcomes in an international network (2020). MedRxiv, 2020.05.26.20112649. https://doi.org/10.1101/2020.05.26.20112649.

24. D. Raví, C. Wong, F. Deligianni, M. Berthelot, J. Andreu-Pèrez, B. Lo, and G. Yang, Deep learning for health informatics, *IEEE J. Biomed. Health Inform.* **21**, 4–21 (2017).

25. J. Tu, Advantages and disadvantages of using artificial neural networks versuslogistic regression for predicting medical outcomes, *J. Clin. Epidemiol.* **49**, 1225–1231 (1996).

26. F. Doshi-Velez and B. Kim. Towards a rigorous science of interpretable machine learning (2017). arXiv:1702.08608v2, https://arxiv.org/abs/1702.08608v2.

27. J. Starkbaum and U. Felt, Negotiating the reuse of health-data: Research, big data, and the european general data protection regulation, *Big Data Soc.* **6**, 2053951719862594 (2019).

28. A. Reiz, M. de la Hoz, and M. Garcia, Big data analysis and machine learning in intensive care units. *Medicina Intensiva* **43**, 416–426 (2019).

29. G. Bhanot, M. Biehl, T. Villmann, and D. Zühlke. Biomedical data analysis in translational research: Integration of expert knowledge and interpretable models. In *Procs. of the 25th European Symposium on Artificial Neural Networks, Computational Intelligence and Machine Learning (ESANN)*, pp. 177–186, Bruges, Belgium (2017).

30. A. Vellido, The importance of interpretability and visualization in machine learning for applications in medicine and health care, *Neural Comput. Appl.* **32**, 18069–18083 (2020).

31. S. Robbins, A misdirected principle with a catch: Explicability for AI, *Minds Mach.* **29**, 495–514 (2019).

32. S. Safdar, S. Zafar, N. Zafar, and N. Khan, Machine learning based decision support systems (DSS) for heart disease diagnosis: A review, *Artif. Intell. Rev.* **50**, 597–623 (2017).

33. A. Vellido, V. Ribas, C. Morales, A. Ruiz-Sanmartín, and J. Ruiz-Rodríguez, Machine learning for critical care: State-of-the-art and a sepsis case study, *BioMed. Eng. OnLine.* **17**, 135 (2018).

34. S. Dreiseitl and M. Binder, Do physicians value decision support? A look at the effect of decision support systems on physician opinion, *Artif. Intell. Med.* **33**, 25–30 (2005).

35. D. Carvalho, E. Pereira, and J. Cardoso, Machine learning interpretability: A survey on methods and metrics, *Electronics* **8**, 832 (2019).

36. M. Ribeiro, S. Singh, and C. Guestrin. "Why Should I Trust You?": Explaining the Predictions of Any Classifier. In *Procs. of the 22nd ACM SIGKDD International Conference on Knowledge Discovery and Data Mining*, pp. 1135–1144 (2016).
37. A. Adadi and M. Berrada, Peeking inside the black-box: A survey on explainable artificial intelligence (XAI), *IEEE Access* **6**, 52138–52160 (2018).
38. D. Alvarez Melis and T. Jaakkola. Towards robust interpretability with self-explaining neural networks. In (eds.) S. Bengio, H. Wallach, H. Larochelle, K. Grauman, N. Cesa-Bianchi, and R. Garnett, *Advances in Neural Information Processing Systems 31*, pp. 7786–7795. Curran Associates, Inc. (2018).
39. A. Arrieta, N. Daíz-Rodríguez, J. Del Ser, A. Bennetot, S. Tabik, A. Barbado, S. García, S. Gil-López, D. Molina, R. Benjamins, R. Chatila, and F. Herrera, Explainable artificial intelligence (XAI): Concepts, taxonomies, opportunities and challenges toward responsible AI, *Inform. Fusion.* **58**, 82–115 (2020).
40. A. Singh, S. Sengupta, and V. Lakshminarayanan, Explainable deep learning models in medical image analysis, *J. Imag.* **6**(6) (2020).
41. B. Shickel, T. J. Loftus, L. Adhikari, T. Ozrazgat-Baslanti, A. Bihorac, and P. Rashidi, Deepsofa: A continuous acuity score for critically ill patients using clinically interpretable deep learning, *Sci. Rep.* **9**, 1879 (2019).
42. E. Tjoa and C. Guan, A survey on explainable artificial intelligence (XAI): Toward medical XAI, *IEEE T. Neur. Net. Lear.* 1–21 (2020).
43. W. Samek, G. Montavon, A. Vedaldi, L. K. Hansen, and K.-R. M. (eds.), *Explainable AI: Interpreting, Explaining and Visualizing Deep Learning*. Springer Nature, Lecture Notes in Artificial Intelligence 11700, Cham, Switzerland (2019).
44. Z. Papanastasopoulos, R. K. Samala, H.-P. Chan, L. Hadjiiski, C. Paramagul, M. A. Helvie, and C. H. Neal. Explainable AI for medical imaging: Deep-learning CNN ensemble for classification of estrogen receptor status from breast MRI. In *Medical Imaging 2020: Computer-Aided Diagnosis*, (eds.) H. K. Hahn and M. A. Mazurowski, Vol. 11314, pp. 228–235, SPIE (2020).
45. A. Singh, A. R. Mohammed, J. Zelek, and V. Lakshminarayanan. Interpretation of deep learning using attributions: Application to ophthalmic diagnosis. In *Applications of Machine Learning 2020*, (eds.) M. E. Zelinski, T. M. Taha, J. Howe, A. A. S. Awwal, and K. M. Iftekharuddin, Vol. 11511, pp. 39–49, SPIE (2020).
46. P. Korfiatis and B. Erickson, Deep learning can see the unseeable: Predicting molecular markers from MRI of brain gliomas, *Clin. Radiol.* **74**(5), 367–373 (2019).

47. G. Futia and A. Vetrò, On the integration of knowledge graphs into deep learning models for a more comprehensible AI—three challenges for future research, *Information* **11**(2) (2020).

48. Z. C. Lipton, The mythos of model interpretability: In machine learning, the concept of interpretability is both important and slippery, *Queue* **16**(3), 31–57 (2018).

49. K. Astromskė, E. Peičius, and P. Astromskis, Ethical and legal challenges of informed consent applying artificial intelligence in medical diagnostic consultations, *AI & SOCIETY* (2020).

Chapter 9

Ethical, Societal and Legal Issues in Deep Learning for Healthcare

Cecilia Panigutti[*,§], Anna Monreale[†,¶], Giovanni Comandè[‡,‖], and
Dino Pedreschi[†,**]

Scuola Normale Superiore, Pisa, Italy
†University of Pisa, Pisa, Italy
‡Scuola Superiore Sant'Anna, Pisa, Italy
§cecilia.panigutti@sns.it
¶anna.monreale@unipi.it
‖giovanni.comande@santannapisa.it
***dino.pedreschi@unipi.it*

The recent availability of massive amounts of personal data that directly
or indirectly describe individuals' health status opened unprecedented
opportunities to develop deep learning models able to leverage them to
provide a wide range of benefits in healthcare. However, the development
and the application of deep learning systems in such a critical domain
raises many ethical and legal concerns. This chapter examines the practical implications of the ethical and legal guidelines for deep learning in
healthcare. First, it provides an overview of the different approaches to
AI ethics across the world. Then, focusing on the EU ethical and legal
framework, it analyzes the pieces of legislation relevant for DL applications in healthcare. Finally, the key ethical values of privacy, fairness and
explainability are mapped to the different stages of the machine learning lifecycle, and several state-of-the-art approaches to inscribe them in
deep learning systems are overviewed.

1. Introduction

The opportunity of learning from big volumes of health data
has brought several new benefits to the healthcare domain. The

effectiveness of Deep Learning (DL) and Machine Learning (ML) has been proven to be valuable in multiple healthcare applications, ranging from medical imaging to predictive algorithms for cancer, Alzheimer's disease and cardiovascular risk factors.[1-3] Some applications could also help manage triage, optimize hospital administration, and reduce physician burnout by relieving them from the burden of medical documentation, allowing them to spend more time with their patients to provide better care. However, the pervasive use of DL algorithms that exploit and combine sensitive data raises several concerns. For example, the increasing use of e-health apps and wearable devices that directly collect "quasi-health" data[4] (e.g., heart-rate and sleep tracking, breathing regularity, steps count) raises *privacy* issues. Indeed, when combined with other information such as weight, height, or genetic illness, this kind of data could allow DL algorithms to make inferences about individuals' lifestyles, health conditions, risks of illness, and much more. Furthermore, health data can contain various *biases* due to an imperfect data collection process or to human biases reflected in the data. These biases are difficult to track or discover when fed into opaque and complex DL models, which raises issues of *transparency* and *explainability*. Furthermore, several *liability* issues arise if the DL system is defective, including *medical malpractice* and healthcare provider's liability due to the negligent reliance on DL systems. The importance of considering the ethical and legal implications of the development and use of DL systems is subject to many national and international organizations' recommendations. Some examples are the OECD's *recommendations on the main five values-based principles for the responsible stewardship of trustworthy Artificial Intelligence*[5] signed up by the OECD's 36 member countries, along with Argentina, Brazil, Colombia, Costa Rica, Peru and Romania, and adopted later, in 2019, by G20 Trade Ministers and Digital Economy Ministers, the ethics guidelines for the development trustworthy AI[6] published in 2019 by the High-Level Expert Group on Artificial Intelligence (AI HLEG) and the recent guidelines on regulation of AI[7] released by US administration. All these documents and recommendations explicitly refer to AI systems and not DL systems. However, we highlight that DL and ML approaches are mechanisms for achieving AI. Since there is still no universal agreement upon the definition of AI, to avoid any confusion, we underline that in this chapter, we use the term AI as defined by the EU Commission in its communication on *Artificial Intelligence for Europe:*[a]

> *Artificial intelligence (AI) refers to systems that display intelligent behaviour by analysing their environment and taking actions — with some degree of autonomy — to achieve specific goals. AI-based systems can be purely software-based, acting in the virtual world (e.g. voice assistants, image analysis software, search engines, speech and face recognition systems) or AI can be embedded in hardware devices (e.g. advanced robots, autonomous cars, drones or Internet of Things applications).*

In this perspective, all the pieces of legislation that refer to AI systems also refer to DL models. In this chapter, we explore the practical implications of the ethical and legal guidelines for DL applications in healthcare. Since the approach to responsible and ethical AI is not homogeneous across the world, we analyse the different ideologies, interpretations and guidelines on AI of three of the most influential world powers. In particular, we discuss the European, Chinese and US approach considering the peculiar societal/ethical issues of the AI-based health applications in each of them. Then, using the EU guidelines as a reference point, we map the ethical concerns to AI technical issues and overview the scientific literature on solutions to inscribe ethical values in DL systems. We focus our analysis on algorithmic transparency, privacy, bias and fairness concerns.

The implementation of the ethical guidelines, together with the compliance with the legal requirements, can help ML researchers and developers to design AI systems that can be easily translated into clinical practices. To support ML developers, we discuss the possible ethical and legal issues to be addressed in any stage of the ML development lifecycle from the design to the deployment and maintenance of DL solutions.

1.1. *On the importance of AI ethics*

Since no research is performed in a social vacuum, there is no such thing as a *value-neutral* technology. What researchers are interested

---

[a]EU Commission: "Artificial Intelligence for Europe" (2018). https://ec.europa.eu/transparency/regdoc/rep/1/2018/EN/COM-2018-237-F1-EN-MAIN-PART-1.PDF.

in studying is an expression of their values and belief system. The technological progress is driven by the cultural, ethical, political and economic interests of society, companies and researchers themselves. Why a certain technology is considered worthy of time and money spending and another one is not? What does a particular technology make it easier to do? There are ethical choices made both in the development phase and in the application phase of any technology. Some choices that might seem harmless and purely technical might not be. Imagine a researcher is designing a DL model to predict the length of time a patient survives after a liver transplant. The goal of the research is to improve the potential recipient ranking system in order to optimize transplant survival. The choice of the loss function that the DL algorithm must optimize for the task is usually considered a purely technical choice. However, the loss function might implicitly give priority to younger patients, which is an ethical choice, whether right or wrong. Now, imagine that the dataset used to train the DL algorithm was collected from a private US-based non-profit organization between 1988 and 1996. The majority of the represented patients are white, furthermore, data show that the graft survival rate of black patients is significantly lower than those of white ones.[8] The algorithm is highly likely to use this correlation in its optimization phase, even if the ethnicity of patients is explicitly removed from the dataset.[9] So, implicitly, the model will choose white patients over black patients for the transplant even if the observed correlation might have nothing to do with a real causal link between ethnicity and graft survival, yet another ethical choice. What is really optimizing the loss function chosen by the developer? The scenario becomes even more complicated if we consider that the dataset is probably outdated since there has been a distribution drift between the last date of data collection (1996) and today. This simple example shows how researchers implicitly embed their beliefs and data biases in the technology they develop. Nevertheless, recent debates have highlighted that many experts on technology feel estranged from the social and policy implications of their work.[10] However, many of the ethical choices listed above are encoded in hard law and therefore are enforceable. Technology development and use are strongly linked to politics and ethical questions on how to advance the good life of individuals or society overall. The field that studies these kinds of ethical questions is *AI ethics*. AI ethics investigates all the ethical questions raised during the development, deployment and use of an AI system. For example, it investigates how values are inscribed into technical artifacts, who is supposed to be held accountable if an AI system fails, and the motives behind research goals and findings. The answers to these questions inform regulators around the world.

2. AI Ethical and Legal Guidelines Around the World

The ethical and legal guidelines for the responsible use of AI vary across the world. In the past few years, a plethora of private and public stakeholders have produced their reports on the requirements for a trustworthy implementation of AI technologies. Five ethical principles emerge across all the recent literature on this topic: transparency, justice, non-maleficence, responsibility, and privacy.[11] However, each country interprets these principles and translates them into its legal system differently. The main dimension along which the different approaches can be distinguished is the *regulatory versus innovation* one. For example, the US tends to favor innovation, whereas the EU has a strong regulatory approach. This and many other ethical and regulatory issues arise because of the different socio-economic and political environments in which these technologies are developed. In this section, we analyze the different value systems of three of the most influential world powers that released an AI policy. Before presenting a detailed discussion, we provide a quick overview of the ideologies driving the different approaches to technological innovation in AI:

- **US:** The American approach to AI ethics is influenced by libertarian values that imply minimal regulation of technology from the government. It promotes a "Silicon valley model"[12] which consists in innovating in the regulatory grey zones, *move fast, break things first, apologize later*. **Conception of human being:** Homo Economicus, individualism.
- **China:** The Chinese approach to AI ethics is influenced by Confucian values and Chinese socialism ideology. There is a focus on social harmony which implies some elements of moral control and surveillance from the government. **Conception of human being:** collectivist, behaviorist, utilitarian.

"Society as a whole should be mobilized to participate in health affairs, thus contributing to the people's health and the country's overall development".[13]

- **EU:** The European Union approach to AI ethics is based on the respect of fundamental rights, democracy, and the rule of law. In particular, four ethical principles are identified as the most relevant for AI policy: *respect for human autonomy, prevention of harm, fairness, and explicability.*[6]
- **Conception of human being:** Kantian conception of the person as autonomous (freedom, autonomy and dignity).

"Human dignity is the fundamental concept that provides the framework within which one needs to interpret[...] European culture and jurisdiction".[14]

These values and ethical principles guide the implementation of the AI policies and explain the different perspectives on the same issue. It is indeed important to note that, even though ethical principles are the basis of law, they are not legally binding and therefore are not enforceable. Still, each legal system has many tools to internalize ethical principles in hard law. We will now focus on each of these three regions of the world to discuss their healthcare policies, their approach to AI, the socio-economic peculiarities of each of them and subsequent ethical issues. Furthermore, we give an overview of the most important pieces of legislation concerning AI applications in healthcare for each of them.

2.1.   *US*

Many US based big-tech companies such as Google[b] and IBM,[c] that develop DL solutions for healthcare, have drafted their ethical policy to address the many concerns about the safe corporate

---

[b]Artificial Intelligence at Google: Our Principles. https://ai.google/principles.
[c]IBM's Principles for Trust and Transparency. https://www.ibm.com/blogs/po licy/trust-principles.

use of healthcare data.[d] Even if their declared goal is to develop healthcare applications which improve the quality of care, reduce healthcare costs, and are beneficial for society overall, some potential conflicts of interests are yet to be acknowledged and enforced by legally binding standards.[15] In 2020, the Trump administration released the draft for the *Guidance for Regulation of Artificial Intelligence Applications.*[7] The memorandum discourages any *"regulatory or non-regulatory actions that needlessly hamper AI innovation and growth"* coherently with the US approach of prioritizing innovation over regulation:

> *Agencies must avoid a precautionary approach that holds AI systems to such an impossibly high standard that society cannot enjoy their benefits. Where AI entails risk, agencies should consider the potential benefits and costs of employing AI, when compared to the systems AI has been designed to complement or replace.*

Note that the approach expressly discourages a "precautionary approach" and relies on a traditional cost–benefit analysis. The document lists 10 principles that federal agencies should consider when they decide how and whether to regulate AI applications. These 10 principles are *Public Trust in AI, Public Participation, Scientific Integrity and Information Quality, Risk Assessment and Management, Benefits and Costs, Flexibility, Fairness and Non-Discrimination, Disclosure and Transparency, Safety and Security* and *Interagency Coordination.* The innovation-oriented approach becomes very apparent in the *Risk Assessment and Management* principle:

> *It is not necessary to mitigate every foreseeable risk; in fact, a foundational principle of regulatory policy is that all activities involve trade-offs.*

---

[d]H. Ledford, Google health-data scandal spooks researchers, *Nature News.* https://www.nature.com/articles/d41586-019-03574-5. R. Casey, IBM's watson supercomputer recommended "unsafe and incorrect" cancer treatments, internal documents show (2018). https://www.statnews.com/2018/07/25/ibm-watson-re commended-unsafe-incorrect-treatments.

These guidelines were following the plan on AI regulation and standards released in February 2019 by the US National Institute of Standards and Technology (NIST) which explicitly addressed the ethical, societal, and legal concerns of the development of AI technologies stating the following:

> While stakeholders in the development of this plan expressed broad agreement that societal and ethical considerations must factor into AI standards, it is not clear how that should be done and whether there is yet sufficient scientific and technical basis to develop those standards provisions.

The regulatory aspects for the DL applications, that are classified as medical devices, are regulated by the US Food and Drug Administration (FDA). In January 2020, the FDA released a discussion paper titled "Proposed Regulatory Framework for Modification to Artificial Intelligence/Machine Learning (AI/ML)-based Software as a Medical Device".[e] [f] While the current regulatory framework is being updated and will be defined in the months to come, the ethical concerns are already known. Indeed, in the US, the biggest ethical concerns derive from the potential health information asymmetry between companies and individuals and from the systemic biases present in the datasets. An information asymmetry creates a power asymmetry in favor of big companies like Google[g] that collected several sensitive data on its users' health through their queries on medical conditions. The combination of this knowledge together with other users' interactions on the Internet could potentially infer very personal and sensitive information, blurring the lines that distinguish health and non-health data.[4] This information was legally collected exploiting HIPAA (Health Insurance Portability and Accountability Act) privacy and security rules limited reach to non-traditional healthcare data.[16] The issue is that many users were unaware that their search history would have been processed to infer their health status and

---

[e]FDA. Proposed Regulatory Framework for Modification to Artificial Intelligence/Machine Learning (AI/ML)-based Software as a Medical Device.

[f]https://www.fda.gov/medical-devices/software-medical-device-samd/artifici al-intelligence-and-machine-learning-software-medical-device.

[g]S. Fussell, Google's totally creepy, totally legal health-data harvesting, *The Atlantic*. https://www.theatlantic.com/technology/archive/2019/11/google-proj ect-nightingale-all-your-health-data/601999/.

have lost the control over this information usage. Potentially, health data could radically change an individual chance of obtaining health insurance or even employment. These concerns are made all more serious by the fact that currently the US does not provide universal healthcare to its citizens. Furthermore, health data contain many biases (see Section 6.1) and also reflect those systemic present in the society. If not properly addressed, the algorithms trained on biased data will learn and perpetrate them in their decision-making process.

2.2. *China*

In late 2016, China released a blueprint of its healthcare strategy, *Healthy China 2030*, intending to set public health as a priority and to shift the focus from disease treatment to disease prevention.[17] In particular, the blueprint states that the healthcare industry efforts should concentrate on early disease detection, diagnosis, and treatment. The blueprint declared goal to prioritize public health is in line with previous efforts of the Chinese government that quadrupled its healthcare budget between 2009 and 2017. These initiatives are a response to the increased number of pollution-related illnesses due to poor air quality, concerns about the health management of the country's aging population,[18] and the inequality of healthcare services access between the rural and urban areas. As declared in the 2017 *New Generation Artificial Intelligence Development Plan (AIDP)*, China plans to use AI as a tool to deal with these health issues. The document, released by the Chinese State Council, outlines China's strategy to become the world leader in the field of AI, among its explicit strategic goals there is the desire to build an *Intelligent Health and Elder Care Systems* and to design an ethical framework for the use of AI to be encoded in hard law.[h] The AIDP guidelines are supposed to be enacted by the private sector. Indeed in the same year of its release, China's Ministry of Science and Technology partnered with the multinational Chinese-based company Tencent to foster AI research in medicine, in particular, to develop computer vision

---

[h]State Council's Plan for the Development of New Generation Artificial Intelligence. http://chinainnovationfunding.eu/dttestimonials/state-councils-planfor-the-development-of-new-generation-artificial-intelligence/.

applications for medical diagnosis.[i] The AI-based applications developed in the last years by Tencent are listed in a recent report written for the 2019 special theme on Medical Innovation of the Global Innovation Index.[19] The document reports China's intention to employ AI technologies for triage, clinical decision-support system, drug discovery, increasing hospital management and operational efficiency. Furthermore, China plans to manage health knowledge diffusion through the medical information platform *Tencent Medipedia* and to monitor users' health conditions through wearable devices. Aside from the potential dangers of centralizing health information on one platform, the main ethical concerns are related to the subtle distinction between health monitoring and surveilling citizens' health behavior in the name of the common good. Similar to the Social Credit System initiative[j] fostered by State Council, AI technology could enhance the remote control power of the Chinese government over citizen behaviors deemed "unhealthy". For example, the lack of physical activity could be monitored using DL applied to inertial sensors data, such as accelerometers and gyroscopes of wearable devices. This danger is relevant to all the so-called *social diseases* (e.g., type II diabetes and obesity).[20] Another episode that exemplifies the surveillance power of the Chinese government on its citizens' health behavior is the recent use of AI technologies to fight the Coronavirus epidemic spread. The government collaborated with Chinese big-tech companies to develop a black-box AI system able to classify each citizen according to his risk of being infected. This classification was used to generate a Q.R. code that helped the police to enforce the quarantine.[k] Furthermore, facial recognition technologies paired with contactless temperature detection helped police to identify potential virus carriers which were breaking the law. A similar trade-off between individual rights and social responsibility affects users' right to share their health data only after informed consent. Indeed, if health data are considered a

---

[i]M. Jing and S. Dai, China recruits Baidu, Alibaba and Tencent to AI 'National Teams', *South China Morning Post* (2017).

[j]R. Creemers, Planning outline for the construction of a social credit system (2014–2020), *China Copyright and Media* (2014).

[k]R. Z. Paul Mozur and A. Krolik: In coronavirus fight, China gives citizens a color code, with red flags, *The New York Times* (2020).

public good, then they might be collected from unaware users to train sophisticated DL algorithms that could benefit society at large.[20]

2.3. *EU*

The European Union is probably the world leader in regulating the ethical principles of AI and in influencing the international discussion on this topic.[l] EU's propensity to code in hard law its ethical principles on AI has raised some concerns about the fact that this regulatory focus might be an obstacle to innovation. However, the European Commission sees the encoding of ethical principles in AI as a competitive advantage that will foster consumers' trust in EU products and as an incentive for companies to create innovative products that satisfy these rules. Indeed, the regulatory approach of the European Commission is believed to foster a trustworthy technology and harmonize its adoption across the Union. The most recent example of hard regulation that also impacts AI application is the *General Data Protection Regulation (GDPR)*.[m] The GDPR came into force in May 2018 and it regulates the processing of personal data in the European Union, protecting EU citizen's privacy and stipulating that every EU citizen has the right *not to be subject to a decision based solely on automated processing, including profiling, which produces legal effects concerning him or her or similarly significantly affects him or her.* In a similar effort to draft new laws for AI regulation, in June 2018, the European Commission appointed a High-Level Expert Group on AI (AI HLEG) to put forward its AI strategy. In the first half of 2019, the group defined seven requirements for trustworthy AI,[6] also containing a pilot version of an assessment list for practical use by companies. This document was well received by companies across Europe that contributed to it with their comments and proposals. In the guidelines, three components for the implementation of trustworthy AI are identified: *lawful, ethical,* and *robust.* The EU approach to ethical and trustworthy AI is fundamental rights-based and human-centered:

---

[l]IBM Statement on EU Ethics Guidelines for Trustworthy AI. https://www.ibm.com/blogs/policy/ai-ethics-eu.
[m]EU General Data Protection Regulation: https://gdpr-info.eu.

> *The human-centric approach to AI strives to ensure that human values are central to the way in which AI systems are developed, deployed, used and monitored, by ensuring respect for fundamental rights, including those set out in the Treaties of the European Union and Charter of Fundamental Rights of the European Union, all of which are united by reference to a common foundation rooted in respect for human dignity, in which the human being enjoy a unique and inalienable moral status.*

This approach promotes research and innovation by putting in place proper safeguards that protect European citizens' rights and freedom. For example, the document explicitly mentions a potential risk of mass surveillance by the Government powered by AI as a critical concern, as opposed to the Chinese approach to surveillance in the name of *social harmony*. It also explicitly mentions the *asymmetries of power or information such as between employers and workers, or between businesses and consumers* as another critical concern. The four ethical principles identified as relevant in the documents are the *principle of respect for human autonomy*, the *principle of prevention of harm*, the *principle of fairness,* and the *principle of explicability*. These principles are further operationalized in the recent white paper, "On Artificial Intelligence — A European approach to excellence and trust".[21] In this document, the European Commission outlines its action plan to foster AI use in the framework of European law and ethical values. The plan includes an increased budget for AI research spending of 70 percent. The white paper specifically addresses the healthcare sector, identifying it as a high-risk sector that needs further legislation refinements.

We consider the ethical framework outlined by the AI HLEG the most complete. Thus in Section 3, we discuss the seven principles identified by the group as foundational for trustworthy AI, highlighting their impact on DL applications in healthcare.

3. EU's Seven Requirements for Trustworthy AI

The foundations that lay the seven requirements of the EU approach to trustworthy AI are the fundamental rights prescribed by the *Charter of Fundamental Rights of the European Union*. We will now go into the details of each requirement and highlight the potential DL scenarios impacted by each of them relevant to the healthcare sector.

3.1. *Human agency and oversight*

This requirement reflects the *principle of respect for human autonomy*, protecting the fundamental rights of EU citizens and laying the foundations for all the other requirements. It is based on three sub-requirements:

- **Fundamental rights:** AI applications should respect fundamental rights. This requires that during the design phase of the application, the developers carry out a *fundamental rights impact assessment*, including the protection of personal data and the right to have these data *processed fairly for specified purposes.*
- **Human agency:** AI applications should promote human autonomy. This requirement is directly linked to the fundamental right of freedom of the individual which implies that *human beings should remain free to make life decisions for themselves.*[6] This means that DL applications in healthcare should be designed as part of a decision-support system, allowing end users to make informed autonomous decisions. This principle is also reflected in Article 22 of the GDPR on *"automated individual decision-making, including profiling"*,[22] stating as follows:

  > The data subject shall have the right not to be subject to a decision based solely on automated processing, including profiling, which produces legal effects concerning him or her or similarly significantly affects him or her.

- **Human oversight:** AI applications should allow the human user to have control over the process. This implies that proper human safeguards should be put in place to prevent unintended adverse effects of the AI system. This requirement is in line with the human-centered design promoted in the guidelines and with the right to obtain human interventions in cases ruled by Article 22 of the GDPR.

3.2. *Technical robustness and safety*

This requirement is perhaps the most relevant for AI application developers. It asks them to operationalize the *prevention of harm* principle by paying attention to four key aspects of technical robustness and safety:

- **Resilience to attack and security:** AI system developers should prevent system hacking and adversarial attacks. Three targets of attacks are identified: the data (data poisoning), the model (model leakage), and the underlying infrastructure (hardware and software).
- **Fallback plan and general safety:** AI system developers should put in place a proper fallback plan to cope with adversarial attacks and unexpected situations. This implies an assessment of potential risks (accidental or malicious use of the technology) and a plan to manage the situation. For example, AI could request human intervention before proceeding. The fallback plan should be tested and proper measures for effective redress in case of adverse outcome should be put in place.
- **Accuracy:** AI systems should have a high accuracy and should report whenever its outcome/prediction is inaccurate. In the context of the guidelines, the term "accuracy" does not refer to the standard metric used to evaluate ML models, it refers to the system ability to perform accurate decisions. This means that the proper definition of system accuracy depends on the task the application is performing.
- **Reliability and reproducibility:** AI systems should be both reliable and reproducible. In the context of the guidelines, AI systems are considered *reliable* if they work properly given a specific set of conditions and are considered *reproducible* if under the same conditions they consistently provide the same outcome. The AI system reliability and reproducibility should be constantly monitored and tested, and if there are scenarios where the AI system does not meet the standards, such conditions should be reported.

3.3. *Privacy and data governance*

This requirement is in line with Articles 7 and 8 of the *EU Charter of fundamental rights* on the "Respect for private and family life" and the "Protection of personal data", which are a reflection of the principle of prevention of harm applied to privacy. Data protection is also regulated by the GDPR, along with other directives, across all EU. The guidelines further prescribe special care for sensitive data (some of them include religious, sexual and political orientation, age and gender) that might be inferred from users' digital traces and used to discriminate them. In order to be compliant to this requirement, two key aspects should be considered:

- **Privacy and data protection:** Since health data are considered among the most sensitive ones, it is of paramount importance to ensure privacy and data protection throughout the entire lifecycle of the AI, eventually performing a data protection impact assessment. We further go into the details on how to deal with health data in Section 5.3 and on privacy attacks in Section 6.4.
- **Data governance — access, quality and integrity of data:** Data governance is the process of managing the data used by an organization. This includes putting in place protocols for *data access* (who can have access to the data), *data quality* (data free of bias, absence of mistakes in the data), and *data integrity* (compromised data, data hacking) assessment. There are several relevant standards for data governance, for example, the ISO and the IEEE standards.

3.4. *Transparency*

This requirement reflects the *principle of explicability* of the EU guidelines for trustworthy AI. Transparency should be applied to every stage of the AI lifecycle, indeed it prescribes the possibility to have a complete view on the whole system. In order to be compliant to this requirement, the following aspects should be considered:

- **Traceability:** All the steps required to implement an AI application should be properly documented. In the context of a DL application for healthcare, this includes documenting the data collection process and how it was labeled, the choice of the DL architecture together with the optimization algorithm used, and how the data was split in order to train, validate and test the model. In the eventuality that the model's wrong outcomes negatively impact a patient's health, it is necessary to understand the reasons behind that decision. In this case, it might be useful to keep track of the model's history of decisions to trace back to a common origin of the mistakes.
- **Explainability:** Two levels of explainability are identified: the first one refers to the technical ability to understand the AI decision-making process, while the second one refers to the ability

to explain how the human decision maker interacts with the AI decision-support system and how (s)he is influenced by it. Their combination contributes to the global transparency of the business model employed. The guidelines prescribe to pay special attention to the AI applications that have a high impact on human lives, for example, in the healthcare context.

- **Communication:** It should always be explicit when a user is interacting with an AI system, and the user should always have the option to opt out. Most importantly, the AI limits and actual capabilities must be appropriately communicated to avoid over-confidence and overreliance on the AI, which can affect both patients and healthcare professionals. Consider, for example, *Babylon Health*,[n] a personalized healthcare service that provides an AI-powered chat-bot that operates a triage of patients through guided questions and redirects them to real physicians or pharmacists. It can also give healthcare advice, e.g., *how to deal with common cold.* However, the user is aware that the initial interaction is with an AI system and (s)he always has the possibility to further continue the conversation with a real physician.

3.5. *Diversity, non-discrimination and fairness*

This requirement is in line with the *principle of fairness* listed in the EU guidelines and with Article 21 of the EU Charter of Fundamental Rights on Non-discrimination that states the following:

> *Any discrimination based on any ground such as sex, race, colour, ethnic or social origin, genetic features, language, religion or belief, political or any other opinion, membership of a national minority, property, birth, disability, age or sexual orientation shall be prohibited.*

The prevention of discrimination entails three main aspects:

- **Avoidance of unfair bias:** Ideally, AI applications in healthcare could facilitate access to better healthcare services increasing societal fairness. However, since these applications hugely rely on the quality of the data they were trained on, they could provide unfair

---

[n]https://www.babylonhealth.com.

and biased outcomes. In Section 6, we discuss in detail the problem of bias and fairness in DL from a technical viewpoint.

- **Accessibility and universal design:** The AI applications should be designed to include the widest possible range of individuals following *Universal Design* principles by taking into account people with diverse abilities, skills, age, and size.
- **Stakeholder participation:** All the relevant stakeholders affected by AI applications should be involved in their design and maintenance.

3.6. *Societal and environmental well-being*

This requirement addresses the environmental costs and the societal risks related to AI applications by extending the principles of fairness and prevention of harm to the broader society. It has been estimated that the carbon footprint of training NLP deep learning models is equivalent to the one of a trans-American flight.[23] This has important consequences on the environment and hence on people health. Three important aspects must be considered to be compliant with this requirement:

- **Sustainable and environmentally friendly AI:** In the design stage of an AI system, there should be an environmental impact assessment (resource usage, energy consumption, carbon footprint). According to a recent study, AI could help realize many *Sustainable Development Goals*,[24] for example, it could enable the third goal of ensuring *healthy lives and promote well-being for all at all ages* through early detection of diseases, treatment personalization, and increasing the quality and accessibility of essential healthcare services.
- **Social impact:** If an AI system directly interacts with humans, a social impact assessment needs to be performed. The end user needs to know that (s)he is interacting with an AI system and the limits of that interaction. In healthcare, a good doctor–patient relationship is crucial to reduce disease-related anxiety, especially for life-threatening diseases.[25] This requires an interaction with a human doctor. The way the AI is embedded in the clinical setting may be the difference between an increased quality of care and a devastating patient experience. For example, if the AI application

interacts directly with the patient giving him or her the diagnosis without an explanation and without the proper communication, this could hurt the patient's mental health.

- **Society and democracy:** AI could potentially increase economic and democratic inequalities. For example, although AI applications in healthcare could enable an easier access to basic healthcare services in rural areas,[26] this could also exacerbate the differences between patients that can afford human care and patients that cannot afford it.

3.7. *Accountability*

The accountability requirement prescribes that appropriate mechanisms to identify the responsibility for AI systems' outcomes are put in place during their whole lifecycle. In particular, it outlines three sub-requirements:

- **Auditability:** It should be possible to assess the algorithms, the data and design processes. This is linked to the previous requirement of transparency and it is a necessary step to ensure the ability to redress.
- **Minimization and reporting of negative impacts:** The ability to safely report the negative outcomes of an AI decision, eventually fostering an algorithm impact assessment proportionate to the risks posed by the AI, should be guaranteed.
- **Trade-offs:** In the design stage of the AI system, it is necessary to acknowledge all the possible trade-offs between the previously listed requirements. This sub-requirement catalyzes, without mentioning it expressly, the only precautionary consideration of the guidelines of the AI HLEG, since they clearly ban the development, deployment and use of an AI system in forms that do not have an ethically acceptable trade-off. An ethically unacceptable trade-off, for instance, is one that undermines the "the essence of the fundamental rights and freedoms" or is not "a necessary and proportionate measure in a democratic society" (see Article 23 of the GDPR).
- **Redress:** The possibility of adequate redress in case of adverse or unfair outcomes should be guaranteed. For example, in accordance with the requirement on diversity, non-discrimination and fairness,

if the AI application fails to address the discrimination bias present in the training dataset, the individual should be enabled to ask for effective redress against the machine decision.

4. The AI Application Lifecycle Stages

Each stage of the journey from prototype to real-world clinical application of the AI system requires attention to be paid to different ethical and legal issues. In the *EU's requirements for trustworthy AI*, the AI HLEG identified three stakeholders who should play a role in the guideline implementation: *developers* (researchers and software engineers), *deployers* (any organization that uses AI in their products) and *end users*.[6] To each of these stakeholders correspond one or more stages of the lifecycle of the AI product. The main four stages for a DL application are as follows:

(1) **Design:** In this stage, the goals of the application are identified, data are acquired, the architecture of the DL model is chosen.
(2) **Development:** In this stage, the DL model is developed, validated and tested. In an academic setting, this might be the final stage before writing a research paper.
(3) **Deployment and maintenance:** In this stage, the DL model is embedded in an application and becomes a product placed in the market. The product needs to be monitored and updated if needed.
(4) **Usage:** In this stage, the final product reaches the end user.

4.1. *Design stage*

In the *design stage*, it is crucial to involve all the relevant stakeholders. For a DL application in healthcare whose final goal is to be deployed in the market, an ideal team would include ML engineers, domain experts such as clinicians and medical researchers, hospital administrators, experts of the legal domain (for regulatory advice) and the future end users of the application. An interdisciplinary team is also essential to identify relevant clinical scenarios and to prevent possible data analysis pitfalls. For example, developing a model that learns to associate end-of-life treatments to a high risk of mortality is not useful in a real-world clinical scenario since the care team already has this information.[27] In this stage, it is also important to consider the ethical implications of the application. It might be useful to go through the *trustworthy AI assessment list* set up by the European Commission[6] to make sure that all the ethical requirements are satisfied upfront. In particular, ML engineers should focus on the *prevention of harm* principle and put in place proper safeguards in case of unintended adverse outcomes and malicious use of the technology they are designing. Since health data is considered to be one of the most sensitive personal data, special attention should be paid to potential privacy risks. We address this issue in Section 6.4. Moreover, in general, the EU Commission prescribes a *X-by-design* (privacy-by-design, security-by-design, ethics-by-design) approach for AI applications. In other words, in this stage, ML engineers should consider both the system's functional requirements and its ethical and legal requirements. The data collection also takes place in the design stage. As previously mentioned, data might contain all sorts of biases (see Section 6.1). To prevent discriminatory or unintended adverse outcomes, the EU Commission envisages the following requirements for data collection:

- Ensure that the DL application is trained on a sufficiently broad and representative dataset.
- Ensure privacy and personal data protection, performing a privacy risk assessment on the data.
- Keep record of how and why the data were selected.

4.2. *Development stage*

The goal of the development stage is to develop, validate and test the model. In this stage, the developers need to implement the strategies defined in the previous design step in order to develop an *ethical ML model*. First of all, *transparency* must be guaranteed during the whole development process. This is crucial to ensure *traceability* and the correct allocation of liability. To this end, it is important to create appropriate technical documentation and to share data and source code of the DL application (accordingly with proprietary rights). This good practice is optimal to also guarantee *reliability* and *reproducibility* of results.

Ensure reproducibility: To ensure the reproducibility of results, it would be optimal to test the model performance against those of benchmark state-of-the-art models. In this regard, there has been a recent effort of the ML community to develop such benchmark models on freely accessible data[28, 29] for many healthcare applications.[3, 30] This aspect is also very important in case the development stage is the last stage before writing an academic paper: if possible, the data and the source code used in the experiments should be shared with the scientific community. We are aware that this is not possible in most of the cases, especially for healthcare applications that perform their experiments on real-world healthcare data that contain sensitive information. However, a recent good practice to solve this issue is emerging in academic works that develop DL applications for healthcare: the performance of model is reported both on private datasets and on freely accessible datasets, and then the preprocessing routines to run the source code and the source code itself are publicly released. The documentation needed to reproduce the results should also include the random seeds as well as the hardware used in the training phase.

Proper evaluation of the model: In the evaluation phase of the model, the developers should carefully choose the appropriate evaluation metric. This metric should take into account if the dataset is unbalanced and if it reflects clinically relevant measures. Consider, for example, a DL application that classifies patients' chest X-ray images as having or not having lung cancer. The choice of the appropriate metric changes if the clinical setting is screening or confirmatory. In a screening setting, i.e., a setting where a large number of asymptomatic people are being tested for potential disease, it might be preferable to have a higher sensitivity in order not to miss a person at risk. However, in a confirmatory setting, i.e., a setting where an individual is being tested for a definite diagnosis, it might be preferable to have high specificity.[31] In any case, the AUC score, one of the most used metrics in ML, does not provide any relevant information in any of the two clinical settings. Furthermore, it is important to prevent *label leakage* when splitting the data into training, validation and test set. Many healthcare application tasks require a patient-level split instead of a random observation-level split. For example, if the DL model must be trained to identify the disease in a chest X-ray image, developers should take into account that one patient may have contributed with more than one image to the dataset, and thus, a patient-level split is needed.[27] Finally, when the model performance is reported, it is important to also specify the context in which the model was trained and validated (e.g., single-center dataset, adult vs pediatric population, etc.), or in other words, the clinical cohort used to develop the model.

Ensure traceability and liability: As suggested by the EU Commission, in order to track back the origin of a potential malfunctioning and to guarantee the determination of liability, the developers should do the following:

- Document the training methodologies as well as the testing and validation techniques.
- Ensure clear information on the application limits and capabilities, for example, information about the system robustness to adversarial attacks and about the reproducibility of its results.
- Report the goal of the application and the conditions under which it is expected to function as intended.
- Report all the relevant metrics employed in the development of the application.

Ensure transparency: As highlighted in Section 3.4, the transparency requirement is strongly connected to the *explainability* requirement that is fundamental when ML models are opaque and incomprehensible to humans. As a consequence, during the development of DL models, it becomes mandatory to take into consideration this aspect by implementing techniques that help in providing tools for explaining the model behavior or the reason of the model decision.[32,33] The problem of explainability is deeply discussed in Section 6.3.

Ensure privacy and fairness: In this stage, it is also necessary to address the *privacy* and *fairness* issues, identified during the *design stage*. To this end, developers should implement protection techniques to mitigate privacy and unfairness risks. As discussed in Sections 6.4 and 6.2, some of them operate data transformations to eliminate risks from training data while others mitigate the risks changing the learning process of the DL model. However, since these techniques can lead to a degradation of the model accuracy, before applying any mitigation strategy, developers should first assess the possible risks of privacy leakage or unfair behavior in order to focus their intervention only where necessary.[34, 35] The combination of risk assessment and mitigation strategies provides the ingredients to define and develop DL-based systems with guarantees of compliance with existing legislation and ethical frameworks.

4.3. *Deployment and maintenance stage*

The goal of the deployment stage is to put the DL model on the market. In this stage, it becomes fundamental to consider all the relevant pieces of legislation that we discuss in Section 5. Note that, even if the EU Commission has not yet analyzed the legal component needed for all possible AI applications (lawful), compliance with the entire regulatory framework is a binding duty with significant consequences. While ethical requirements are difficult to enforce without relying on legal rules, legal rules entail enforcing mechanisms by definition. Thus, for instance, a violation of the GDPR rules in the ML process opens to civil and criminal liability and sanctions while biases embedded in the ML product might make it defective and/or illegal to put in the market. Furthermore, some new forms of evaluation of the model might be necessary to prove the clinical utility of the final tool. For example, a recent work argues that a DL model that has just been tested using the training–validation–test set split lack proof of clinical validity.[31] This claim is mainly due to two reasons: first, because the dataset might contain all sorts of biases that prevent the model from generalizing well in clinical practices (we go into the details in Section 6.1) and second, because such an application should prove to be useful to the patients' health outcomes. In particular, the authors suggest an evaluation of the entire patient treatment strategy involving the DL application through randomized controlled trials. Moreover, once deployed, the DL application should be monitored to allow for system maintenance. In 2016, the World Health Organization (WHO) released its first guidelines on *Monitoring and Evaluating Digital Health Interventions*.[36] Even if the focus of these guidelines is on digital health intervention at a national level, the considerations they set out are also relevant to smaller-scale applications (up to the penultimate stage of the application maturity). In particular, the WHO guidelines states that, as the digital health application matures over time, the monitoring activity also needs to evolve. Indeed, in the context of a DL application, the monitoring activity has to verify that such an application is working as intended by continuously assessing if there is a degradation of the system performance over time. At the same time, the monitoring activity should also take into account the system's compliance with the ethical requirements. In other words, *deployers* should put in place auditing processes able to assess both the system's technical performance and the system's ethical and legal requirement compliance. Indeed, some features of the dataset describing a certain population might undergo a significant data distribution drift over time. This means that the relationship between the inputs and outputs of the model changed due to external factors, e.g., the relationship between patients' features and their probability of survival to a renal transplant might change because of medical innovations. Such a kind of drift might affect both medical and ethical aspects. Therefore, they might lead to the degradation of the DL model performance (e.g., accuracy degradation[37]) and degradation of the ethical risk mitigation, such as privacy protection degradation or fairness degradation. This monitoring is essential because, based on the result of this assessment, the *deployers* might need to retrain the model.

4.4. *Usage stage*

In the case of DL applications that directly interact with end users, they should be aware that it is not an interaction with a human being. Users should also be informed and aware about possible ethical and legal risks derived from the use of that application. For example, user should have the opportunity to know if data used to make a prediction are stored and/or used to update the learning model by continuous learning techniques.[38]

5. Relevant EU Legislation

In its white paper on Artificial Intelligence,[21] the EU Commission sets out its policy objectives regarding regulation. AI applications in healthcare are often cited in the document, in particular, the EU

Commission highlights how its regulatory focus will be on *high-risk* AI applications,[o] explicitly mentioning AI applications in healthcare as one high-risk example.

5.1. Medical devices in EU

Under the EU law, software intended to be used in a medical device needs to fulfill some requirements to be compliant with the *EU Medical Device Regulation* (MDR).[p] In this section, we refer to the MDR legal rules.[q] A first innovation MDR entails that all software intended to be used for medical purposes by the manufacturer is considered a medical device under its regime.[r] This means that DL applications for healthcare are also considered to be medical devices and are subject to the same regulation. In particular, the software applications, that fall under the definition of a medical device, are all the applications developed for the following:

- diagnosis, prevention, monitoring, prediction, prognosis, treatment or alleviation of disease;
- diagnosis, monitoring, treatment, alleviation of, or compensation for, an injury or disability;
- investigation, replacement or modification of the anatomy or of a physiological or pathological process or state;
- providing information by *in vitro* examination of specimens derived from the human body, including organ, blood and tissue donations.

However, the regulation specifies that *software intended for general purposes, even when used in a healthcare setting, or software intended for life-style and well-being purposes, is not a medical device.* A clear example is a wearable device that tracks vital signs (e.g., blood pressure, heartbeat, oxygen saturation) and offers advice on lifestyle and sleep habits, as opposed to a device performing exactly

---

[o]High-risk applications are identified with two criteria: the sector of application and if the application is employed in a way that significant risk is likely to arise.
[p]Council Regulation 2017/745 of 5 April 2017.
[q]Amending Directive 2001/83/EC, Regulation (EC) No. 178/2002 and Regulation (EC) No. 1223/2009 and repealing Council Directives 90/385/EEC and 93/42/EEC.
[r]Regulation (EU) 2017/745.

the same tasks and functions and developed the same way but that is intended for the above-mentioned medical uses. The latter is subject to MDR legal and safety rules, whereas the former is not (even if they are created out of the same dataset and methods).[s]

Annex I of MDR "General safety and performance requirements" requires that such software

> shall be designed to ensure repeatability, reliability and performance in line with their intended use. In the event of a single fault condition, appropriate means shall be adopted to eliminate or reduce as far as possible consequent risks or impairment of performance.

Furthermore, the regulation requires a document containing detailed information regarding *test design, complete test or study protocols, methods of data analysis, in addition to data summaries and test conclusions.* In particular, the regulation mentions the need for information regarding stability, performance, and safety. These requirements guarantee accountability in the medical device monitoring systems. Also, according to this information and characteristics, the MDR classifies medical devices into different risk classes (the higher the class, the higher the risk it entails): **Class I** — *Low risk*; **Class IIa** — *Low to medium risk*; **Class IIb** — *Medium to high risk*; **Class III** — *High risk*.

In general, software is classified under Class I. However, software intended to provide information which is used to take decisions with diagnosis or therapeutic purposes and software intended to monitor physiological processes are classified under Class IIa. Finally, if such decisions have an impact that may cause respectively serious deterioration of a person's state of health/surgical intervention and death or an irreversible deterioration of a person's state of health, they are classified under medium-to-high (Class IIb) or high-risk devices (Class III). If the nature of variations of the monitored vital

---

[s]Note that the MDR also applies to the provision of a diagnostic or therapeutic service offered by Information Society (IT) services, as defined in point (b) of Article 1(1) of Directive (EU) 2015/1535 or by other means of communication (Article 6, MDR). Thus, an ML-based software offering a diagnostic or therapeutic service is subject to the same regulation.

physiological parameters is such that it could result in immediate danger to the patient, it is classified under Class IIb.

It then becomes apparent that it is essential to consider the intended use of the developed medical device together with the information regarding its stability, performance, and safety. These are indeed the bases of the risk–benefit analysis needed to obtain and maintain marketability and to eventually investigate liability for defective medical devices. This risk–benefit analysis is also vital to secure sufficient financial coverage for the eventual malfunctioning of the medical device, which should be proportionate to its risk class, type of device, and size of the enterprise.

5.2. *Medical device malfunction*

The legal definition of a medical device malfunction must be sought in the coordination of the two definitions given by the MDR and by the *Product Liability Directive* (Article 6, Council Directive 85/374/EEC). The MDR defines *device deficiency* (Article 2, No. 59) in terms of *any inadequacy in the identity, quality, durability, reliability, safety or performance of an investigational device, including malfunction, use errors or inadequacy in information supplied by the manufacturer*, while according to the Product Liability Directive, *a product is defective when it does not provide the safety which a person is entitled to expect, taking all circumstances into account, including: (a) the presentation of the product; (b) the use to which it could reasonably be expected that the product would be put; (c) the time when the product was put into circulation.*

In case of a malfunction, current EU legislation on liability for defective products (Directive 85/374/EEC) states that *if a defective product causes any physical damage to consumers or their property, the producer has to provide compensation irrespectively of whether there is negligence or fault on their part.* Therefore, the producer of the medical device is the subject that should be held accountable if the consumer is harmed.

However, in the case of medical devices that use DL, it might be difficult to identify the origin of the defect and hold accountable the device manufacturer or the developer if they are different.[33] Note that, in principle, the manufacturer of a complex device, that incorporates more components, is usually considered to be the solely liable entity for a defective product. There is an ongoing discussion on this allocation of liability in products where the ML component constitutes the greatest part of the material good. Finally, note that the safety level requested is high for medical devices.[t] Accordingly, stability, performance and safety information are particularly relevant for developers since the reference to inadequacy of performance widens the notion of defective device.

Even though the EU laws for medical devices still fully apply to DL-fueled devices, the EU Commission wants to update some of them to make them easily enforceable and to avoid different treatments of software and software-based devices among different EU Countries.[39] This intent is explicitly specified in the EU white paper on AI.[21] Even if the health-related DL application does not fall under the definition of medical device, some other relevant laws still apply. Consider, for example, the case of a DL application trained on "unrepresentative health data",[40] i.e., data containing features that describe only a particular ethnic group and that does not generalize well outside of that ethnic group. The *EU Race Equality Directive*[u] might apply to this kind of application if their scope remains in the protected domains. The fact that training datasets should be sufficiently representative is also directly mentioned in the white paper.[21] Another health-related example of this kind is a DL model which targets the wrong dietary advice[41] to a consumer that has a chronic pathology such as diabetes or has a mental illness such as Anorexia nervosa, the *Unfair Commercial Practices Directive*[v] and the *Consumer Rights Directive*[w] might apply. Similarly, the Products Liability Directive applies, although the notion of defectiveness can have a smaller scope for non-medical device health-related products. Note, again, that less regulated ML-based products might remain on a higher slippery slope for possible unethical uses.

5.3. *Handling health data under the GDPR*

The GDPR has a significant — non-negative — practical impact on the activities of ML. First, in the EU, a fundamental right to data

---

[t]EUCJ Joined Cases C-503/13 and C-504/13, of 5 March 2015.

[u]Directive 2000/43/EC.

[v]Directive 2005/29/EC.

[w]Directive 2011/83/EC.

protection goes hand in hand with the right to privacy. It is worth noting that the right to the protection of personal data (Article 8) and the right to privacy (Article 7) do not coincide in the EU Charter of Fundamental Rights. The notions of privacy and data protection in the GDPR are directly connected to those of "personal data" and "processing" (Article 4, Paras 1 and 2), expanded with respect to the previous EU rules.

Personal data *means any information relating to an identified or identifiable natural person ("data subject"); an identifiable natural person is one who can be identified, directly or indirectly, in particular by reference to an identifier such as a name, an identification number, location data, an online identifier or to one or more factors specific to the physical, physiological, genetic, mental, economic, cultural or social identity of that natural person.*

This definition adds objective "identifiers" (location data, name), which are mixed with subjective/personal "factors", and the association of "genetic identity" with physical, physiological, mental, economic, cultural or social factors, increasing the spectrum of data considered as personal data affected by the research, especially in case of data-intensive research as it happens in ML.

Processing *means any operation or set of operations which is performed on personal data or on sets of personal data, whether or not by automated means, such as collection, recording, organisation, structuring, storage, adaptation or alteration, retrieval, consultation, use, disclosure by transmission, dissemination or otherwise making available, alignment or combination, restriction, erasure or destruction.* Consequently, almost all forms of processing of personal data within ML fall within the scope of the right to data protection, regardless of whether the right to privacy is impaired. If the ML procedures are carried out for research purposes, they enjoy simplifications. From now on, we will refer to the standard regime for ML and to the exemptions it enjoys when it is carried out in the research field. The GDPR also imposes to data processing for ML, the establishment of a real governance structure for personal data: obligation to demonstrate compliance (Articles 5, 13, and 30); hypothesis of appointment of a data protection officer (Articles 37–39); rules on data breaches (Articles 33 and 34); and sanctions, including fines of up to 20 million EUR or 4% of total turnover (Article 83). The GDPR does not apply to anonymous data, while Recital 26 offers a reidentifiability test:

> To determine whether a natural person is identifiable, account should be taken of all the means reasonably likely to be used, such as singling out, either by the controller or by another person to identify the natural person directly or indirectly. To ascertain whether means are reasonably likely to be used to identify the natural person, account should be taken of all objective factors, such as the costs of and the amount of time required for identification, taking into consideration the available technology at the time of the processing and technological developments.

In case data are not anonymous, the GDPR requires a *legal basis* for any data processing, i.e., it is necessary to identify the scenario where data processing is legally permitted. We will now identify the different possible legal bases (Articles 6 and 9 GDPR) for the processing of personal data in the ML activities in the (research) medical field.

Consent: The consent of the data subject, although sometimes problematic, has always been a very important legal basis also for research. It is *any freely given, specific, informed and unambiguous indication of the data subject's wishes*(Article 4.11 GDPR) by which data subjects accept the processing of their personal data. It must be given for one or more specific purposes (Article 6 (1)(a)). This general requirement of the GDPR is problematic for data-intensive activities and for data reuse also within ML. However:

> Data subjects should have the opportunity to give their consent only to certain areas of research or parts of research projects to the extent allowed by the intended purpose.

Therefore, it is necessary to verify the correspondence of the activity itself with the scope and aims of consent as well as with the requirements of the consent (Article 7). Nonetheless, consent is not always an appropriate legal basis; it can be a problematic one since it (a) is always withdrawable (Article 7, Para 3) and, in the absence of another legitimate legal basis, (b) any further processing after the withdrawal of consent would be unlawful, (c) requiring the immediate erasure of personal data (*European Data Protection Board*). Recital 33 contributes to the greater flexibility of consent in the context of scientific research. Its practical consequence appears to be the legitimacy of broad consensus formulas possibly covering reuse provided that (a) they cover specific areas of research and (b) the relevant ethical standards are respected. ML developers should check the applicable national ethical rules and follow them. Regarding sensitive data, Article 9 includes consent as a legal basis along with other alternative legal bases. Note that data deletion following the withdrawal of consent affects the model developed, the training implemented, and the technical choices made. Thus, the whole development and deployment stages of the lifecycle of the ML application need to be reviewed accordingly, taking into consideration that the assessment of privacy, bias, and fairness should also be influenced.

Special categories of personal data: Given these difficulties, other legal bases for data processing for ML in the health domain can be more suitable. For instance, Article 9(2)(h) and (i) allow the use of special categories of personal data in health research without consent, only when the law provides for an exception, respecting the essence of the right to data protection.

Public interest and legitimate interests: Article 9 GDPR establishes that Union or Member States law may provide alternative legal bases such as the public interest (Article 6 (1)(e)) and the legitimate interests of the holder (Article 6 (1)(f)). However, to rely on the public interest, there must be a statutory basis found in the Member States or the EU for which ML developers need to find out.

5.3.1. *Further processing*

A central issue for ML is that of legitimate further processing and therefore the reuse of personal data. Concerning this aspect, we need to distinguish two scenarios:

Research context: Article 5.1(b) explicitly states that further processing of personal data for scientific or historical research or statistical purposes is compatible with the initial purposes if aligned with Article 89(1) that relaxes some constraints. Further elaboration, a presumption of non-incompatibility for research, is therefore allowed. To benefit from it, the safeguards set out in Article 89 and Recital 156 must be respected, including the demonstration that it was not possible to use anonymous data.

Non-research context: In case the further processing in the ML processing is not for research purposes, there is no presumption of compatibility with the original processing. The developer must positively evaluate (in a demonstrable way for accountability purposes) the provisions of Article 6.4.

6. Technical Focus on Bias, Fairness, Explainability and Privacy in Deep Learning

6.1. *Biases in the data*

Healthcare data might contain some biases that can impact the model performance beyond its predictive accuracy. These biases are usually due to a lack of cohort diversity that might originate due to technical and non-technical reasons. Technical reasons that generate lack of cohort diversity are as follows:

- **Clinical study exclusion criteria:** This happens when data used to train the DL model were collected for a specific target clinical population study, e.g., some studies focus only on adult population.
- **Poor data collection design:** This generally applies every time the population used to train, validate and test the model does not reflect the target population of the clinical setting in which the model will be deployed. This mismatch might generate a wide range of biases. A comprehensive list of all these biases is outside the scope of this chapter, however, the main ones are *temporal biases*[37] (there is a concept drift between the time the model was developed and the time the model is deployed), *geographical biases* (the model was developed using only one-site data), *bias due to confounding or omitted variables* (for example, one missing variable such as the aggressivity of the treatment might mislead the model to wrongly classify high-risk patients as low-risk ones),[42] and *spectrum bias* (the population of the dataset used to develop the model does not have a real representation of the spectrum of disease states — severity, stage, etc. — of the target population).[31]
- **Secondary use of data collected with other purposes:** An example of such practice is the use of ICD (International Classification of Diseases) codes for predictive diagnosis purposes in DL

applications. These codes were originally intended for billing purposes and might not properly describe the real health status of the patient.[43]

- **Lack of high-quality human labeling:** This might happen for two reasons: the first one is the general low quality of the dataset being used, and the second one is specific to healthcare data. The problem arises from the fact that different doctors might give different diagnoses to the same patient. Furthermore, sometimes a lack of high-quality labeling might reflect a lack of knowledge: this is, for example, the case of sepsis prediction, there is no agreed upon definition of what sepsis is, and thus, there is no universal ground truth.[44]

Non-technical reasons of bias are due to the historic omission of certain populations from clinical studies[40,45] and due to the reflection of human biases and discrimination into the dataset. These two aspects are linked to the fundamental right of non-discrimination and to the *fairness principle* that lay the foundation of the related requirement of the EU guidelines. The requirement of *diversity, non-discrimination, and fairness* prescribes that training data should include all potentially vulnerable categories of individuals relevant to the study. Several examples in the literature show how discriminatory biases influence ML outcomes. For example, Sayyed-Kalantari *et al.*[45] studied the bias of state-of-the-art Deep Convolutional Neural Network (CNN) on assigning the right diagnosis to chest X-ray images. They trained the CNN on three different large open datasets and showed that the underdiagnosis rate was consistently higher for women, minorities, and those with low socio-economic status. Another work by Obermeyer *et al.*[46] exposes the racial bias of a risk-prediction algorithm used to rank patients according to their healthcare needs. They found out that using healthcare costs as a proxy label to identify patients that would benefit the most from targeted intervention was discriminating black patients. This result was due to the fact that white patients generated higher healthcare costs conditional on health conditions with respect to black patients, so the algorithm was favoring white patients.

Even though most of the time fairness studies focus on legally protected groups, other forms of biases in healthcare could still be detrimental if ignored. For example, it is proven that many healthcare providers hold strong biases against people with obesity. This attitude influences the quality of care provided and the healthcare outcomes of treatments.[47] Even if weight bias is still not regulated, it could still be very harmful if silently perpetrated by ML applications in healthcare. Lastly, it is important to note that removing sensitive features do not prevent discrimination since there might be other features correlated with the sensitive ones. We illustrate some techniques to mitigate known biases in Section 6.2.

6.2. *Fairness*

The *fairness* notion is strongly linked to the *discrimination*[9] and *bias*[48] notions because, as explained in Section 6.1, unfair DL outcomes could result from the human biases and the existing demographic inequalities reflected in the training data. Proposals for solving the problem of algorithmic fairness have been put forward within different fields, such as computer science, economics, philosophy, and organizational psychology.[49] However, these answers are fragmented and offer only partial solutions to the problem. Either their technical nature tends to ignore the social context of the decision-making, or they are unconcerned with the normative aspects of fairness decisions. The problem of algorithmic fairness has also sparked intensive research in the technical field of ML,[50] and several techniques to address this problem have been suggested.

In any case, in order to fight against discrimination and achieve fairness, it is mandatory first to define the notion of *fairness*. In the literature, there exist different definitions of fairness; this is because the problem of fairness may be viewed from different perspectives and the definitions strongly depend on the existing differences among various cultures.[50,51] Thus, finding a single definition that fits all the different notions of fairness is hard. A high-level categorization of the fairness definitions is as follows:

- **Individual fairness,** involving definitions that require similar treatment for similar individuals;
- **Group fairness,** involving definitions that require similar treatment for protected and non-protected groups.

There are two main lines of research on fairness in ML: the first one studies methods to audit ML models for discrimination discovery, typically by investigating how decisions vary across social groups that differ with respect to sensitive variables.[49,52] The second one studies how to embed fairness into the design of ML models (*fairness-by-design*). In the following, we focus our discussion on this last research line.

Fairness-by-design approach: Approaches for embedding fairness in ML can be categorized into methods reaching fairness by focusing on training data transformations and methods reaching fairness by acting on the ML algorithm.

- **Debiasing training data:** The first category involves methods that modify the training data distribution changing the class labels of selected instances close to the decision boundary by assigning different weights to instances based on their group membership or by carefully sampling from each group.[53] The main goal is to balance the protected and unprotected groups in the training data.
- **Reformulation of the classification problem:** This second category of approaches reformulate the classification task incorporating fairness (or non-discrimination) requirements *by design* into the model. The fairness goal is considered in the overall model objective function. This regularization also needs to know featurewise annotations that specify whether each feature within the input correlates with protected attributes or not.[54] Another approach exploits the adversarial training to eliminate information about protected attributes from the intermediate representation of the deep neural networks.[55] Typically, these approaches are based on the simultaneous learning of a predictor and an adversarial classifier. The role of the last one is to minimize the ability of the predictor to correctly classify the protected attribute.

An additional underinvestigated line of research regards the relationships between privacy and fairness. Even if data are protected, the predictions and classifications obtained by ML-based decision systems can lead to categorization of people and possibly to deduction of other private information. Moreover, this categorization can lead to unfair discrimination and treatment for which often it is hard to understand the reasons due to the opacity of most of the ML models. People may thus be inclined to provide the data themselves to ensure more fair decisions. In the scientific literature, only few works addressed the challenge of developing data mining and ML models that provide both privacy and fairness safeguards.[56, 57]

We highlight that although a large number of researchers have studied the fairness problem in ML, there are still no conclusive results regarding what the state-of-the-art method is. As discussed by Ntoutsi *et al.*,[48] a systematic evaluation of the existing methods is mandatory to understand their potentialities and limitations. However, we underline that a comparative evaluation is hard because of the heterogeneity of the fairness notions, which led to the design and development of methods working for different fairness definitions. The challenge of inscribing fairness values in ML is still open and will require multidisciplinary studies since fairness is a dynamic concept that may vary across countries, cultures and domains of application.[51]

6.3. *Interpretable and explainable AI*

The need to understand the reasoning behind AI decision-support systems, i.e., *explicability*, is listed as one of the four ethical imperatives of the EU guidelines for trustworthy AI. This principle is strongly linked to the *transparency requirement*. Most of state-of-the-art AI models are not transparent and are often referred to as *black boxes*. An AI system might be considered a black box for two reasons:

(1) The AI system is based on a complex ML model whose outcomes cannot be understood and interpreted just by looking at its internal parameters. In this case, the lack of transparency reflects a lack of knowledge or understanding of the model's inner knowledge representation.

(2) The AI system is based on proprietary software. The source code of the model, its specifications and the data used to train it are not available. In this case, the lack of transparency might have nothing to do with the inherent characteristic of the ML model.

We will now focus on the first case. DL models fall into this first category of black boxes since the increasing complexity of their hierarchical layer structure is not straightforwardly interpretable to human beings. Some ML researchers have compared the black-box reasoning of DL application in healthcare to the black-box reasoning of many doctors, claiming that it is impossible to explain all the factors which led a physician to his diagnosis. However, being able to explain clinical decisions to patients and to be held accountable for adverse outcomes of their diagnosis are key ethical responsibilities of every doctor. Furthermore, it has been argued that Article 22 of the GDPR establishes a right to explanation, making explicability a legal requirement.

There are two ways of reaching the level of transparency mandated by the GDPR and suggested by the EU guidelines. The first way is to avoid the use of black boxes and to use inherently interpretable models instead, and the second way is to apply techniques from the field of explainable AI.

Interpretable models for healthcare: Saying that a model is interpretable means that it has the *ability to explain or to present in understandable terms to a human.*[58] In this context, we say that a model is interpretable if the user can understand and interpret how the inputs are mathematically mapped into the outputs. In the literature, there is a small number of models that are recognized as inherently interpretable: linear models, decision trees and rules.[32] DL models are usually preferred to inherently interpretable ones because they capture highly nonlinear relationships between the variables without requiring a feature engineering process and therefore yield higher accuracy with less effort. However, there are some examples of high-performance interpretable models in healthcare. For example, Caruana *et al.* used generalized additive models with pairwise interactions (GA^2M) to predict pneumonia risk and hospital 30-day readmission, generating high-performance interpretable models.[42] Since GA^2M allows visualizing single and pairwise feature interactions with the outcome, the authors were able to identify a dangerous omitted-variable bias present in the real-world dataset used to train the algorithm. More specifically, the model was classifying asthma patients as having low risk of dying for pneumonia complications because the dataset did not contain information on the type of treatment these patients received. This highlights, even more, the dangers of using black boxes that do not allow for such exploration of the model's learned biases in healthcare applications. Furthermore, in her work, Rudin[59] claims that the accuracy interpretability trade-off is a myth.

This claim is based on the fact that Data Science is an iterative process that involves many back-and-forths between problem definition, data analysis and modeling. During this knowledge discovery process, it becomes easier to find a good data representation that allows simpler models to have the same level of performance of the black-box ones.

Explainable AI: EXplainable AI (XAI) is a sub-field of ML that studies the techniques that explain in human-understandable terms the logic that a black-box model uses to solve its task. These techniques are particularly useful if it is not possible to develop a high-performance transparent model for the task at hand or to understand the reasoning behind a black box of the second type (proprietary software). In the last few years, there has been a surge in the academic literature related to this field[32] and a complete review of all the methods applicable to DL techniques is outside the scope of this section. However, we list here some examples of relevant XAI techniques used for DL applications in the healthcare domain. One of the most common techniques used to explain medical DL applications is the use of attention weights[60] as an explanation of the model behavior.[61] However, recent works have highlighted how this kind of explanation might lack consistency[62] and that attention should not be used as an explanation. Another approach to explaining black-box decisions is through the use of an inherently interpretable proxy model (such as a linear model or a decision tree) able to mimic its local or global behavior.[63-66] Among the vast literature of XAI, one emerging trend might be particularly relevant for applications in healthcare: the use of medical ontologies in the explanation process.[67, 68] In general, when deciding the XAI technique to be applied to the DL model, it is important to consider several dimensions of the problem.[69] First, it is important to consider the functional requirements of our system. For example, what kind of data is the model using (tabular, images, sequential)? What kind of problem is it solving (classification, regression)? What kind of model architecture are we using? According to the answers to these questions, we can filter out the XAI methods that cannot be applied to our model for technical reasons. Second, it is important to decide what kind of explanation we want to provide from a user-centric perspective. Who is the end user of our application? We should answer these questions with the first requirement of trustworthy AI on *human agency and oversight* in mind. The kind of explanation needed for the final end user varies according to his expertise. For example, consider a DL application that is designed to advise a physician on the best medications for a specific patient. In this case, the end user is the physician, for this reason, the explanation provided should not require extensive knowledge of ML to be understood. However, a recent study on the use of XAI techniques in deployment found that the majority of users of such methods are ML engineers using them as a debugging tool.[70] For this reason, further research is needed to bridge the gap between current explanation techniques and real-world clinical scenarios of application.

6.4. *Privacy*

Healthcare data is one of the most *sensitive* kind of data; as a consequence, it is often segregated and its potential for insightful analytics is limited. Moreover, the US HIPAA and the European GDPR restrict access to health data. Learning from this kind of data while being compliant with data protection regulations poses some challenges. In such a sensitive context, it becomes mandatory to apply the *privacy-by-design* principle introduced by Ann Cavoukian[71] in the 1990s and successively elaborated by Monreale *et al.*[72] The main idea is to inscribe the privacy requirements in the design of the knowledge discovery process to balance privacy protection and data utility. This goal is important in any task but is fundamental in the medical field where data and model quality, often reduced by privacy-preserving techniques, should be preserved as much as possible to avoid a negative impact on patients. In DL, the privacy risks can arise in two different phases: during the *development stage* of the deep learning-based system, since the training phase of the model requires access to the data which have to be anonymized to avoid patients reidentification[73] and during the *deployment stage* when the model is used to predict or classify new unknown instances. In this chapter, we focus our discussion on privacy attacks on predictive models and corresponding mitigation techniques.

During the *deployment stage*, a *privacy breach* occurs if the adversary can infer sensitive information about *specific individuals* represented in the training data of the ML model. Some ML algorithms generate models that explicitly store feature vectors representing data used during the learning phase. This kind of models (e.g., SVM) should be avoided without considering a protection strategy against the *reconstruction attacks*. This kind of attack aims at reconstructing the raw private data by using *a priori* knowledge of the feature vectors and accessing the model. However, this kind of privacy issues may arise even if no explicit feature vector is stored in the learned model (e.g., neural networks). In this case, we can have two different attack settings: the adversary can access the ML model and its parameters, or the adversary can only query the model without having access to it. Two attack models can act in these settings: *model inversion attacks* and *membership attacks*. In the former, the goal of the adversary is to infer some sensitive features used in the learning phase by knowing a set of features and observing the output of the queried model. This attack however does not necessarily entail a privacy breach of a specific individual represented in the training data, but allows the adversary the inference of sensitive information about a specific population. For example, this attack was used in the case of pharmacogenetics analyzed by Fredrikson *et al.*[74] that shows as a model inversion attack, without accessing the prediction model but only querying it, is able to learn sensitive genomic information about individuals. In particular, the model is able to detect the correlation between the patient's genotype and the dosage of a medicine. In this context, it is evident that the correlation is not valid only for a specific person, but it is a scientific fact that holds for *all* patients. Moreover, this correlation is also valid for patients that are not included in the training data used for learning the ML model. McSherry[75] observed that it is hard to avoid this kind of collective *breach* if the model is based on statistics about a specific population. This because given a record and a model, a model inversion attack provides the same result in case the record was used to train the model and when it was not used. Advanced model inversion attacks were proposed to recover images from deep neural networks in both centralized learning setting[76] and collaborative learning setting.[77]

An attack that infers the presence or not of an individual's record in the training data of an ML model is the *membership inference attack*.[78] This attack can directly lead to a privacy breach because, for example, knowing that a certain patient is represented in the training data of an ML model associated with a specific disease can reveal that the individual under analysis has that disease. The typical assumptions of this attack are that the adversary's knowledge is the individual's record and the adversary can only query the ML model and receive the model's output. The membership inference attack exploits ML to attack an ML model. In particular, it is based on the learning of an ML model that distinguishes the target model's behavior on the training inputs from its behavior on the inputs that it did not contain in the training data. The main idea is to create multiple *shadow models*, i.e., ML models that imitate the target model's behavior on known training datasets (typically synthetically generated). By using these models, it is possible to construct a set of data labeled as "in" or "out" of the training dataset. The "in" value derives from the high confidence of the prediction of the target model for an instance. On the labeled dataset, it is possible to train the attack model.

Most of the privacy-preserving techniques for DL are focused on differentially private approaches, sometimes combined with a collaborative training of a model, allowing multiple parties to contribute to the learning process without releasing their private data in its original form. Differential privacy is especially effective in preventing membership inference attacks and limiting the effect of model inversion attacks.

Differential privacy[79] requires that the presence or not of a record in the data does not significantly affect the outcome of any analysis. It ensures an individual in the data that any privacy breach will not be due to his/her participation in the dataset because anything that is learnable from the data with his/her record is also learnable from the one without his/her record. For any two datasets D and D' differing in a single record and any output O of function f, $\mathrm{Prob}\{f(D) \in O\} \leq e^{\epsilon} \times \mathrm{Prob}\{f(D') \in O\}$. The parameter ϵ is the privacy budget and controls the trade-off between the accuracy of the differentially private f and the privacy loss. A smaller ϵ means more noise and stronger privacy level. A fundamental concept of differential privacy is the global sensitivity of the function f that helps in determining the utility of the function f. Techniques for achieving differential privacy are based on randomization of their input. Some approaches first learn a model on original data and then use either the exponential or Laplacian mechanism to generate a noisy model. As an example, Arachchige *et al.*[80] proposed to apply a local differentially private algorithm redesigning the training process of a convolutional neural network (CNN). In particular, the CNN architecture is divided into three layers: (1) convolutional module, (2) randomization module, and (3) fully connected module. Abadi *et al.*[81] instead developed a DP-deep learning system that achieves differential privacy, modifying the stochastic gradient descent algorithm to have Gaussian noise added in each of its iterations. Shokri *et al.*[82] proposed the combination of differential privacy protection with a distributed multi-party learning mechanism for a neural network without sharing input datasets. They parallelized the learning process, which is based on the stochastic gradient descent optimization algorithm. Each party only shares a subset of parameters of the local model with the other parties to reduce communication costs, and differential privacy is achieved by inserting noisy values to truncated weights. The drawback is that the total privacy budget depends on the number of parameters, which may be in the tens of thousands in DL models. Zhao *et al.*[83] addressed a similar problem, but, instead of injecting noise directly to the gradients, they apply a functional mechanism to perturb the objective function of the neural network and obtain the sanitized parameters by minimizing the perturbed objective function. The process considers that each party, e.g., a medical institution, maintains a local neural network model and the local high-sensitive data. It shares with a central server only the updated parameters of the local model generated from the local data. The central server derives the global parameters for the collective model exploiting the contributions from all parties. To avoid possible disclosure of sensitive information, differential privacy is used to sanitize the parameters and minimize the privacy leakage.

7. Concluding Remarks

AI systems have the power to improve the healthcare sector thanks to more and more effective deep learning models. In this chapter, we discussed the ethical and legal implications of the development and deployment of such applications in the healthcare domain, which is very critical from an ethical perspective. We provided an overview of the different approaches to AI ethics across the world, and we mapped some ethical values to the different stages of the ML development lifecycle. Additionally, we analyzed the literature covering the different approaches to inscribe the ethical values of privacy, fairness and explainability in DL systems.

Our legal, ethical and technical analysis highlighted some important challenges and issues. First of all, the approach to AI ethics across the world is deeply heterogeneous. In the era of globalization, this could be an obstacle to the regulatory harmonization of such technologies that can, in turn, result in a fragmented global market. Furthermore, this could undermine the trust in AI-based systems and slow down their adoption in real-world clinical scenarios. Often, such different approaches to AI ethics depend on cultural differences, which can also have an impact on the definition of some values such as *fairness*, which is one of the most difficult ethical values to be uniquely defined across the world.

Second, our analysis of the technical solutions showed that most of them are designed to address only one particular ethical issue. There is no solution to integrate more than one value, such as privacy, fairness, and explainability with a holistic approach. We argue that the study of the interplay between the different values could be beneficial for the development of human-centric AI systems.

Finally, our technical analysis highlighted that the human component is, at the same time, too present in the biases often discovered in the data and too far removed from the decision-making process. Future research should focus on finding the right balance between AI and the human component to enhance their complementary strengths and allow AI technology to develop to its full beneficial potential.

References

1. E. Gibson, W. Li, C. Sudre, L. Fidon, D. Shakir, G. Wang, Z. Eaton-Rosen, R. Gray, T. Doel, Y. Hu, T. Whyntie, P. Nachev, D. Barratt, S. Ourselin, M. J. Cardoso, and T. Vercauteren, Niftynet: A deep-learning platform for medical imaging, *Comput. Methods Programs Biomed.* **158**, 113–122 (2017).
2. R. Poplin, A. Varadarajan, K. Blumer, Y. Liu, M. McConnell, G. Corrado, L. Peng, and D. Webster, Predicting cardiovascular risk factors from retinal fundus photographs using deep learning, *Nat. Biomed. Eng.* **2**, 158–164 (2018).
3. J. D. V. Oriol, E. E. Vallejo, K. Estrada, J. G. T. Peña, A. D. N. Initiative, *et al.*, Benchmarking machine learning models for late-onset

alzheimer's disease prediction from genomic data, *BMC Bioinformat.* **20**(1), 1–17 (2019).

4. G. Malgieri and G. Comandé, Sensitive-by-distance: Quasi-health data in the algorithmic era, *Inf. Commun. Technol. Law.* **26**(3), 229–249 (2017).

5. OECD. Recommendation of the council on artificial intelligence, oecd/legal/0449 (2019).

6. High-Level Expert Group on AI. The Ethics Guidelines for Trustworthy Artificial Intelligence (AI). https://ec.europa.eu/futurium/en/ai-allian ce-consultation (2019).

7. White House's Office of Science and Technology Policy. Guidance for regulation of artificial intelligence applications. https://www.whitehouse.gov/wp-content/uploads/2020/01/Draft-OMB-Me mo-on-Regulation-of-AI-1-7-19.pdf (2019).

8. S. Nair, J. Eustace, and P. J. Thuluvath, Effect of race on outcome of orthotopic liver transplantation: A cohort study, *Lancet.* **359**(9303), 287–293 (2002).

9. S. Ruggieri, D. Pedreschi, and F. Turini, Data mining for discrimination discovery, *TKDD* **4**(2), 9:1–9:40 (2010).

10. H. Jones, Geoff hinton dismissed the need for explainable AI: 8 experts explain why he's wrong, *Forbes,* Dec. **20** (2018).

11. A. Jobin, M. Ienca, and E. Vayena, The global landscape of ai ethics guidelines, *Nat.Mach. Intell.* **1**(9), 389–399 (2019).

12. A. Armitage, A. Cordova, and R. Siegel, Design-thinking: The answer to the impasse between innovation and regulation, *UC Hastings Research Paper* (250) (2017).

13. P. Zhang and Y. Liang, China's national health guiding principles: A perspective worthy of healthcare reform, *Prim. Health Care. Res. Dev.* **19**(1), 99–104 (2018).

14. L. Floridi, On human dignity as a foundation for the right to privacy, *Philos. Technol.* **29**(4), 307–312 (2016).

15. J. Morley, M. Taddeo, and L. Floridi, Google health and the NHS: Overcoming the trust deficit, *Lancet Digit. Health.* **1**(8), e389 (2019).

16. I. G. Cohen and M. M. Mello, Hipaa and protecting health information in the 21st century, *JAMA* **320**(3), 231–232 (2018).

17. X. Tan, X. Liu, and H. Shao, Healthy China 2030: A vision for health care, *Value Health Reg. Issues* **12**, 112–114 (2017).

18. S. L. Myers, J. Wu, and C. Fu, China's looming crisis: A shrinking population, *New York Times* (2019).

19. M. Huateng. Application of artificial intelligence and Big Data in China's healthcare services. In *Global Innovation Index 2019 Creating Healthy Lives — The Future of Medical Innovation*, pp. 103–109

(2019). https://www.wipo.int/edocs/pubdocs/en/wipo_pub_gii_2019-c hapter5.pdf.

20. H. Roberts, J. Cowls, J. Morley, M. Taddeo, V. Wang, and L. Floridi, The chinese approach to artificial intelligence: An analysis of policy and regulation, *Available at SSRN 3469784* (2019).

21. European Commission. White paper: On Artificial Intelligence — A European approach to excellence and trust. https://ec.europa.eu/info/ sites/info/files/commission-white-paper-artificial-intelligence-feb2020_ en.pdf (2020).

22. G. Comandé and G. Malgieri, Why a right to legibility of automated decision-making exists in the general data protection regulation, *Int. Data Priv. Law* **7**(4), 243–265 (2017).

23. E. Strubell, A. Ganesh, and A. McCallum, Energy and policy considerations for deep learning in nlp, *arXiv preprint arXiv:1906.02243* (2019).

24. R. Vinuesa, H. Azizpour, I. Leite, M. Balaam, V. Dignum, S. Domisch, A. Felländer, S. D. Langhans, M. Tegmark, and F. F. Nerini, The role of artificial intelligence in achieving the sustainable development goals, *Nat. Commun.* **11**(1), 1–10 (2020).

25. L. J. Fallowfield, Treatment decision-making in breast cancer: The patient–doctor relationship, *Breast Cancer Res. Treat.* **112**(1), 5–13 (2008).

26. V. Bellemo, Z. W. Lim, G. Lim, Q. D. Nguyen, Y. Xie, M. Y. Yip, H. Hamzah, J. Ho, X. Q. Lee, W. Hsu, *et al.*, Artificial intelligence using deep learning to screen for referable and vision-threatening diabetic retinopathy in africa: A clinical validation study, *Lancet Digit. Health.* **1**(1), e35–e44 (2019).

27. J. Wiens, S. Saria, M. Sendak, M. Ghassemi, V. X. Liu, F. Doshi-Velez, K. Jung, K. Heller, D. Kale, M. Saeed, *et al.*, Do no harm: A roadmap for responsible machine learning for health care, *Nat. Med.* **25**(10), 1627–1627 (2019).

28. A. E. Johnson, T. J. Pollard, L. Shen, H. L. Li-wei, M. Feng, M. Ghassemi, B. Moody, P. Szolovits, L. A. Celi, and R. G. Mark, Mimic-iii, a freely accessible critical care database, *Sci. Data* **3**, 160035 (2016).

29. C. R. Jack Jr, M. A. Bernstein, N. C. Fox, P. Thompson, G. Alexander, D. Harvey, B. Borowski, P. J. Britson, J. L. Whitwell, C. Ward, *et al.*, The alzheimer's disease neuroimaging initiative (adni): Mri methods, *J. Magn. Reson. Imag.: An Official J. Int. Soc. Magnet. Reson. Med.* **27**(4), 685–691 (2008).

30. H. Harutyunyan, H. Khachatrian, D. C. Kale, G. Ver Steeg, and A. Galstyan, Multitask learning and benchmarking with clinical time series data, *Sci. Data* **6**(1), 1–18 (2019).

31. S. H. Park and K. Han, Methodologic guide for evaluating clinical performance and effect of artificial intelligence technology for medical diagnosis and prediction, *Radiology* **286**(3), 800–809 (2018).

32. R. Guidotti, A. Monreale, S. Ruggieri, F. Turini, F. Giannotti, and D. Pedreschi, A survey of methods for explaining black box models, *ACM Comput. Surv.* **51**(5), 93:1–93:42 (2019).

33. G. Comandé. Multilayered (accountable) liability for artificial intelligence. In *Liability for Artificial Intelligence and the Internet of Thing*, (ed.) D. Staudenmayer, S. Lohsse, R. Schulze, pp. 165–187 (2019).

34. F. Pratesi, A. Monreale, R. Trasarti, F. Giannotti, D. Pedreschi, and T. Yanagihara, Prudence: A system for assessing privacy risk vs utility in data sharing ecosystems, *Trans. Data Priv.* **11**(2), 139–167 (2018).

35. P. Saleiro, B. Kuester, A. Stevens, A. Anisfeld, L. Hinkson, J. London, and R. Ghani, Aequitas: A bias and fairness audit toolkit, *CoRR.* **abs/1811.05577** (2018). http://arxiv.org/abs/1811.05577.

36. W. H. Organization *et al.*, Monitoring and evaluating digital health interventions: A practical guide to conducting research and assessment (2016).

37. J. A. Casey, B. S. Schwartz, W. F. Stewart, and N. E. Adler, Using electronic health records for population health research: A review of methods and applications, *Ann. Rev. Pub. Health* **37**, 61–81 (2016).

38. G. I. Parisi, R. Kemker, J. L. Part, C. Kanan, and S. Wermter, Continual lifelong learning with neural networks: A review, *Neural Netw.* **113**, 54–71 (2019).

39. P. Machnikowski, *European Product Liability: An Analysis of the State of the Art in the Era of New Technologies*. Intersentia, Cambridge, UK (2016).

40. I. Y. Chen, S. Joshi, and M. Ghassemi, Treating health disparities with artificial intelligence, *Nat. Med.* **26**(1), 16–17 (2020).

41. J.-W. Baek, J.-C. Kim, J. Chun, and K. Chung, Hybrid clustering based health decision-making for improving dietary habits, *Technol. Health Care.* (Preprint), 1–14 (2019).

42. R. Caruana, Y. Lou, J. Gehrke, P. Koch, M. Sturm, and N. Elhadad. Intelligible models for healthcare: Predicting pneumonia risk and hospital 30-day readmission. In *ACM SIGKDD International Conference on Knowledge Discovery and Data Mining*, pp. 1721–1730 (2015).

43. P. Yadav, M. Steinbach, V. Kumar, and G. Simon, Mining electronic health records (ehrs): A survey, *ACM Comput. Surv. (CSUR)* **50**(6), 85 (2018).

44. M. Sendak, M. C. Elish, M. Gao, J. Futoma, W. Ratliff, M. Nichols, A. Bedoya, S. Balu, and C. O'Brien. The human body is a black box supporting clinical decision-making with deep learning. In *Conference on Fairness, Accountability, and Transparency*, pp. 99–109 (2020).

45. L. Seyyed-Kalantari, G. Liu, M. McDermott, and M. Ghassemi, Chexclusion: Fairness gaps in deep chest x-ray classifiers, *arXiv:2003.00827* (2020).

46. Z. Obermeyer, B. Powers, C. Vogeli, and S. Mullainathan, Dissecting racial bias in an algorithm used to manage the health of populations, *Science* **366**(6464), 447–453 (2019).

47. S. M. Phelan, D. J. Burgess, M. W. Yeazel, W. L. Hellerstedt, J. M. Griffin, and M. van Ryn, Impact of weight bias and stigma on quality of care and outcomes for patients with obesity, *Obes. Rev.* **16**(4), 319–326 (2015).

48. E. Ntoutsi, P. Fafalios, U. Gadiraju, V. Iosifidis, W. Nejdl, M.-E. Vidal, S. Ruggieri, F. Turini, S. Papadopoulos, E. Krasanakis, *et al.*, Bias in data-driven artificial intelligence systems — an introductory survey, *Wiley Interdiscip. Rev.: Data Min. Knowl. Discov.* p. e1356.

49. A. Romei and S. Ruggieri, A multidisciplinary survey on discrimination analysis, *Knowl. Eng. Rev.* **29**(5), 582–638 (2014).

50. N. Mehrabi, F. Morstatter, N. Saxena, K. Lerman, and A. Galstyan, A survey on bias and fairness in machine learning, *arXiv:1908.09635* (2019).

51. M. Schäfer, D. B. M. Haun, and M. Tomasello, Fair is not fair everywhere, *Psychol. Science* **26**(8), 1252–1260 (2015).

52. C. Panigutti, A. Perotti, A. Panisson, P. Bajardi, and D. Pedreschi, Fairlens: Auditing black-box clinical decision support systems, *arXiv preprint arXiv:2011.04049* (2020).

53. F. Kamiran and T. Calders, Data preprocessing techniques for classification without discrimination, *Knowl. Inf. Syst.* **33**(1), 1–33 (2011).

54. M. Du, N. Liu, F. Yang, and X. Hu. Learning credible deep neural networks with rationale regularization. In eds. J. Wang, K. Shim, and X. Wu, *IEEE International Conference on Data Mining, ICDM*, pp. 150–159 (2019).

55. B. H. Zhang, B. Lemoine, and M. Mitchell. Mitigating unwanted biases with adversarial learning. In *AAAI Conference on AI, Ethics, and Society*, pp. 335–340, ACM (2018).

56. S. Hajian, J. Domingo-Ferrer, A. Monreale, D. Pedreschi, and F. Giannotti, Discrimination- and privacy-aware patterns, *Data Min. Knowl. Discov.* **29**(6), 1733–1782 (2015).

57. S. Ruggieri, Using t-closeness anonymity to control for non-discrimination, *Trans. Data Priv.* **7**(2), 99–129 (2014).

58. F. Doshi-Velez and B. Kim, Towards a rigorous science of interpretable machine learning, *arXiv preprint arXiv:1702.08608* (2017).

59. C. Rudin, Stop explaining black box machine learning models for high stakes decisions and use interpretable models instead, *Nat. Mach. Intell.* **1**(5), 206–215 (2019).

60. A. Vaswani, N. Shazeer, N. Parmar, J. Uszkoreit, L. Jones, A. N. Gomez, L. Kaiser, and I. Polosukhin. Attention is all you need. In *Advances in Neural Information Processing Systems*, pp. 5998–6008 (2017).

61. E. Choi, M. T. Bahadori, J. Sun, J. Kulas, A. Schuetz, and W. Stewart. Retain: An interpretable predictive model for healthcare using reverse time attention mechanism. In *Advances in Neural Information Processing Systems*, pp. 3504–3512 (2016).

62. S. Jain and B. C. Wallace, Attention is not explanation, *arXiv:1902.10186* (2019).

63. M. Craven and J. W. Shavlik. Extracting tree-structured representations of trained networks. In *Advances in Neural Information Processing Systems*, pp. 24–30 (1996).

64. S. M. Lundberg and S.-I. Lee. A unified approach to interpreting model predictions. In *Advances in Neural Information Processing Systems*, pp. 4765–4774 (2017).

65. M. T. Ribeiro, S. Singh, and C. Guestrin. "why should i trust you?" explaining the predictions of any classifier. In *ACM SIGKDD International Conference on Knowledge Discovery and Data Mining*, pp. 1135–1144 (2016).

66. R. Guidotti, A. Monreale, F. Giannotti, D. Pedreschi, S. Ruggieri, and F. Turini, Factual and counterfactual explanations for black box decision making, *IEEE Intell. Syst.* **34**(6), 14–23 (2019).

67. C. Panigutti, A. Perotti, and D. Pedreschi. Doctor xai: An ontology-based approach to black-box sequential data classification explanations. In *Conference on Fairness, Accountability, and Transparency*, pp. 629–639 (2020).

68. R. Confalonieri, F. M. del Prado, S. Agramunt, D. Malagarriga, D. Faggion, T. Weyde, and T. R. Besold, An ontology-based approach to explaining artificial neural networks, *arXiv preprint arXiv:1906.08362* (2019).

69. K. Sokol and P. Flach. Explainability fact sheets: A framework for systematic assessment of explainable approaches. In *Conference on Fairness, Accountability, and Transparency*, pp. 56–67 (2020).

70. U. Bhatt, A. Xiang, S. Sharma, A. Weller, A. Taly, Y. Jia, J. Ghosh, R. Puri, J. M. Moura, and P. Eckersley. Explainable machine learning in deployment. In *Conference on Fairness, Accountability, and Transparency*, pp. 648–657 (2020).

71. A. Cavoukian, Privacy design principles for an integrated justice system. Working paper (2000). www.ipc.on.ca/index.asp?layid=86%26;fidl=318.

72. A. Monreale, S. Rinzivillo, F. Pratesi, F. Giannotti, and D. Pedreschi, Privacy-by-design in big data analytics and social mining, *EPJ Data Sci.* **3**(1), 10 (2014).

73. L. Sweeney, k-anonymity: A model for protecting privacy, *Int. J. Uncertain. Fuzziness Knowl.-Based Syst.* **10**(5), 557–570 (2002).

74. M. Fredrikson, E. Lantz, S. Jha, S. Lin, D. Page, and T. Ristenpart. Privacy in pharmacogenetics: An end-to-end case study of personalized warfarin dosing. In *USENIX Security Symposium*, pp. 17–32 (2014).

75. F. McSherry, Statistical inference considered harmful, see https://github. com/frankmcsherry/blog/blob/master/posts/2016-06-14. md (2016).

76. M. Fredrikson, S. Jha, and T. Ristenpart. Model inversion attacks that exploit confidence information and basic countermeasures. In *ACM Conference on Computer and Communications Security*, pp. 1322–1333, ACM (2015).

77. B. Hitaj, G. Ateniese, and F. Perez-Cruz. Deep models under the gan: information leakage from collaborative deep learning. In *ACM SIGSAC Conference on Computer and Communications Security*, pp. 603–618 (2017).

78. R. Shokri, M. Stronati, C. Song, and V. Shmatikov. Membership inference attacks against machine learning models. In *IEEE Symposium on Security and Privacy*, pp. 3–18 (2017).

79. C. Dwork. Differential privacy. In eds. M. Bugliesi, B. Preneel, V. Sassone, and I. Wegener, *Automata, Languages and Programming, 33rd International Colloquium, ICALP 2006, Proceedings, Part II*, Vol. 4052, *Lecture Notes in Computer Science*, pp. 1–12, Springer (2006).

80. P. C. M. Arachchige, P. Bertok, I. Khalil, D. Liu, S. Camtepe, and M. Atiquzzaman, Local differential privacy for deep learning, *IEEE Internet Things J.* pp. 1–1 (2019).

81. M. Abadi, A. Chu, I. J. Goodfellow, H. B. McMahan, I. Mironov, K. Talwar, and L. Zhang. Deep learning with differential privacy. In *ACM Conference on Computer and Communications Security*, pp. 308–318, ACM (2016).

82. R. Shokri and V. Shmatikov. Privacy-preserving deep learning. In *ACM Conference on Computer and Communications Security*, pp. 1310–1321 (2015).

83. L. Zhao, Q. Wang, Q. Zou, Y. Zhang, and Y. Chen, Privacy-preserving collaborative deep learning with unreliable participants, *IEEE Trans. Inf. Foren. Sec.* **15**, 1486–1500 (2020).

Index

www.ingramcontent.com/pod-product-compliance
Lightning Source LLC
Chambersburg PA
CBHW050539190326
41458CB00007B/1843